STATISTICS FOR THE ALLIED HEALTH SCIENCES

Richard J. Larsen
Vanderbilt University

CHARLES E. MERRILL PUBLISHING COMPANY
A Bell & Howell Company
Columbus, Ohio

Published by
CHARLES E. MERRILL PUBLISHING CO.
A Bell & Howell Company
Columbus, Ohio 43216

This book was set in Times Roman.
The Production Editor was Frances Margolin.
The cover was designed by Will Chenoweth.

Copyright © 1975 by *Bell & Howell Company*. All rights reserved. No part of this book may be reproduced in any form, electronic or mechanical, including photocopy, recording, or any information storage and retrieval system, without permission in writing from the publisher.

Library of Congress Catalog Card Number: 74-28908

International Standard Book Number: 0-675-08782-1

Printed in the United States of America

1 2 3 4 5 6 7 8 — 80 79 78 77 76 75

PREFACE

If a statistics course is to be of any real value, it must leave a student with more than just a list of formulas and a collection of methods. Statistics, after all, is a way of thinking and that, more than anything else, is what needs to be emphasized.

Unfortunately, this is precisely what students find most difficult about the subject. Learning *how* to use a given method is easy — you start with Step A, follow that with Step B, continue with Step C, and when you finally reach Step H the problem is solved. But learning *when* to use that method is a far more difficult task, one that requires a much deeper understanding of what statistics and statistical thinking are all about.

It is the author's firm conviction that there is only one way to convey effectively this "spirit" of statistics — by showing, through the use of substantive and *real* examples, how all the various formulas and methods are actually put into practice. The important word here is "real." It is simply not sufficient to work with numbers out of context or with data that are hypothetical. When statistics is taught as an exercise in mathematics, or when its relationship to the real world is hinted at but never truly explored, it becomes a subject in limbo, having no relevancy and generating no interest.

Throughout the eight chapters in this book, there are almost 100 sets of data, all taken from recently published books and journals. To the extent that space permits, background information is provided with each set — what the experiment was intended to prove, who the subjects were, and how the measurements were recorded.

All of this material was specifically designed for a one-semester, three-hour course at Vanderbilt University for students in the School of Nursing. The objective was to focus on the principles of statistics as they apply — and *are* applied — to the medical sciences. As a general policy, it was felt that presenting a smaller number of techniques thoroughly would be more preferable than surveying a larger number superficially. For this reason, and because of the time restrictions imposed by a one-semester course, certain "standard" topics have been omitted, including combinatorics, small sample binomial theory, and nonparametrics. At the same time, certain medical topics, like rates and titers, not appearing in most introductory texts have been added. As much as possible, the *unity* of statistical thinking has been stressed, so that what motivates a procedure in one chapter is shown to be simply a restatement of a principle that appeared in another context in an earlier chapter.

The format of the book, particularly the first chapter, deserves a word of comment. It has been the author's experience as a teacher that, for most students, learning to recognize the statistical structure of a set of data is not an ability that comes automatically. It does not follow, for example, that a student who is able to carry out the calculations required for, say, a t-test necessarily has any appreciation for the two-sample problem in general, or for how such a problem might arise in an experimental setting.

Therefore, the first chapter is devoted to problem recognition. The purpose is to teach the student, at the very outset, how to distinguish the more common types of experimental designs — two-sample problems, paired-data problems, correlation problems, and so on. This chapter also serves another purpose: it affords the student an opportunity to think about data from a common sense point of view, without being immediately burdened with any formal methodology.

The remainder of the book is organized around the six different models profiled in Chapter 1. One chapter develops the two-sample problem, another, the paired-data problem, and so on. If the student comes away from all of this with a genuine understanding of the role that statistics plays in medical research, and with the ability and confidence to apply these various techniques to his own problems, this book will have been a success.

Needless to say, no project of this sort can be accomplished without many different people helping in many different ways — my colleagues with their encouragement, Prof. Jean Hensel of The Ohio State University with her many helpful comments, the secretaries in the Mathematics Department with their manuscript assistance, and the Vanderbilt nursing students with their patience. And, above all, my sincerest appreciation goes to my teaching assistants — Linda Daniel, Sylvia Flippin, Joanne Roman, and, especially, Donna Stroup. Without all of this support, what has taken three years to complete would still not be finished.

R.J.L.
Nashville

CONTENTS

CHAPTER 1 STATISTICAL MODELS 2

1.1	Introduction	3
1.2	Samples and Populations	4
1.3	Notation	9
1.4	Data Structures	9
1.5	Model One: Total-Population Problems	10
1.6	Model Two: One-Sample Problems	12
1.7	Model Three: Two-Sample Problems	14
1.8	Model Four: Paired-Data Problems	16
1.9	Model Six: Correlation Problems	19
1.10	Model Six: k-Sample Problems	23
1.11	Summary	26
	Definitions	27
	Review Exercises	29

CHAPTER 2 MODEL ONE — DESCRIPTIVE STATISTICS 36

2.1	Introduction	37
2.2	Scales of Measurement	38
2.3	Rates	40
2.4	Adjusted Rates	44
2.5	Descriptive Statistics for Nominal and Ordinal Data	47
2.6	Descriptive Statistics for Interval Data	52
2.7	Special Techniques	61
2.8	Logarithmic Scaling	65
2.9	Summary	68
	Definitions	70
	Review Exercises	71

CHAPTER 3 PRINCIPLES OF INFERENCE — 76

3.1	Introduction	77
3.2	The Sample Mean	78
3.3	Sigma Notation	81
3.4	Alternatives to the Sample Mean	85
3.5	The Sample Standard Deviation	87
3.6	The Sampling Distribution of $\bar{X}$	92
3.7	Introduction to Hypothesis Testing	96
3.8	Probability and Area	101
3.9	Areas Under Normal Curves	108
3.10	Summary	117
	Definitions	118
	Review Exercises	120

CHAPTER 4 MODEL TWO — THE ONE-SAMPLE PROBLEM — 124

4.1	Introduction	125
4.2	Large Sample Hypothesis Tests for μ	126
4.3	Small Sample Hypothesis Tests for μ	146
4.4	Confidence Intervals	153
4.5	Binomial Data	159
4.6	Type I and II Errors	164
4.7	Summary	170
	Definitions	172
	Review Exercises	173

CHAPTER 5 MODEL THREE — THE TWO-SAMPLE PROBLEM — 176

5.1	Introduction	177
5.2	The Two-Sample t-Test for Means (Equal Standard Deviations)	179
5.3	The Two-Sample t-Test for Means (Unequal Standard Deviations)	186
5.4	Confidence Intervals for $\mu_X - \mu_Y$	194
5.5	Summary	198
	Definitions	200
	Review Exercises	200

CHAPTER 6 MODEL FOUR — THE PAIRED-DATA PROBLEM — 206

6.1	Introduction	207
6.2	A Student t-Test for Paired Data	210
6.3	Titer Data: Acute and Convalescent Sera	215
6.4	Summary	220
	Definitions	222
	Review Exercises	222

Contents vii

CHAPTER 7 MODEL FIVE — THE CORRELATION PROBLEM   226

7.1 Introduction — *227*
7.2 The Least Squares Line — *229*
7.3 The Correlation Coefficient — *235*
7.4 Testing H: $\rho = 0$ — *240*
7.5 Time χ^2 Test: 2×2 Contingency Tables — *245*
7.6 The χ^2 Test: $R \times C$ Contingency Tables — *251*
7.7 Summary — *257*
Definitions — *259*
Review Exercises — *259*

CHAPTER 8 MODEL SIX — THE k-SAMPLE PROBLEM   264

8.1 Introduction — *265*
8.2 Double Subscript Notation — *266*
8.3 Hypothesis Testing in the k-Sample Problem — *269*
8.4 Computing Formulas for the Analysis of Variance — *279*
8.5 Summary — *285*
Definitions — *287*
Review Exercises: Chapter 8 — *288*

Bibliography   291

Appendix I   Areas Under Standard Normal Curve   297
Appendix II   Areas Under the Student t-Curve   299
Appendix III   Critical Values for the F-Test   301
Appendix IV   Areas Under the χ^2 Curve   304
Appendix V   Critical Values for the Analysis of Variance   306
Appendix VI   Answers to Selected Questions and Review Exercises   309

Index   325

STATISTICS FOR THE ALLIED HEALTH SCIENCES

1

Statistical Models

Mathematicians are like Frenchmen;
Whatever you say to them,
They translate into their own language
And forthwith it is something entirely different.
                                                    Goethe

1.1
INTRODUCTION

As a subject, statistics is not very old. Unlike mathematics, which has a heritage reaching back thousands of years, statistics is based on principles laid down less than a century ago. Its earliest practitioners came from the life sciences — biology, genetics, agriculture, and medicine. But today that clientele has grown to include almost all the sciences, from astronomy to zoology.

This is not to say that what the astronomer and the zoologist, the economist and the psychologist, demand of statistics is exactly the same. Each discipline has its own unique problems. And in response to those problems, statistics has evolved in a number of different directions. In some cases, there has been so much specialization that whole new subjects have been created — such as statistics for the psychologist, statistics for the economist, statistics for the engineer, and statistics for the social scientist.

Here we look at still another variation, statistics for the medical scientist. Actually, statistics and the health sciences go together very well — maybe because in many ways analyzing an experiment is like treating a patient. Both require the same two steps: (1) identify the problem and (2) decide on a course of action. Chapter 1 is concerned with the *first* step — problem recognition. That is, given a set of data and details about how those data were collected, what sort of statistical analysis would be most appropriate?

Fortunately, "statistical diagnosing" is far simpler than medical diagnosing, largely because the number of alternatives is so much smaller. In fact, almost all medical experiments belong to one of only six different statistical types (or "models"):

> Model One: Total population problems
> Model Two: One-sample problems
> Model Three: Two-sample problems
> Model Four: Paired-data problems
> Model Five: Correlation problems
> Model Six: k-sample problems

Thus even though experiments in, say, pharmacology or geriatrics or nutrition are entirely different medically, they may be completely identical statistically. It also means that we need to develop the ability to see past the superficial aspects of an experiment and to focus on its underlying structure. The purpose of this chapter is to develop that ability.

Beginning in Section 1.5 with Model One and continuing through Section 1.10 with Model Six, each of these six statistical prototypes is profiled, first in general terms and then in specific examples.

Comment

The medical details of these examples are not important for our purposes. All that needs to be gained from this chapter is an awareness of structural differences. Try to recognize what it is that makes a particular set of data belong to, say, Model Four as opposed to Model Five.

The first part of Chapter 1 is both general and introductory. Sections 1.2 and 1.4 define some of the basic terminology shared by all the models, and Section 1.3 discusses subscript notation, a mathematical shorthand for writing statistical variables.

1.2
SAMPLES AND POPULATIONS

Every discipline is rooted in just a few basic concepts. In statistics, probably nothing is more basic than the idea of a *sample* and a *population*, and the distinction between the two. Generally speaking, a *population* is a (large) group of individuals with certain characteristics in common. A *sample* is a usually smaller group, thought of as having been "selected" from a particular population; the total number of individuals in a sample is referred to as the *sample size*.

As a case in point, we might define as a population all those individuals who have had heart transplants; as the sample, all the ones whose operations were performed at Stanford University. (As of January 1, 1971, the sample size was 26.)

Comment

Populations can be either *real* or *hypothetical*. For instance, if the problem of acute lymphocytic leukemia in the United States were to be studied, the population of greatest interest would be "all children, fourteen years and under." This would be a real population, meaning that every single child included could be identified by name.

On the other hand, suppose an experiment was done with 100 persons to see how often two aspirins can relieve a headache. Unless these particular sample members were chosen in some biased way, the "success" rate that they experienced would, hopefully, be a good indicator of how effective aspirin will be in the hypothetical population of *all* persons who, sometime in the future, might take two aspirins for similar reasons. Here the population can be characterized — that is, "people with headaches" — but its members cannot be enumerated.

Taken collectively, the set of measurements made on the members of a sample is known as the *sample distribution*. Likewise, the *population distribution* is the set of observations that would be obtained if a measurement were recorded for each and every member of the population. It might be reasonable, for example, to evaluate the feasibility of heart transplants on the basis of how long the recipients live. In that case, a listing of the post-operative survival times of the 26 Stanford patients would constitute the sample distribution. (What would be the population distribution?)

For reasons of time and money, it is usually impossible to consider separately every individual in even a real population; instead, we need to rely on the sample measurements to represent all those population individuals that are not directly observed. The theory and methodology for doing this — that is, for generalizing about population characteristics on the basis of sample information — make up the subject of *statistical inference*. Most of the material covered in this book is related, either directly or indirectly, to various applications of this particular topic.

Comment

The word "measurement" is given a broad interpretation in statistics. Any observed attribute of an individual qualifies as a measurement. We are already accustomed to thinking of *quantitative* observations — red blood cell count, length of hospital stay, cholesterol level, etc. — as bona fide measurements, but the word also applies to *qualitative* observations — a person's eye color, a doctor's medical specialty, whether a patient lives or dies, etc.

6   Statistical Models

The next three examples illustrate some of the concepts introduced in this section.

EXAMPLE 1.2.1.   Disease and the Civil War

Contrary to what war movies might lead us to believe, infectious diseases, rather than combat wounds, often inflict the heaviest losses on military personnel. In the Civil War, for example, the Union armies sustained 195,627 casualties. Of that number, only 38,115 were due to wounds, accidents, or injuries; the remainder, 157,512 (approximately 80% of the total), were the result of various diseases (Steiner, 1968).

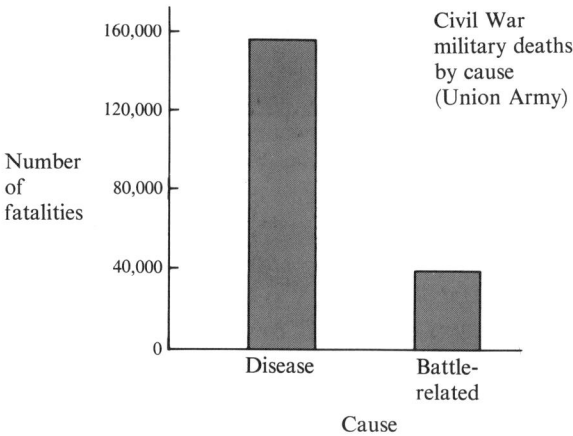

FIGURE 1.1

Comment

The sample described in these data is the group of Union soldiers who died during the Civil War. Cause of death, whether "battle trauma" or "disease," is the (qualitative) information recorded. The sample distribution — that is, the number of times each measurement was observed — is shown by the graph. The sample size is 195,627.

EXAMPLE 1.2.2.   Effects of Marihuana on Pulse Rate

Marihuana smoking has been the target of many research projects in recent years. Some have focused on its psychological effects; others, on its physiological effects. So far, very few conclusions have been reached.

The problems encountered in doing marihuana research are formidable. First of all, the true dose that a subject receives cannot be measured accurately. Secondly, the effect of the drug seems to be closely linked to the effect the subject wants it to have. And, finally, it produces a reverse tolerance — prolonged usage lessens the amount required to induce the same level of intoxication.

In one study recently published (Weil et al., 1968), eight regular marihuana users each smoked 18 mg of tetrahydracannabinol (THC) for 15 minutes. Among the measurements recorded were their changes in pulse rate (pulse rate "after" minus pulse rate "before").

Subject	Change in pulse rate (After 15 min.)
1	+32
2	+36
3	+20
4	+ 8
5	+32
6	+54
7	+24
8	+60

Comment

Here the sample (of "size eight") consists of eight regular marihuana users, and the sample distribution is the set of recorded pulse rate changes.

Comment

With most data, and this set is no exception, a precise "definition" of the population being represented is difficult to make. Suppose, for example, a group of mice is irradiated and the mutation rates of their progeny recorded. Should it be assumed that the observed dosage level–mutation rate relationship holds true only for mice? Or might it apply to all rodents? Or even to humans? Needless to say, questions like these are extremely difficult to answer, but when it comes time to interpret the results of an experiment, *some* answer has to be given, either implicitly or explicitly.

Subjects for drug experiments are often recruited from advertisements run in college newspapers. In this particular study, all eight subjects were college-affiliated males, between the ages of 21 and 26. Knowing that, to what population should we generalize? All marihuana users? Definitely not, for extent of usage is an important factor. All regular marihuana users? Probably not, for age and sex might have an effect. Most likely, we would think of these eight individuals as representing the population of all "young, male, adult regular marihuana users."

EXAMPLE 1.2.3. Cigarette Smoking and Coronary Heart Disease

By late 1971, all cigarette packs had to be labeled with the words "Warning: The Surgeon General Has Determined That Cigarette Smoking Is Dangerous to Your Health." The case against smoking rested heavily on statistical, rather than laboratory, evidence. Extensive surveys of smokers and nonsmokers had revealed the former to have much higher risks of dying from a variety of causes, including heart disease.

8   Statistical Models   [1.2]

The table below shows (1) the annual cigarette consumption and (2) the mortality rate due to coronary heart disease for 21 countries (Mulcahy, McGilvray, and Hickey, 1970). Looking at the graph that follows, we can see a definite relationship between these two characteristics — countries with high cigarette consumptions tend to have high CHD mortality rates.

Cigarettes and coronary heart disease

Year	Country	Cigarette consumption per adult per year	CHD mortality per 100,000 (Ages 35–64)
1962	United States	3900	256.9
1962	Canada	3350	211.6
1962	Australia	3220	238.1
1962	New Zealand	3220	211.8
1963	United Kingdom	2790	194.1
1962	Switzerland	2780	124.5
1962	Ireland	2770	187.3
1962	Iceland	2290	110.5
1962	Finland	2160	233.1
1963	West Germany	1890	150.3
1962	Netherlands	1810	124.7
1962	Greece	1800	41.2
1962	Austria	1770	182.1
1962	Belgium	1700	118.1
1962	Mexico	1680	31.9
1963	Italy	1510	114.3
1961	Denmark	1500	144.9
1962	France	1410	59.7
1962	Sweden	1270	126.9
1961	Spain	1200	43.9
1962	Norway	1090	136.3

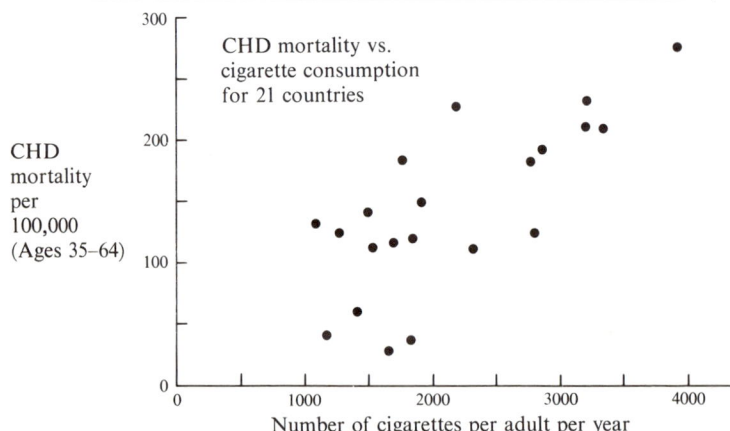

FIGURE 1.2

Comment

Note that the structure of these data is quite different from that of the first two examples. First of all, the members of the sample are countries rather than people; secondly, each sample member has been "measured" twice, instead of once.

1.3
NOTATION

The purpose of statistical notation is to identify measurements in a sample distribution with symbols that are mathematically convenient. In general, sample measurements are denoted by a letter, usually x or y, followed by a subscripted numeral (x_1, x_2, y_6, etc.). The subscript refers to the *order* in which the observation was recorded. In Example 1.2.2, x_1 would be the symbolic representation of $+32$, and we would write "$x_1 = +32$"; also, $x_2 = +36$, $x_3 = +20$, etc.

In Example 1.2.3, where two measurements have been taken on each sample member, an x might be used to denote the cigarette consumption of a country and a y, its CHD mortality rate. Then, for the United States, $x_1 = 3,900$ and $y_1 = 256.9$; for Canada, $x_2 = 3,350$ and $y_2 = 211.6$, etc.

Two extensions of this notation will prove useful in later chapters:

(1) If a sample size is not specified numerically, the sample is referred to as being "of size n." To indicate symbolically the set of measurements made on a sample of size n, we write $x_1, x_2, \ldots, x_n$. The three dots are an abbreviation meaning "and so on."

(2) The symbol x_i is used to denote an *arbitrary* member of the sample distribution.

1.4
DATA STRUCTURES

It was mentioned in the introduction to this chapter that the vast majority of medical studies can be classified into one of six statistical models. The next six sections contain a series of examples showing how this classification is accomplished. In every instance, there are two factors that determine to which model a given set of data belongs: (1) the nature of the measurements and (2) the relationship between the sample and the population.

Comment

Having pointed out earlier (Example 1.2.2) the arbitrariness in defining populations, it may seem inconsistent to base a classification system on the sample-population "structure." However, the freedom we have in specifying a population seldom extends beyond the limits of a particular sample-population type. That is, there may be many ways to define precisely an appropriate population

10 Statistical Models

for, say, a Model Three problem but none of these alternatives would transform it into a Model Four problem.

In reading the examples in Sections 1.5 through 1.10, think about who or what the sample members are and whether the measurements are quantitative or qualitative. And in each case, try to characterize the populations that the samples might accurately represent.

1.5
MODEL ONE: TOTAL-POPULATION PROBLEMS

Total-population problems are distinguished by the characteristic that the sample observed is actually the entire population being considered. The mortality figures discussed in Example 1.2.1 are of this type: there the population to be described was the entire set of Union soldiers who died during the Civil War, and the sample included all the 195,627 individuals who shared that particular characteristic.

Of the six models, the total-population problem is the one most uniquely medical. This is because so many medical events — like births, deaths, and the occurrences of certain diseases — are reportable, either by law or by agreement. Therefore, when the Public Health Service says that there were 81 deaths in the United States in 1967 due to measles, it can be assumed for all intents and purposes that *every* death in the U.S. in 1967 was, in fact, "sampled" and that out of that sample a total of 81 could be attributed to measles.

The statistical analysis appropriate for a Model One problem is descriptive rather than inferential (since the entire population has been sampled there is nothing to be inferred). For this reason, our discussion of total-population problems will concentrate on some of the many graphic and numerical methods that can be used to summarize data.

EXAMPLE 1.5.1. Suicide

Ever since Emile Durkheim published *Suicide: A Study in Sociology* in 1897, the phenomenon of suicide has been widely studied as a means of evaluating the levels of stress prevailing in a society. Relationships between suicide rates and a host of social factors have been proposed, tested, and verified. For example, suicide rates decline during wars and rise during depressions. They are high for the aged, the unmarried, and the childless — in short, for any group alienated from the society that surrounds it. In recent years, suicide has been the second or third leading cause of death among college students. Figure 1.3 shows suicide rates by race and sex for the United States in 1965 (Susser and Watson, 1971).

Population. All 1965 U.S. suicides.

[1.5] Model One: Total-Population Problems 11

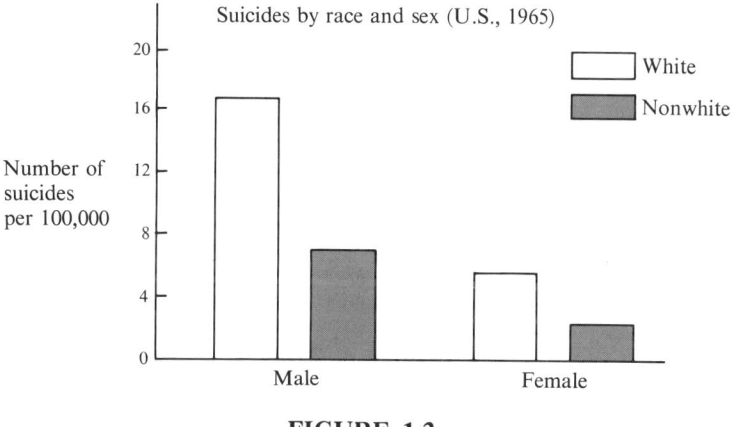

FIGURE 1.3

Question 1.5.1. The bar representing "white male suicides" is approximately twice as high as the one representing "nonwhite male suicides." Does this mean that in the United States in 1965 there were twice as many white male suicides as nonwhite male suicides? Explain.

Question 1.5.2. What might explain the considerable differences between suicide rates for males and females?

EXAMPLE 1.5.2. Male–Female Ratios

For a given area, the male–female ratio is defined as

$$\frac{\text{Number of males}}{\text{Number of females}} \times 100$$

In 1966, the overall male–female ratio in the United States was 97.0, indicating a deficit in the number of males. (This was, in fact, the lowest value recorded for the male–female ratio in the history of the United States.) At that same time, however, there was a surplus of *single* males. The next table gives the 1966 male–female ratio for single persons, ages 14 and over, in the four geographical sections of the United States (Petersen, 1969).

U.S. male-female ratio; Single, age 14+

Region	Ratio
Northeast	109.9
North central	122.7
South	124.5
West	149.1
Total U.S.	123.4

12 Statistical Models [1.6]

> *Population.* All single U.S. citizens, 14 years and older.

Question 1.5.3. The average of the four regional ratios,

$$\frac{109.9 + 122.7 + 124.5 + 149.1}{4}$$

equals 126.6 rather than the national average of 123.4 shown at the bottom of the table. Why are these two averages not equal?

1.6 MODEL TWO: ONE-SAMPLE PROBLEMS

In a Model Two problem, the sample selected does *not* include every individual in the population. With data of this type, the usual objective is to "estimate" some property of the population distribution on the basis of the sample distribution. Suppose, for example, a new toothpaste is being tested by a sample of 50 adults, and after six months a total of 40 (or 80%) have no new cavities. On that information alone, how successful might we expect the toothpaste to be in the population of *all* adults? Will it continue to be 80% effective? Or could its "true" effectiveness actually be as high as 90% — or as low as 70%?

Needless to say, any statement that might be made about the effectiveness of a product among people who have never even used it can be nothing more than a conjecture. Nevertheless, there are good conjectures, and there are bad conjectures. The objective in a one-sample problem is to make more of the former and fewer of the latter.

Actually, the one-sample problem serves a dual role. As already mentioned, it is the appropriate model for describing experiments where a single treatment is involved and where the sample size is less than the population size. At the same time, it serves as a prototype for the other four models involving inference (Three through Six). As later chapters will bear out, the basic concepts and principles of statistical inference are much the same from model to model. Yet these same concepts are easiest to understand when developed within the context of the one-sample problem.

EXAMPLE 1.6.1. X-Rays and Color TV

In the home, the amount of radiation emitted by a color television set does not pose a health problem of any consequence. But the same may not be true in department stores, where as many as fifteen or twenty sets may be turned on at the same time in a relatively confined area.

The following readings were taken at ten different department stores, each having at least five sets in their display areas. The figure shown for each store is an "average" radiation level based on readings taken at several different locations within each area (James and Moncada, 1969). In three of the ten stores, the radiation level exceeded the recommended safety limit of 0.5 milliroentgens per hour set by the National Council On Radiation Protection.

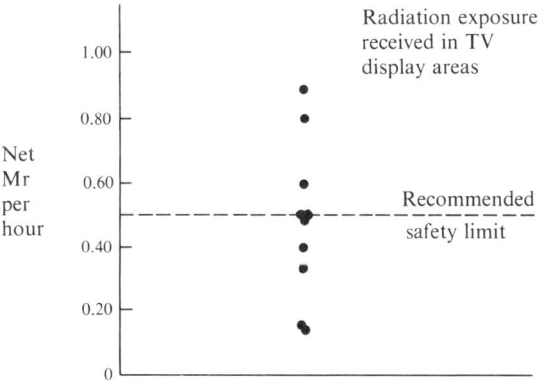

FIGURE 1.4

Population. All department store areas where color TV's are sold.

Question 1.6.1. How could these ten quantitative observations be "reduced" to ten qualitative observations?

EXAMPLE 1.6.2. Mosquito Bites

Aedes aegypti is the scientific name of the mosquito that transmits yellow fever. Although it is no longer a major health problem in this part of the world, there was a period of almost 200 years when yellow fever was possibly the most devastating communicable disease in the United States.

In a recent experiment (Jones and Pilitt, 1973), young *Aedes aegypti* females were allowed to bite an exposed human forearm. One of the variables measured was the total length of time it took the mosquito to complete the bite.

Mosquito	Bite duration (sec)
1	176.0
2	202.9
3	315.0
4	374.6
5	352.5

Population. See Question 1.6.2.

Question 1.6.2. Do these five observations accurately represent the population distribution of bite durations that would occur in a nonlaboratory environment? Explain.

1.7
MODEL THREE: TWO-SAMPLE PROBLEMS

In a one-sample problem we measure and try to characterize the effects of a single treatment on a given sample of subjects. In many situations, though, a more natural objective is to *compare* the effects of Treatment A with those of a second treatment, B. The makers of Anacin, for example, are probably more concerned with how their product measures up to Bufferin than they are about its performance relative to any arbitrarily self-imposed standards.

Studies involving the comparison of two treatments are classified as two-sample problems if (1) the individuals in the sample representing the first population are unrelated to those in the sample representing the second population and (2) the measurements recorded for both samples are "similar" (i.e., both are pulse rates, platelet counts, etc.).

Comment

In general, two measurements x and y are considered similar if their difference $(x - y)$ has physical meaning. The two measurements referred to in Example 1.2.3, for instance, would *not* be considered similar.

Pay particular attention in the next two sections to what it is in the sample-population structures that distinguishes Model Three from Models Four and Five. All three models are very common and can easily be confused.

EXAMPLE 1.7.1. Raynaud's Syndrome

Raynaud's syndrome is characterized by the sudden impairment of blood circulation in the fingers, resulting in discoloration and heat loss. The causes of this condition are not known, but the magnitude of the heat loss can be seen in the following data, where 20 subjects (10 "normals" and 10 with Raynaud's syndrome) immersed their right forefingers in water kept at 19° C. The heat output (in cal/cm²/minute) of that finger was then measured with a calorimeter (Lottenbach, 1971).

Normal subjects		Raynaud's syndrome	
Patient	Heat output (cal/cm²/min)	Patient	Heat output (cal/cm²/min)
W.K.	2.43	R.A.	.81
M.N.	1.83	R.M.	.70
S.A.	2.43	F.M.	.74
Z.K.	2.70	K.A.	.36
J.H.	1.88	H.M.	.75
J.G.	1.96	S.M.	.56
G.K.	1.53	R.M.	.65
A.S.	2.08	G.E.	.87
T.E.	1.85	B.W.	.40
L.F.	2.44	N.C.	.31

> (*First*) *Population.* All normal persons.
>
> (*Second*) *Population.* All persons with Raynaud's syndrome.

Question 1.7.1. Ideally, the *control group* (the normal subjects) in any two-sample problem should be as similar as possible to the treatment group, except with respect to the treatment. Given a set of ten patients with Raynaud's syndrome, how might they be "matched," as a group, with ten normal subjects?

EXAMPLE 1.7.2. Splenectomies

Thrombocytopenia is a condition marked by a chronically lowered blood platelet count. One of its most effective treatments is a splenectomy, the surgical removal of the spleen. But an operation of this sort is not always successful. To better understand when it *will* be, a comparison was made between the spleen weights of 5 patients for whom a splenectomy did not work and those of 14 patients for whom it did (Orringer, et al., 1970). The results are shown in Figure 1.5.

> (*First*) *Population.* All adults with thrombocytopenia whose conditions *would not be* alleviated by a splenectomy.
>
> (*Second*) *Population.* All adults with thrombocytopenia whose conditions *would be* alleviated by a splenectomy.

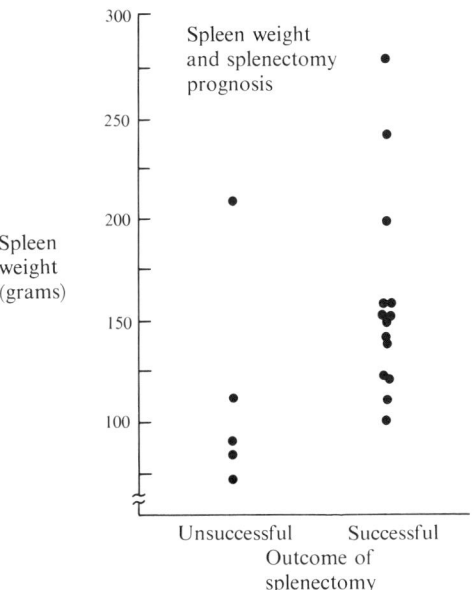

FIGURE 1.5

Spleen weights (grams)

Splenectomy was unsuccessful	Splenectomy was successful
70	150
110	142
85	160
90	110
210	120
	240
	152
	136
	122
	200
	160
	102
	152
	280

Question 1.7.2. How might these data be helpful to a physician?

1.8
MODEL FOUR: PAIRED-DATA PROBLEMS

The paired-data problem is a modification of the two-sample problem. What distinguishes the two is the identity of the individuals in the two samples. In Model Four the individuals included in the first sample (and given the first treatment) are carefully "matched," *one-by-one*, with those making up the second sample (and given the second treatment). As in the two-sample problem, the measurements recorded for the two samples must be similar.

Figure 1.6 illustrates this fundamental difference between Model Three and Model Four. In Model Three, the data consist of a set of x's and a set of y's, each measured on a set of nonhomogeneous subjects (as represented by the different geometrical shapes). In Model Four, the subjects are paired off in such a way that the members within a pair are as similar as possible. As we will see in Chapter 6, there is often much that can be gained by analyzing the d_i's of Model Four rather than the x_i's and y_i's of Model Three.

"Paired" experiments take on many forms. In medical research, pairing is often done on the basis of age, sex, and overall physical condition. A common practice in animal experiments is to form pairs out of litter mates. And, of course, any study done on a "before" and "after" basis is automatically paired.

EXAMPLE 1.8.1. Bee Stings

There are many factors that predispose a bee to sting. A person wearing dark clothing, for example, is more likely to get stung than someone wearing light clothing. Someone whose movements are quick and jerky runs a higher risk than a person who moves more slowly. Still another factor — one particularly

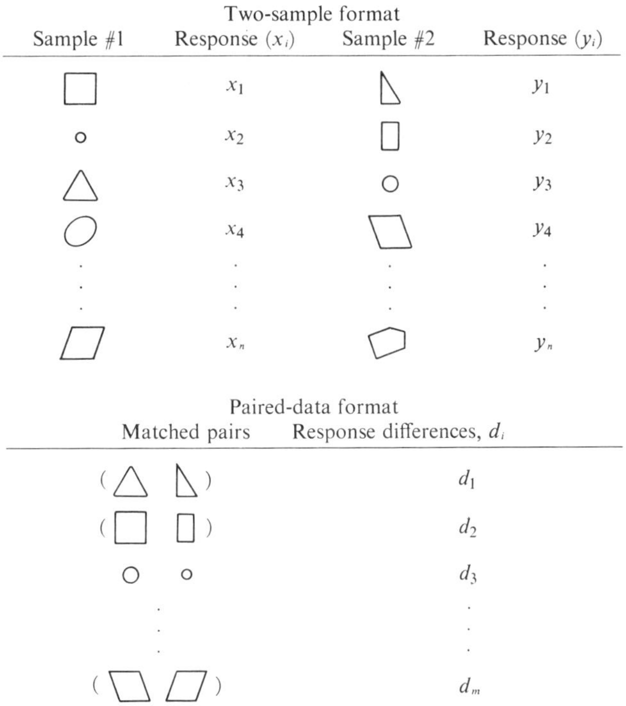

Model Four: Paired-Data Problems

Two-sample format
Sample #1   Response (x_i)   Sample #2   Response (y_i)

x_1 y_1
x_2 y_2
x_3 y_3
x_4 y_4
. . . .
. . . .
. . . .
x_n y_n

Paired-data format
Matched pairs   Response differences, d_i

d_1
d_2
d_3
.
.
.
d_m

FIGURE 1.6

important to beekeepers — is whether or not the person has just been stung by another bee.

This latter effect was simulated in an experiment (Free, 1961) by dangling eight cotton balls wrapped in muslin up and down in front of the entrance to a hive. Four of the balls had just been exposed to a swarm of angry bees and were filled with stingers; the other four were "fresh." After a specified length of time the number of new stingers in each of the balls was counted. The entire procedure was repeated eight more times.

Trial	Number of times stung Cotton balls with stings already present	Fresh cotton balls
1	27	33
2	9	9
3	33	21
4	33	15
5	4	6
6	21	16
7	20	19
8	33	15
9	70	10

18 Statistical Models [1.8]

Most likely, the disposition of the bees at any given time will be subject to a variety of more or less transient factors in addition to the cotton balls. As a result, the overall experimental environment may be quite different from trial to trial. Nevertheless, in any one trial, all eight balls are tested under the same conditions, so the two measurements in each replication can be thought of as a pair.

(First) Population. See Question 1.8.1.

(Second) Population. See Question 1.8.1.

Question 1.8.1. What two populations are represented by these data?

EXAMPLE 1.8.2. Lithium Salts and Manic-Depressives

In recent years there has been renewed interest in the use of lithium salts as a treatment for the manic phase of manic-depressive psychoses. The following study is typical of the research being done (Fieve, Platman, and Fleiss, 1969).

Six manics were observed before and after being put on a lithium regimen. Their behavior was evaluated with the Psychiatric Evaluation Form (PEF), a standard test covering six criteria (elation, hyperactivity, etc.). Each criterion was scaled from 1 to 6 in such a way that low scores would be considered good.

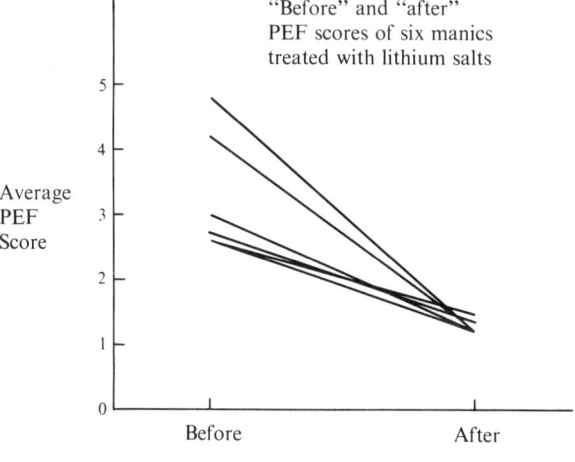

FIGURE 1.7

(First) Population. All manic depressives *before* being treated with lithium.

(Second) Population. All manic depressives *after* being treated with lithium.

Question 1.8.2. "Double blind" experiments are ones where neither the subject nor the experimenter knows which treatment the subject has been given. In that way no biases can be introduced, even if the measurements are subjective. The experiment just described was done double blind. Was that necessary? Explain.

1.9 MODEL FIVE: CORRELATION PROBLEMS

The correlation model is probably the single most common sample-population structure in medical statistics. Even newspapers feature story after story about the latest correlations found between cigarette smoking and lung cancer or coffee drinking and heart attacks. In problems of this sort, two (usually) dissimilar traits are measured for each of the members in the sample. The objective is to determine how the two are related. For the data of Example 1.2.3, the two dissimilar measurements were (1) a country's per capita cigarette consumption and (2) its CHD mortality rate. The relationship between the two has already been commented on: when one was high, the other tended to be high; when one was low, the other tended to be low.

We will consider two kinds of correlation models — those where both measurements are quantitative (such as Example 1.9.1) and those where both measurements are qualitative (such as Examples 1.9.3 and 1.9.4). The latter are known as *chi-square* (χ^2) problems and are especially important in the life sciences.

EXAMPLE 1.9.1. Health Problems and Social Change

Not long ago, Alvin Toffler wrote a best-seller called *Future Shock* in which he speculated about the cultural, medical, and moral effects of change. To what extent, for example, should change be considered a health hazard? Or is it a health hazard at all? And if it is, how might its impact best be measured?

A recent study (Wyler, Masuda, and Holmes, 1971) has provided researchers with some preliminary answers to these questions. A group of patients hospitalized for a number of chronic illnesses were asked to fill out a Schedule of Recent Experience (SRE) questionnaire. The questions related to 42 different life-change situations (a new job, another child, etc.). A composite score was computed that summarized the degree of change each person had experienced in the preceding two years. Also, each patient's health condition was graded according to the Seriousness of Illness Rating Scale (SIRS). Figure 1.8 indicates a strong association between these two variables — patients having undergone the greatest change (high SRE scores) tended to have more serious health problems (high SIRS scores).

Population. Everyone hospitalized with a chronic health problem.

Statistical Models

Life-style changes (SRE)
and health evaluations (SIRS)

Admitting diagnosis	SIRS	Average SRE
Dandruff	21	26
Varicose veins	173	130
Psoriasis	174	317
Eczema	204	231
Anemia	312	325
Hyperthyroidism	393	816
Gallstones	454	563
Arthritis	468	312
Peptic ulcer	500	603
High blood pressure	520	405
Diabetes	621	599
Emphysema	636	357
Alcoholism	688	688
Cirrhosis	733	443
Schizophrenia	776	609
Heart failure	824	772
Cancer	1020	777

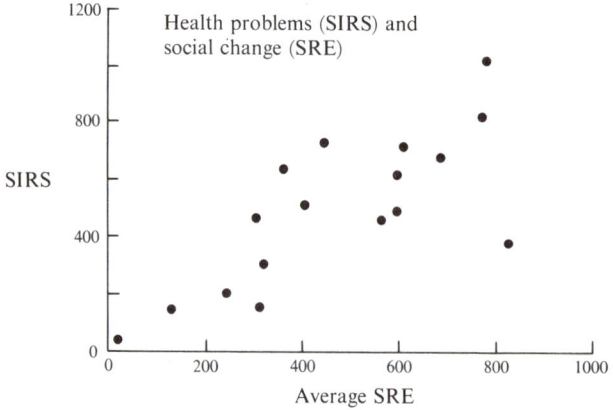

FIGURE 1.8

Question 1.9.1. When two variables (like SIRS and SRE) have a noticeable straight-line relationship, they are said to be *correlated*. It does not follow, though, that one of the variables "causes" the other. What explanation might be given to account for the observed relationship between SRE and SIRS scores other than the obvious one that more excessive life-style changes tend to precipitate more serious health problems?

Comment

Linear (that is, straight-line) relationships of the sort described in Example 1.9.1 are very important in medical research. As we will see, they provide a more than adequate description for a wide variety of phenomena. There are occasions, however, when the relationship between two variables is *nonlinear*. Example 1.9.2 is one such instance.

EXAMPLE 1.9.2. Concealing Drug Usage

A study was done at Northwestern University (Schaps and Sanders, 1970) to characterize patterns of drug usage among full-time students. A total of 38 subjects were interviewed. Their levels of usage were divided into five categories, ranging from "light" (those having only limited experience with marihuana) to "heavy" (those who regularly used a variety of drugs). A second variable of interest was the extent to which each person sought to conceal his (or her) drug habit. As a measure of this variable, each person was assigned a value on a nine-point secrecy rating scale that ranged from "not at all secretive" (1) to "highly secretive" (5). Figure 1.9 shows how the 38 subjects were eventually classified.

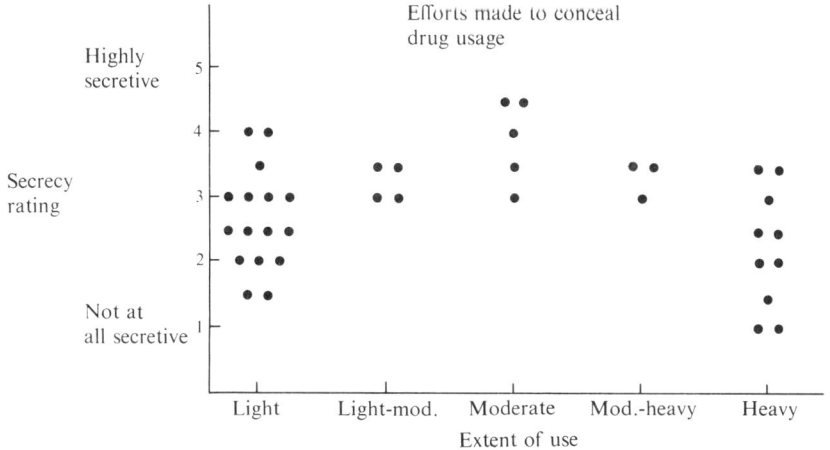

FIGURE 1.9

Population. All college drug users.

Question 1.9.2. What would explain the pattern revealed in these data — namely, that moderate users tend to be more secretive than either light or heavy users?

EXAMPLE 1.9.3. Religion and Being a Good Patient

If asked "What makes a good patient?" we would probably respond by reciting a list of personality traits — trust, perseverance, a positive attitude, etc. Maybe a better answer, though, would be a list of biological and cultural traits.

A group of 57 elderly persons visiting a certain clinic on an outpatient basis were labeled as being either "compliers" or "noncompliers" according to whether or not they followed their doctor's orders in taking medication. Typical of the data collected is the following breakdown showing that Catholics tended to be compliers and Protestants, noncompliers (Vincent, 1971). This study also revealed that, according to the same criterion, whites make better patients than nonwhites and women make better patients than men.

	Religion	
	Catholic	Protestant
Compliers	10	15
Noncompliers	7	25

Population. All elderly Catholic and Protestant patients.

Question 1.9.3. What is there about the Catholic and Protestant religions that might explain this apparent difference in patient compliance?

EXAMPLE 1.9.4. Rubella and Birth Defects

Certain viral infections contracted during pregnancy — particularly during the early part of a pregnancy — can cause birth defects. By far the most dangerous of these are Rubella infections (German measles) because of both their virulence and the frequency with which they occur.

In one study documenting this problem (Fishbein, 1962) a total of 578 pregnancies, each complicated by a Rubella infection, were classified in retrospect as having been either normal or abnormal. The abnormal group included abortions, stillbirths, all deaths within two years, and all babies with birth defects. As the accompanying table shows, a Rubella infection is especially dangerous when it occurs during the first trimester.

	When did rubella occur?	
	First 3 months	Last 6 months
Abnormal births	59	27
Normal births	143	349

Population. All pregnancies complicated by German measles.

[1.10] Model Six: *k*-Sample Problems   23

Question 1.9.4. Suppose a woman gets German measles on the seventieth day of her pregnancy. Estimate the chances that her pregnancy will be otherwise "normal."

1.10 MODEL SIX: *k*-SAMPLE PROBLEMS

Model Three problems (Section 1.7) compare two treatments on the basis of two independent samples: the individuals receiving the first treatment are different from, and unrelated to, those receiving the second treatment. The *k*-sample problem extends Model Three to include situations where three or four or, in general, *k* treatments are to be compared.

In many areas drawing heavily on applied statistics, the *k*-sample problem is the most important of the six models. This is true in psychology, biology, and the agricultural sciences. But in medicine only limited use is made of the many variations of this model. We will restrict our attention to the type shown in Examples 1.10.1 and 1.10.2.

Comment

On paper, Model Five and Model Six data sometimes look very much alike. To decide which is which, it is necessary to know *how* the data were collected. If the total sample is first divided up into treatment groups and then some response (*y*) is measured for each member in each group, the data belong to

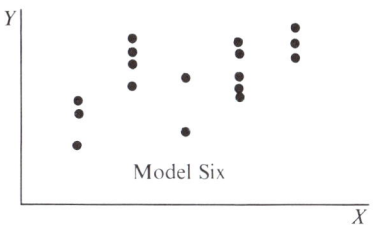

Treatment groups (a)

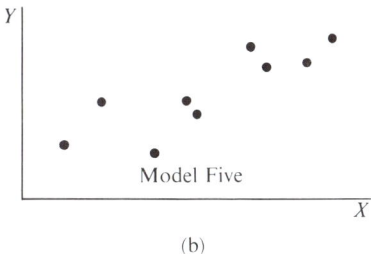

(b)

FIGURE 1.10

24   Statistical Models   [1.10]

Model Six. But if both the *x* and *y* measurements are taken simultaneously, with no attempt being made to predetermine one or the other, the data belong to Model Five. When graphed, Model Six data usually looked "grouped," whereas Model Five data generally do not.

Question 1.10.1. The data of Example 1.9.2 seem to be like the first of the diagrams in Figure 1.10. Why was it classified as a correlation problem?

EXAMPLE 1.10.1.   Mental Problems and the Full Moon

In folklore, the full moon is always portrayed as something sinister, a kind of evil force that suppresses the Dr. Jekyll and brings out the Mr. Hyde in all of us. But what happens in real life? Are there really any changes that can be measured in the way people behave when the moon is full? According to the following study, the answer may be yes.

During the 12-month period from August, 1971, to July, 1972, records were kept of the average daily admissions to the emergency room of a Virginia mental health clinic (Blackman and Catalina, 1973). Three groups were singled out: (1) admissions occurring from 4 to 13 days *prior* to the full moon, (2) admissions occurring *during* the full moon, and (3) admissions occurring from 4 to 13 days *after* the full moon. The graph below shows the average daily admissions for each of these periods during the 12 months in question.

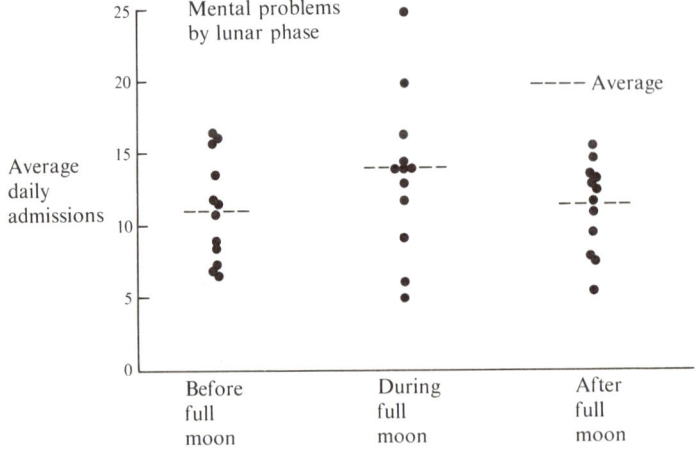

FIGURE 1.11

(*First*) *Population.* Everyone *before* a full moon.

(*Second*) *Population.* Everyone *during* a full moon.

(*Third*) *Population.* Everyone *after* a full moon.

Question 1.10.2. What other theories might explain the pattern in these data?

EXAMPLE 1.10.2. Walking Exercises for the Newborn

Normally, infants are not able to walk by themselves until they are almost 14 months old. But, as the following experiment suggests, it may be possible to substantially reduce that time by giving newborn babies special walking exercises.

A total of 23 infants were used in this study. All were white males, one week old. They were randomly divided into four groups, and for seven weeks each group followed a different "training" program. Group A received special walking and placing exercises for 12 minutes each day. Group B had similar 12-minute sessions, but without these same exercises. Groups C and D received no special instruction. The progress of Groups A, B, and C was checked every week; the progress of Group D was checked only once, at the end of the study.

After seven weeks the formal training ended and the parents were told they could continue with whatever procedure they desired. Shown below are the ages (in months) at which each of the 23 children first walked alone (Zelazo, Zelazo, and Kolb, 1972).

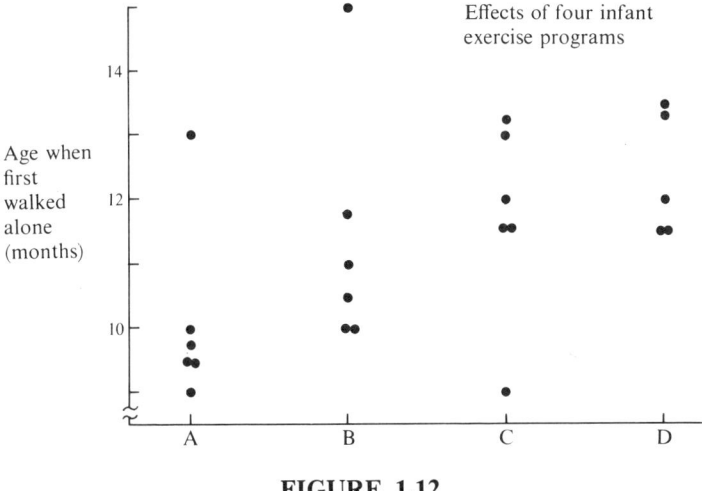

FIGURE 1.12

Populations. See Question 1.10.4.

Question 1.10.3. Why did the children in Groups C and D walk at an earlier age than the 14-month "norm" even though they received no special exercises during the training period?

Question 1.10.4. What populations are represented by these samples?

1.11 SUMMARY

Chapter 1 has two objectives — one formal, the other informal. The formal objective is to provide the guidelines necessary for distinguishing between the statistical models most frequently encountered in medical research. There are six of these, each having a different sample–population structure:

> Model One: The total-population problem
> Model Two: The one-sample problem
> Model Three: The two-sample problem
> Model Four: The paired-data problem
> Model Five: The correlation problem
> Model Six: The k-sample problem

In almost all cases, the particular model to which a given experiment belongs will be fairly obvious, once it is known what the data represent and how they were collected.

The informal objective of Chapter 1 is probably just as important as learning to distinguish Model Three from, say, Model Four. Students taking their first course in statistics almost never have a clear idea of what the subject is all about. This chapter has tried to give a first indication, in very specific terms, of the domain of statistics. Counting the exercises following this section, there are 30 applications of statistics to medicine discussed in this chapter. Areas represented include physiology, radiology, pediatrics, pharmacology, gerontology, immunology, psychiatry, and epidemiology. It should be clear from these examples, and from those in later chapters, that making sense out of numbers is a problem faced by *all* medical researchers, whatever their field.

Definitions

Control group. An "untreated" sample, whose purpose is to provide baseline responses against which the effects of the treatment(s) in the other sample(s) can be compared.

Correlation problems (*Model Five*). Experiments involving two (usually dissimilar) measurements taken on each sample member; the objective is to determine how the two are related.

Double blind studies. Experiments in which neither the subject nor the evaluator knows which treatment the subject received; helps prevent the introduction of biases.

Independent samples. Two or more samples whose members have no influence on one another, with respect to the characteristic being measured.

k-sample problems (*Model Six*). Problems involving single (and similar) measurements taken on each member of k (greater than 2) independent samples; an extension of Model Three.

Linear relationship. A particular type of association between two characteristics that can be "described" mathematically by a straight line.

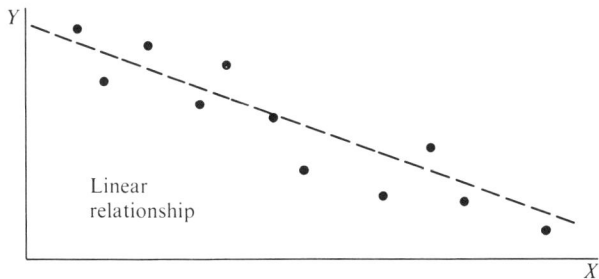

FIGURE 1.13

Matched sample. A sample whose members share many of the characteristics of another sample, but receive a different treatment.

Nonlinear relationship. Any association between two characteristics that cannot be adequately summarized by a straight line.

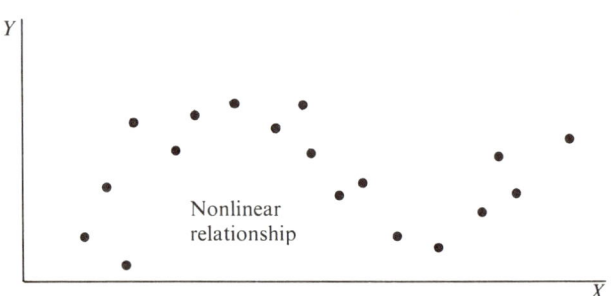

FIGURE 1.14

One-sample problems (Model Two). Experiments where a single measurement is recorded for each member of the sample; furthermore, the sample does not include every member of the population.

Paired-data problems (Model Four). Experiments where the sample subjects are matched to form pairs; each of two treatments is then applied to one member of each pair.

Population. A usually large group of individuals or objects with certain specified characteristics in common; the group about which we seek to make inferences (in Models Two through Six).

Population distribution. The collection of measurements that could be made on the members of a population; usually hypothetical.

Qualitative measurement. A nonnumerical measurement.

Quantitative measurement. A numerical measurement.

Random sample. A sample selected by any process that affords each individual in the population an equal chance of being included.

Sample. Any group of individuals or objects on which data are collected.

Sample distribution. The collection of measurements made on members of a sample.

Sample-population structure. Those characteristics of the sample and the relationship between the sample and the population that determine to which "model" a set of data belongs.

Sample size. The number of individuals (or objects) in a sample.

Statistical inference. The theory and methodology for generalizing about the properties of a population distribution on the basis of information contained in the sample distribution.

Total-population problems (Model One). Studies where the sample and the population are identical.

Two-sample problems (Model Three). Experiments involving single (and similar) measurements taken on each member of two independent samples.

Review Exercises

The data in Exercises 1.1 through 1.13 are examples of various sample-population structures. In each instance (1) decide which model is appropriate and (2) describe the population(s) represented.

1.1 Since the end of World War II, plutonium for nuclear weapons has been produced at an AEC facility in Hanford, Washington. One of the major problems encountered there has been the storage of radioactive waste. Certain of the fission by-products — most notably, Strontium 90 and Cesium 137 — have seeped into the nearby Columbia River and been carried into the Pacific Ocean. The public health consequences of these "incidents" were made apparent in a recent survey (Fadeley, 1965). Each Oregon county bordering on either the Columbia River or the Pacific Ocean was assigned an exposure index based on, among other factors, its water frontage and its stream distance from Hanford. The table below lists the index of exposure and the mortality rate from cancer for the nine counties involved. (Larger values of the index represent higher degrees of nuclear contamination.)

County	Index of exposure	Cancer mortality*
Umatilla	2.49	147.1
Morrow	2.57	130.1
Gilliam	3.41	129.9
Sherman	1.25	113.5
Wasco	1.62	137.5
Hood River	3.83	162.3
Portland	11.64	207.5
Columbia	6.41	177.9
Clatsop	8.34	210.3

*Cancer deaths per 100,000 man years from 1959 to 1964.

1.2 Fabrics washed without bleach or without any special sanitizing additives may look clean and smell clean and yet not be "bacteriologically clean." Swatches cut from 10 colored napkins, commercially laundered and ironed, were soaked in water, shredded with a blender, and poured over Petri dishes filled with a growth medium. Listed in the table are the estimated bacteria counts (per sq in. of fabric) recorded 48 hours later (Nicholes, 1970).

Napkin	Bacteria/sq in.
1	1,600,000
2	96,500
3	407,000
4	185,000
5	34,400
6	5,200
7	33,300
8	21,000
9	3,740,000
10	259,000

30   Statistical Models

1.3 In the past several years there have been two epidemics of acute mercury poisoning in Japanese fishing villages. Since then the subject has become a hotly-debated ecological issue all over the world. Much of the mercury released into the environment originates as a by-product of coal burning and other industrial processes. It does not become really dangerous until it falls into large bodies of water where microorganisms change it into methylmercury, an organic form that is particularly toxic to humans. Methylmercury is ingested and absorbed by fish which are then eaten by humans. Figure 1.15 shows, for three different age groups, the mercury uptake (in ppm) measured in 12 walleyed pike caught in Lake Erie (Pillay et al., 1972).

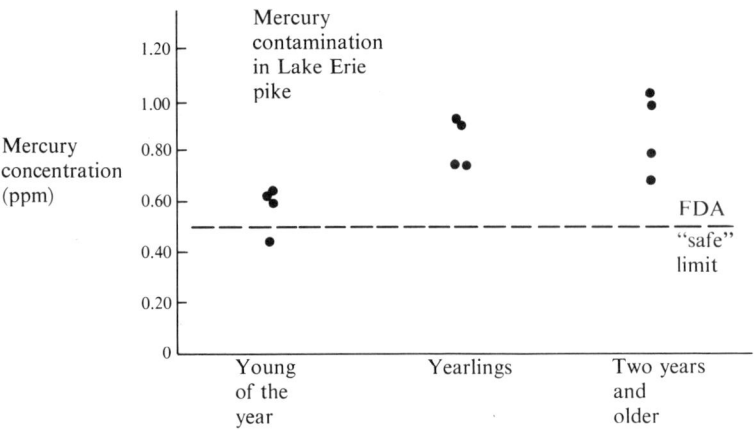

FIGURE 1.15

1.4 In general, suicide rates are much higher for men than for women (see Example 2.3.1). But that pattern is apparently reversed for members of the American Chemical Society (Li, 1969). Death certificates were obtained for 3,637 members of the ACS who died during the period from April, 1948, to July, 1967. Of that total, 3,522 were males and 115 were females. While only 3.0% of the male deaths were attributed to suicide, the corresponding figure for the female deaths was 11.3%.

	Males	Females
Suicides	106	13
Nonsuicides	3416	102
Total deaths	3522	115
Suicide %	3.0	11.3

1.5 Anyone exposed to an infectious agent, either naturally or by a vaccination, will normally develop antibodies to that agent. These antibodies are proteins carried in the blood that have the capability of inactivating the infectious agents. Presumably, the severity of an infection is related to the number of antibodies produced. The "degree" of antibody response is indicated by saying that the person's serum has a certain *titer* — the higher the titer, the greater the concentration of antibodies. In the table are the titers of 22 persons involved in a 1968 tularemia epidemic in Vermont (Buchanan, Brooks, and Brachman, 1971). Of the 22, 11 had been very ill with the disease while the other 11 were asymptomatic.

Severely ill		Asymptomatic	
Subject	Titer	Subject	Titer
1	640	12	10
2	80	13	320
3	1280	14	320
4	160	15	320
5	640	16	320
6	640	17	80
7	1280	18	160
8	640	19	10
9	160	20	640
10	320	21	160
11	160	22	320

1.6 In the United States the two leading causes of death for persons between the ages of 50 and 80 are heart disease and malignant neoplasms (cancer, leukemia, etc.). After age 80, vascular lesions (arteriosclerosis, aneurysms, etc.) rank as the second principle cause. This pattern, however, is not repeated in all countries. Figure 1.16 shows the percentage of all deaths due to either heart disease or vascular lesions, in both the U.S. and Japan (Abse, 1967). The differences are striking. For example, while heart disease accounts for 40% of all U.S. deaths at age 70, it causes only 10% of all Japanese deaths at the same age.

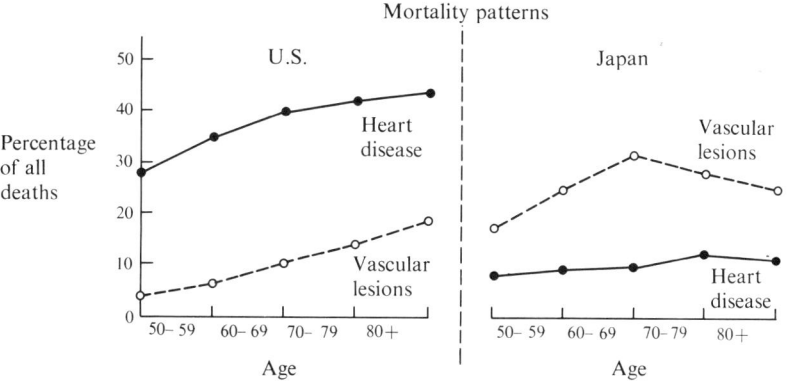

FIGURE 1.16

These data show clearly the potential hazards of overgeneralizing. Knowing only the U.S. mortality figures, we might be tempted to assume that the Japanese experience would be similar. But differences in diet, life style, genetic make-up, and so on, prove to be very important.

1.7 Radioactive gold (^{195}Au-aurothiomalate) has an affinity for inflamed tissue and is sometimes used as a tracer to help diagnose arthritis. The following data came

32 Statistical Models

from an experiment (Gerber et al., 1972) investigating the length of time, and in what concentrations, ^{195}Au-aurothiomalate is retained in a person's serum. Figure 1.17 shows serum gold concentrations found in 11 blood samples taken from patients given 50 mg of aurothiomalate. Readings were made at various times, ranging from one to nine days after injection. In each case, the retention is expressed in terms of the patient's day zero serum gold concentration. Estimate the effective half-life of ^{195}Au-aurothiomalate. That is, how long does it take for half of the gold to disappear from a person's serum?

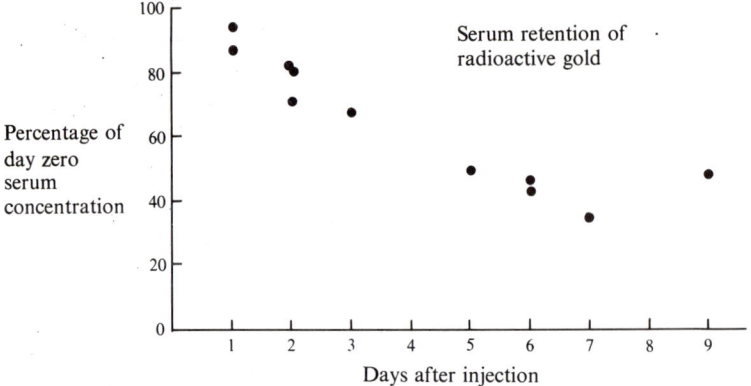

FIGURE 1.17

1.8 Methadone is a widely-used drug in the treatment of heroin addiction, another is cyclazocine. The data given here (Resnick, Fink, and Freedman, 1970) were part of a study designed to see how effective a cyclazocine program can be in eliminating an addict's psychological dependence. Two groups were examined, both were made up of chronic, male heroin addicts. Members in one group had remained on cyclazocine therapy continuously for fairly long periods of time.

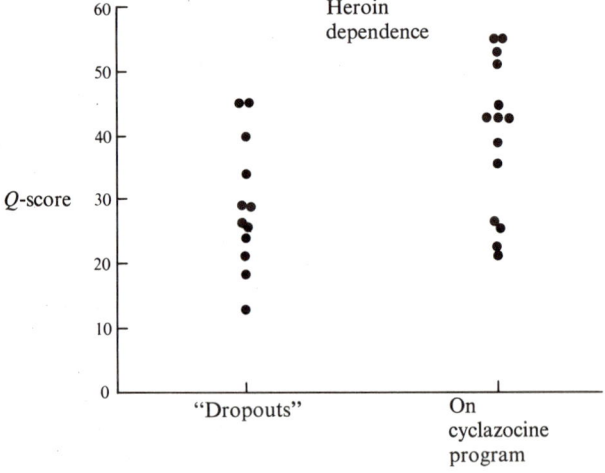

FIGURE 1.18

Members in the second group had started the program but dropped out shortly afterwards. Each of the subjects was given a psychological test that measured how he felt when he was using heroin compared to when he was "clean." The resultant Q-scores ranged from a possible minimum of 11 to a possible maximum of 55. (Higher scores represent less dependence on heroin.)

1.9 The production of a nationally-marketed detergent results in certain workers receiving prolonged exposures to *Bacillus subtilis* enzyme. Nineteen workers were tested to determine the effects of these exposures on various respiratory functions (Shore, Greene, and Kazemi, 1971). One such function, air-flow rate, was measured by computing the ratio of a person's forced expiratory volume (FEV_1) to his vital capacity (VC). (Vital capacity is the maximum volume of air a person can exhale after taking as deep a breath as possible. FEV_1 is the maximum volume of air a person can exhale in one second.) In persons with no lung dysfunction, the "norm" for the FEV_1/VC ratio is 0.80.

Subject	FEV_1/VC	Subject	FEV_1/VC
RH	.61	WS	.78
RB	.70	RV	.84
MB	.63	EN	.83
DM	.76	WD	.82
WB	.67	FR	.74
RB	.72	PD	.85
BF	.64	EB	.73
JT	.82	PC	.85
PS	.88	RW	.87
RB	.82		

1.10 Studies attempting to link water hardness with hypertension have been largely unsuccessful, but a survey done in Colorado revealed a strong relationship between hypertension and one particular constituent of water hardness, NO_3 concentration. All 63 Colorado counties were grouped according to elevation. For each of the six groupings, the 1959–1961 mortality rates from hypertension and hypertensive heart disease were compared to the average NO_3 concentration in the municipal water supplies (Morton, 1971). This finding may have important ecological significance because the current trend towards increased usage of nitrogenous fertilizers will cause NO_3 concentrations to rise in ground waters all over the country.

County elevations	Mortality rate per 100,000*	NO_3 (ppm)
8000+	24	0.1
7000–7999	24	0.8
6000–6999	22	0.4
5000–5999	24	1.9
4000–4999	24	4.1
<3999	66	10.2

*Age-adjusted 3-year mortality rate per 100,000 from hypertension and hypertensive heart disease.

34   Statistical Models

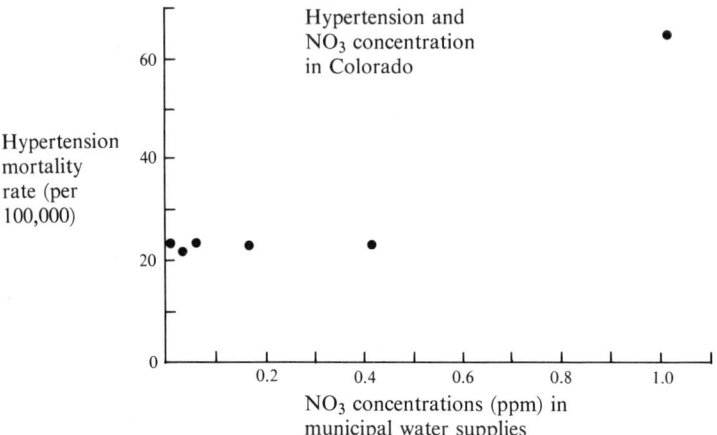

FIGURE 1.19

1.11 Oxygen deficiency is a common problem for people living at high altitudes. Its effects are varied. Some sensory functions — for example, vision — are substantially impaired; others, like hearing, are relatively unaffected. The following study examined the effect of oxygen deficiency on memory. A word association test designed to measure memory was administered to groups of people living at different altitudes. The results, scaled against normal sea-level scores, are shown below (McFarland, 1969).

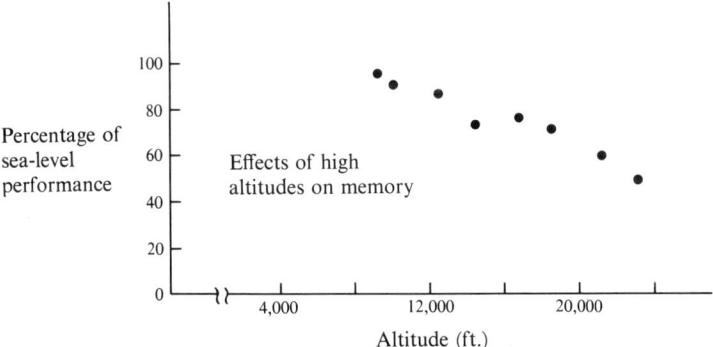

FIGURE 1.20

1.12 The average daily energy expenditures for eight elderly women were estimated on the basis of information received from a battery-powered heart rate monitor that each subject wore. Two overall averages were calculated for each woman, one for the summer months and one for the winter months (Salvosa, Payne, and Wheeler, 1971).

	Average daily energy expenditures (kcal)	
Subject	Summer	Winter
1	1458	1424
2	1353	1501
3	2209	1495
4	1804	1739
5	1912	2031
6	1366	934
7	1598	1401
8	1406	1339

1.13 As recently as the middle of the nineteenth century, the mortality associated with amputations was extremely high. For example, out of 13,000 amputations performed on soldiers injured in the Franco-Prussian War, there were 10,000 fatalities. The major problem was infection. It wasn't until 1870 that Joseph Lister, a British physician, provided the answer. The work of Louis Pasteur in demonstrating the part played by yeasts and bacteria in fermentation suggested to Lister that human infections may have a similar organic origin. He began to use carbolic acid as a wound disinfectant and achieved dramatic results. His records showed a total of 16 fatalities in 35 amputations performed *without* carbolic acid (or 46%), as compared to 6 out of 40 (or 15%) performed *with* carbolic acid (Winslow, 1943).

Lister's work was an important breakthrough in medicine on several fronts. It not only drastically reduced the risk of surgery but it also helped to firmly establish the "germ theory" as the accepted model for the nature of disease.

2

MODEL ONE
Descriptive Statistics

*A pinch of probably is
worth a pound of perhaps.*
                              Thurber

2.1
INTRODUCTION

Everyone knows how important "packaging" is in selling a product. In the short run, a little bit of tinsel, a catchy slogan, or a glossy cover can be more important to the success of a product than its own inherent quality. For better or for worse, salesmanship of this same kind has its counterpart in statistics. Ultimately, content is the most important attribute of a set of data; but what matters most to someone seeing that data for the first time is the *way* it is presented.

The many techniques, both tabular and graphical, for summarizing and displaying data are known collectively as *descriptive statistics*. In order to be effective, they must be accurate, easy to understand, and, if possible, attractive.

Of course, with only three criteria to serve as guidelines, there will necessarily be a large number of techniques to choose from. Furthermore, the generality of the criteria makes it impossible to single out any one technique as *the* method that would be best for a given set of data. Most descriptive methods, though, are variations on one of five basic formats:

(1) Frequency distributions
(2) Bar graphs
(3) Histograms
(4) Frequency polygons
(5) Scatterdiagrams

Where each of these is used and how each is constructed are the topics of Sections 2.5 and 2.6. But not every set of data lends itself to one of these five formats. In Sections 2.7 and 2.8 we look at some of the alternatives. The first part of this chapter introduces *scales* and *rates*. These are concepts related to the underlying properties of measurements and the ways those measurements can best be expressed.

Comment

While the material in this chapter is intended primarily for data belonging to Model One, much of what is covered is also applicable to the other five models. It cannot be overemphasized that a thorough statistical analysis for *any* problem should begin with a good look at the data, using whatever descriptive methods may be helpful. Only then, after getting an idea of what the numbers mean, should more quantitative methods be brought to bear.

2.2
SCALES OF MEASUREMENT

To the nonstatistician, numbers are numbers; but to the statistician, there are different *kinds* of numbers. In Example 1.9.3 a sample of 57 clinic patients was polled and found to include 17 Catholics; in Example 1.7.1 the caloric output of the right forefinger of R. A., one of the persons with Raynaud's disease, was found to be 0.81 cal/cm^2/min. Clearly, the numerical properties of these two observations are not entirely similar. The first was a count; the second, an actual laboratory measurement. The first couldn't possibly have equaled, say, 25.4 but the second could have been 0.814 or 0.8143875 . . . , depending on the precision of the calorimeter.

What makes one measurement different from another are the properties of the *scales* on which the two are recorded. Here it will be sufficient to distinguish three types of scales: nominal, ordinal, and interval.

A *nominal* scale is the most primitive. It consists of a set of possible outcomes having no particular order. For instance, suppose a family tree is traced back for several generations, with each decedent's cause of death being noted. We could record that information on a scale like the one in Figure 2.1, showing, in this case, two deaths from tuberculosis and one from diphtheria.

Clearly, there is no order relationship among these outcomes. "TB" is not, in any sense, "less than influenza" or "greater than cancer." This means that the possible outcomes could just as easily have been listed in some other way, as in Figure 2.2.

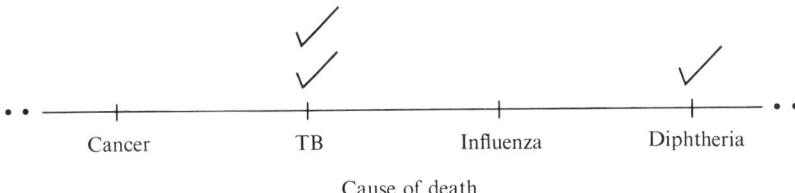

FIGURE 2.1

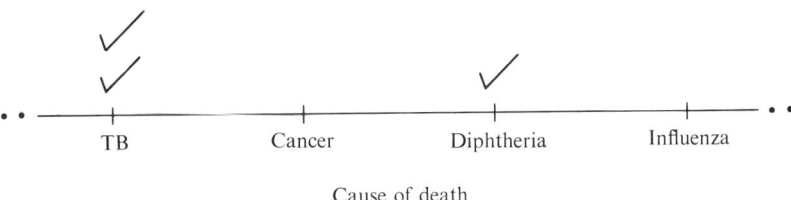

FIGURE 2.2

Ordinal scales are one step more "advanced"; their outcomes *are* ordered. For instance, suppose we test an antihistamine by giving it to a person suffering from hay fever and recording, one hour later, the degree of his discomfort. A suitable scale might be Figure 2.3. In this case the four outcomes making up the scale are definitely ordered: "none" < "mild" < "moderate" < "severe." It would not make sense to list the outcomes in any other arrangement, say Figure 2.4.

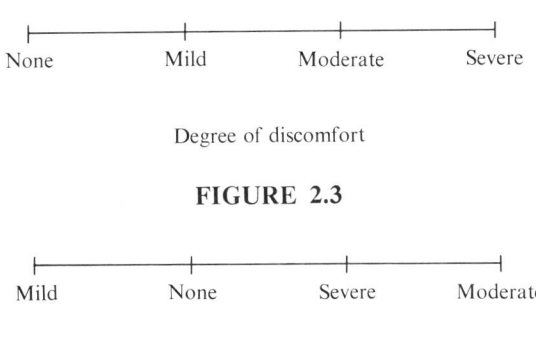

FIGURE 2.3

FIGURE 2.4

With an ordinal scale, there is the concept of "less than" but not the concept of "interval." That is, moderate is less than severe, and mild is less than moderate; but it does not follow that the difference (or interval) between moderate and severe is equivalent to the difference between mild and moderate, even though the three classes are separated by equal distances along the scale.

40 Model One — Descriptive Statistics

The highest level in the hierarchy of measurements combines the properties of differences with those of the "less than" relationship. Scales of this type are called *interval*. Height is an example of a measurement whose scale is interval.

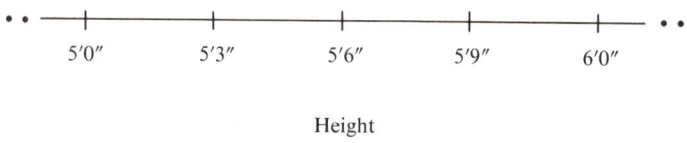

Height

FIGURE 2.5

Consider for example, four equally spaced points along the scale — say, 5'0", 5'3", 5'6", and 5'9". Not only can it be said that a person who is 5'6" is shorter than (i.e., "less than") a person who is 5'9", but it also follows that the difference between persons who are 5'6" and 5'9" is the same as the difference between persons who are 5'0" and 5'3" — namely, three inches.

Comment

As the preceding discussion would indicate, finding the scale of a set of measurements is fairly straightforward. The quickest way is to think of the possible outcomes for a single observation and ask the following two questions:
(1) Are the outcomes ordered?
(2) Does the difference between any two possible outcomes have a numerical meaning?

Positive responses to both questions imply the scale is interval; a yes to only (1) signifies an ordinal scale; two no's mean the scale is nominal.

In Chapter 1 data are classified as being either *qualitative* or *quantitative*; in this section we use the terms *nominal, ordinal*, or *interval*. The difference is basically one of refinement. In most cases, measurements recorded on either nominal or ordinal scales could also be called qualitative, and those recorded on interval scales, quantitative.

2.3 RATES

In studying medical phenomena, it helps to be able to describe numerically the "rate" at which events occur. For example, in 1968 there were 260 cases of diphtheria reported in the United States. Since the U.S. population at that time was estimated to be 201,166,000 (at midyear), it could be said that the *annual rate* at which diphtheria occurred was

$$\frac{260 \text{ cases}}{201{,}166{,}000 \text{ persons}} = .0000129 \text{ cases per person}$$

[prevalence — handwritten annotation]

But this is not entirely satisfactory because most rates encountered in medicine are so small when expressed as "cases per person" that they become difficult to interpret. A better approach is to compute the rate as, say, "cases per 10,000 persons" or "cases per 100,000 persons." For example,

$$\frac{0.0000129 \text{ cases}}{\text{person}} \times \frac{100,000}{100,000} = 1.29 \text{ cases per } 100,000 \text{ persons}$$

or

$$\frac{0.0000129 \text{ cases}}{\text{person}} \times \frac{1,000,000}{1,000,000} = 12.9 \text{ cases per } 1,000,000 \text{ persons}$$

Comment

The denominator for any rate will always be a power of 10, but the choice of a *particular* power is, to some extent, arbitrary. As a rule of thumb, we choose a denominator that will force the numerator to lie somewhere between 1 and 999. For diphtheria, any of the forms

1.29 cases per 100,000 persons

12.9 cases per 1,000,000 persons

129 cases per 10,000,000 persons

would be acceptable, but we would not express the rate as, say,

0.0129 cases per 1,000 persons

Comment

Almost all the rates we will consider describe some aspect of either natality, mortality, or morbidity. *Natality rates* refer to births, *mortality rates* to deaths, and *morbidity rates* to the occurrences of diseases.

Rates take on many different forms within each of the broad headings of natality, mortality, and morbidity. What distinguishes one form from another are the restrictions imposed on the population base. For example, the quotient formed by dividing *all* the reported cases of diphtheria by the *entire* population at risk is called a *crude morbidity rate*. Here the term "crude" refers to the fact that the population being considered — namely, everyone in the United States — is composed of individuals whose chances of contracting the disease are widely different. First of all, diphtheria occurs almost exclusively in the South. Secondly, it occurs predominantly among young children. This means that the overall rate of 1.29 cases per 100,000 persons is an inaccurate (or crude) assessment of the risk that diphtheria poses to, say, a child living in Louisiana or a senior citizen living in Maine. (It underestimates the former and overestimates the latter.)

A clearer picture of the epidemiological features of diphtheria is obtained by computing a *series* of morbidity rates, each referring to, perhaps, a particular age group and state. For instance, we might consider the quotient:

$$\frac{\text{Number of diphtheria cases among children, ages 0–14, in Louisiana}}{\text{All children, ages 0–14, in Louisiana}}$$

This is an example of a *specific morbidity rate* — in this case, age- and state-specific. By comparing similarly constructed rates for different states and different age groups we would begin to get an idea of the relative, as well as the absolute, likelihoods of various kinds of people, in various situations, contracting diphtheria.

Rates can be made specific in several ways, depending on how the denominator population is restricted. Two of the more common ways involve the age group and state of residence criteria. Two other classifications widely used are race and sex.

The next example shows how suicide rates are calculated.

EXAMPLE 2.3.1.   Suicide in the United States (1968)

(a) *Crude suicide rate in 1968*

$$\text{Total number of suicides} = 21{,}372$$

$$\text{Total U.S. population (midyear)} = 201{,}166{,}000$$

$$\begin{aligned}\text{Crude suicide rate} &= \frac{21{,}372 \text{ suicides}}{201{,}166{,}000 \text{ persons}} \\ &= \frac{0.000106 \text{ suicides}}{\text{person}} \\ &= \frac{10.6 \text{ suicides}}{100{,}000 \text{ persons}}\end{aligned}$$

(b) *Sex-specific suicide rates in 1968*
    (1) *Males*

$$\text{Total number of male suicides} = 15{,}379$$

$$\text{Total number of males (midyear)} = 98{,}869{,}000$$

$$\begin{aligned}\text{Male suicide rate} &= \frac{15{,}379 \text{ suicides}}{98{,}869{,}000 \text{ males}} \\ &= \frac{0.000155 \text{ suicides}}{\text{male}} \\ &= \frac{15.5 \text{ suicides}}{100{,}000 \text{ males}}\end{aligned}$$

(2) *Females*

$$\text{Total number of female suicides} = 5993$$
$$\text{Total number of females (midyear)} = 102{,}296{,}000$$
$$\text{Female suicide rate} = \frac{5993 \text{ suicides}}{102{,}296{,}000 \text{ females}}$$
$$= \frac{0.0000586 \text{ suicides}}{\text{female}}$$
$$= \frac{5.9 \text{ suicides}}{100{,}000 \text{ females}}$$

(c) *Sex- and age-specific suicide rates*

(1) Males

Age	Number of males	Number of suicides	Rate (per 100,000)
0–14	30,384,000	97	0.3
15–24	17,223,000	1789	10.4
25–44	23,502,000	4515	19.2
45–64	19,566,000	5893	30.1
65+	8,194,000	3085	37.6

(2) Females

Age	Number of females	Number of suicides	Rate (per 100,000)
0–14	29,286,000	21	0.1
15–24	16,761,000	568	3.4
25–44	24,111,000	2149	8.9
45–64	21,201,000	2481	11.7
65+	10,937,000	774	7.1

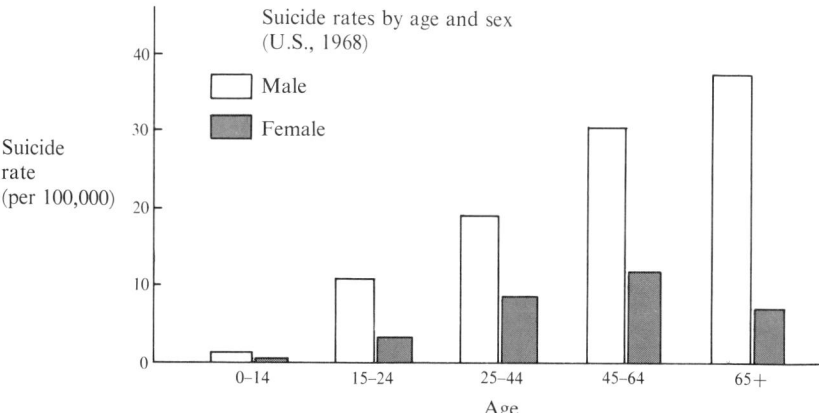

FIGURE 2.6

Notice that by breaking down suicides into age and sex categories, it was possible to retrieve certain information that was lost in the crude suicide rate. Not only are the suicide rates for males higher than those for females at *every* age group, but they follow a different pattern. The male rate increases with age; the female rate increases until it reaches a peak in the 45–64 age group. Then it declines sharply.

Question 2.3.1. In 1968, Tennessee had an estimated population of 3,878,000 and recorded a total of 415 suicides. Florida had 879 suicides among a population of 6,433,000. Compute the state-specific suicide rates for Tennessee and Florida. Why are the two so different?

Question 2.3.2. In 1970, the female population of Nashville, Tennessee, had the following age structure:

Age	Number of females
0–14	73,388
15–24	50,795
25–44	70,787
45–64	57,715
65+	29,424

Using the 1968 rates of Example 2.3.1, estimate the "expected" number of female suicides for Nashville in 1970.

2.4 ADJUSTED RATES

As demonstrated in Section 2.3, one way to characterize the occurrence pattern of a particular kind of event is to compute a series of rates, where the numerator and denominator populations have been restricted in various ways — by age, by race, by age and sex, etc. Another way is to recombine some of the, say, age-specific rates to form a single "adjusted" rate — one that is free of certain population biases.

As an example, consider the following tables showing tuberculosis mortality in Arizona and New York over the three-year period from 1959 to 1961.

TB deaths in Arizona (1959–1961)

Age	Number of deaths	1960 population	Percent	Annual rate (per 100,000)
0–24	25	560,000	48	1.5
25–44	81	313,000	27	8.6
45+	387	297,000	25	43.3
	493	1,170,000	100	14.0

Comment

When computing an *annual* mortality rate, it is necessary to account for the number of years spanned by the data. Here the total of 493 deaths in a population of 1,170,000 gives a three-year mortality rate of

$$\frac{493 \text{ deaths in 3 years}}{1{,}170{,}000 \text{ persons}} = \frac{42.1 \text{ deaths}}{100{,}000 \text{ persons per 3 years}}$$

Dividing by 3 converts this to an annual rate,

$$\frac{493 \text{ deaths in 3 years}}{1{,}170{,}000 \text{ persons}} \times \frac{1}{3} = \frac{14.0 \text{ deaths}}{100{,}000 \text{ persons}}$$

The three age-specific mortality rates listed in the last column were calculated the same way.

TB deaths in New York (1959–1961)

Age	Number of deaths	1960 population	Percent	Annual rate (per 100,000)
0–24	83	6,655,000	40	0.4
25–44	736	4,548,000	27	5.4
45+	2,929	5,579,000	33	17.5
	3,748	16,782,000	100	7.4

Suppose we wanted to characterize TB mortality in each of these states with a single number. Which number would we choose? Our first inclination might be to use the two state-specific mortality rates, 14.0 deaths per 100,000 for Arizona and 7.4 deaths per 100,000 for New York. But notice the relationship between age and the TB mortality rate: as people get older, their chances of dying from TB increase sharply. This is an important consideration because the age structures of these two states are not the same. New York is "older" in the sense that 33% of its population is made up of persons 45 or over, compared to a figure of 25% for Arizona. This means that, relative to Arizona's, New York's state-specific mortality rate is inflated, simply because its population is older.

State-specific mortality rates can be adjusted to compensate for differences in age structures by applying the already calculated age-specific rates to a standard population. For this example (and, in general), the entire United States population will be taken as the standard.

The tables on p. 45 show each state's age-specific mortality rates for TB applied to the 1960 U.S. population. The results are listed in the "Putative Deaths" columns, which give the number of TB deaths we would *expect* to occur in the entire United States in a certain age group if, say, the Arizona rate for that age group were operative throughout the entire country. For example, if all 80,653,000 persons in the United States between the ages of 0 and 24 were exposed to the Arizona 0–24 age-specific rate of 1.5 TB deaths/100,000 persons, a total of

$$80{,}653{,}000 \text{ persons} \times \frac{1.5 \text{ TB deaths}}{100{,}000 \text{ persons}} = 1{,}209.8 \text{ TB deaths}$$

would be expected in that age group, nationwide.

Arizona rates applied to the
United States population

Age	U.S. population (1960)	Rate (per 100,000)	Putative deaths
0–24	80,653,000	1.5	1,209.8
25–44	47,157,000	8.6	4,055.5
45+	52,867,000	43.4	22,944.3
	180,677,000		28,209.6

New York rates applied to the
United States population

Age	U.S. population (1960)	Rate (per 100,000)	Putative deaths
0–24	80,653,000	0.4	322.6
25–44	47,157,000	5.4	2,546.5
45+	52,867,000	17.5	9,251.7
	180,677,000		12,120.8

For each state, the *age-adjusted TB mortality rate* is defined to be the total number of putative deaths divided by the total U.S. population. For Arizona,

$$\text{Age-adjusted TB mortality rate} = \frac{28{,}209.6 \text{ deaths}}{180{,}677{,}000 \text{ persons}} \times \frac{100{,}000}{100{,}000}$$

$$= \frac{15.6 \text{ deaths}}{100{,}000 \text{ persons}}$$

For New York,

$$\text{Age-adjusted TB mortality rate} = \frac{12{,}120.8 \text{ deaths}}{180{,}677{,}000 \text{ persons}} \times \frac{100{,}000}{100{,}000}$$

$$= \frac{6.7 \text{ deaths}}{100{,}000 \text{ persons}}$$

Having negated the biases introduced by age differences in the two states' populations, the rates 15.6 and 6.7 deaths per 100,000 should provide a better assessment of the risk of TB in Arizona and in New York than do their unadjusted counterparts, 14.0 and 7.4 deaths per 100,000. (This same approach can be followed to adjust rates for other factors, or combinations of factors. See Exercise 2.4.2.)

Question 2.4.1. Common sense would tell us that, with regard to respiratory diseases, Arizona should be a healthier place to live than New York. How can this be reconciled with the fact that the age-adjusted TB mortality rate is more than twice as great in Arizona as it is in New York?

Question 2.4.2. Shown below are the frequencies of leukemia deaths, by race, for Tennessee in 1960.

Race	Number of leukemia deaths	Tennessee population
White	213	2,977,753
Nonwhite	29	589,336

Compute the race-adjusted mortality rate for leukemia in Tennessee. As a standard, use the total 1960 U.S. population, which included 158,837,671 whites and 20,487,986 nonwhites. Compare this with the unadjusted leukemia mortality rate for Tennessee.

2.5 DESCRIPTIVE STATISTICS FOR NOMINAL AND ORDINAL DATA

Recall the antihistamine example of Section 2.2 and the four-class ordinal scale ("none," "mild," "moderate," "severe") suggested for the responses. Now suppose, in fact, the drug was actually tested on five individuals.

Subject	Degree of discomfort
O.A.	Mild
N.L.	None
L.N.	Moderate
H.D.	Moderate
O.E.	None

A first step, when confronted with data like these, would be to *count* the number of times each of the possible outcomes occurred.

Degree of discomfort	Number of subjects
None	2
Mild	1
Moderate	2
Severe	0
	5

A tally of this sort is called a *frequency distribution*.

EXAMPLE 2.5.1. Changes in Mortality Patterns

Advances in medical science during the twentieth century have profoundly changed the way we are likely to die. No longer can infectious diseases, such as pneumonia and tuberculosis, be considered major killers; for the most part, their places on the mortality scale have been taken over by various degenerative diseases associated with senescence (heart attacks, strokes, etc.). The accompanying table gives an indication of the magnitude of this shift for the period from 1900 to 1965 (Susser and Watson, 1971).

Crude death rates (per 100,000) for the ten leading causes of death in 1900 and rates for these same causes in 1965

Cause	1900	1965
Influenza and pneumonia, except pneumonia of the newborn	202.2	31.9
Tuberculosis, all forms	194.4	4.1
Gastroenteritis	142.7	4.1
Diseases of the heart	137.4	367.4
Cerebral hemorrhage and other vascular lesions affecting the central nervous system	106.9	103.7
Chronic nephritis	81.0	*
All accidents	72.3	55.7
Cancer and other malignant neoplasms	64.0	153.5
Certain diseases of early infancy**	62.6	28.6
Diphtheria	40.3	0.0

*Not comparable because of change in classification.
**Birth injuries, asphyxia, infections of the newborn, ill-defined diseases, immaturity, etc.

Comment

This is an example of *two* frequency distributions, one pertaining to 1900; the other, to 1965. In both instances, the numbers of times each of the ten classes occurred have been converted to rates.

Question 2.5.1. Is the crude death rate for cancer in a typical underdeveloped country more likely to be higher or lower than it is in the United States?

Question 2.5.2. Does the fact that the crude death rate for diphtheria in 1965 was 0.0 per 100,000 mean that no one died of diphtheria in 1965?

EXAMPLE 2.5.2. Nurses and Marihuana

In 1970, over 2,000 persons attending conventions of the National Student Nurses' Association (NSNA) and the American Nurses' Association (ANA) participated in a survey studying the extent of marihuana usage within the nursing profession. Since members of the NSNA tend to be younger than members in the ANA, it was anticipated that the two groups would respond differently. The results are shown below (Lipp, Benson, and Allen, 1971).

NSNA

Past usage	Number of respondents
Have used marihuana	152
Have never used marihuana	1019
	1171

ANA

Past usage	Number of respondents
Have used marihuana	29
Have never used marihuana	933
	962

As suspected, the two groups *do not* share the same attitude towards marihuana: 13% [= (152/1171) × 100] of the NSNA members reported having had at least one experience with marihuana as compared to 3% [= (29/962) × 100] for the ANA.

Question 2.5.3. Even though survey questionnaires are filled out anonymously, there are some people who feel compelled to give answers they would *like* to be true or think *should* be true. In which "direction," if any, will false answers regarding marihuana usage tend to go?

Note that in the structure of frequency distributions we find only two of the three components necessary for the effective presentation of data (see page 37). To their credit, they are both accurate and easy to understand; unfortunately, they lack the visual impact needed to get a reader's attention. A more graphical, and hence "attractive," version of the frequency distribution is a *bar graph*, where the number of times each of the possible outcomes occurred is represented by the height of a bar.

EXAMPLE 2.5.3. A Nurse's Day

Much has been written about the shortage of medical personnel and its ultimate effect on the delivery of community health services. But numbers are only part of the problem. In many cases, the personnel that *are* available are used in inefficient ways, doing time-consuming tasks that could just as easily be handled by nonmedical assistants.

The role of the public health nurse is probably typical of this situation. Over one-third of all nurses working in public health are employed by boards of education and assigned to schools, where their duties include audiovisual testing, immunizations, and general health care. A recent survey, though, showed that school nurses spend almost as much time doing clerical and housekeeping chores as they do nursing (Doster, 1970).

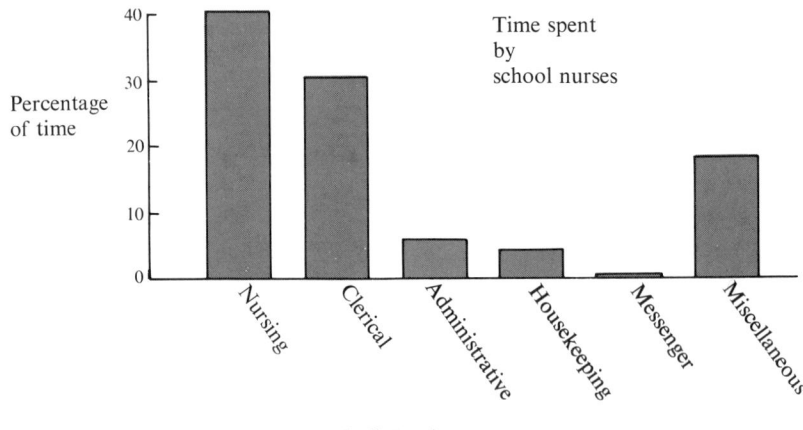

FIGURE 2.7

Question 2.5.4. How might this same information be presented using a circle?

Comment

There are certain conventions that should be followed when drawing a bar graph:

(1) Each axis should be labeled clearly and with enough detail that the reader can easily understand what the graph represents.
(2) A space should be left between each of the bars.
(3) A space should be left between the leftmost bar and the vertical axis.
(4) Whenever possible, the vertical axis should begin at zero. The lone exception to this is when all the frequencies or rates being graphed are much larger than zero. For example, the frequency distribution:

Outcome	Frequency
A	920
B	910
C	960

would be graphed with a "broken" vertical axis as in Figure 2.8(a), rather than with a continuous axis beginning at zero as in Figure 2.8(b). It would be wrong, though, simply to begin the vertical axis at, say, 900, and not even indicate the number zero. The reason for making such an issue of what may seem to be a small point is that data can easily be

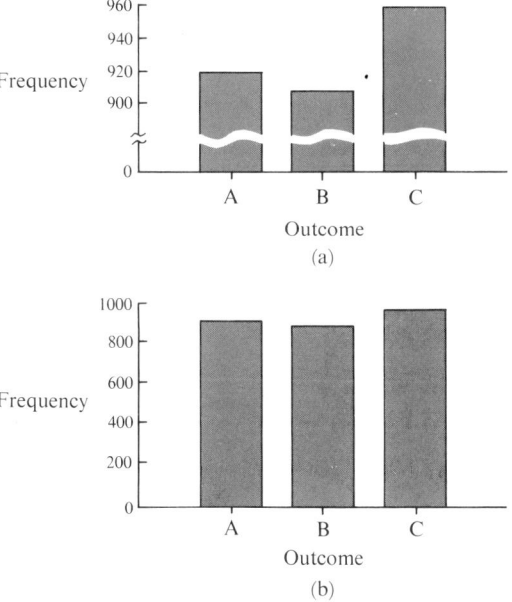

FIGURE 2.8

distorted with a vertical scale that does not begin at zero. But when the symbol:

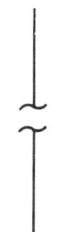

is used, the reader is at least warned to proceed with caution.

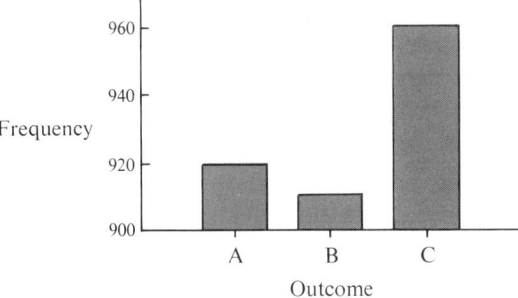

FIGURE 2.9

EXAMPLE 2.5.4. **Infections during Pregnancy**

Estimates show that more than 5% of all pregnancies are complicated by viral infections. Some of these can have very serious consequences. For example, if a woman gets German measles (Rubella) during the first month of her pregnancy, there is a 50–50 chance that the baby will be born with a birth defect.

The bar graph in Figure 2.10 shows the six viral infections occurring most frequently during pregnancy (Sever, 1970). Of these particular six, however, only the Rubella virus increases the likelihood of a birth defect.

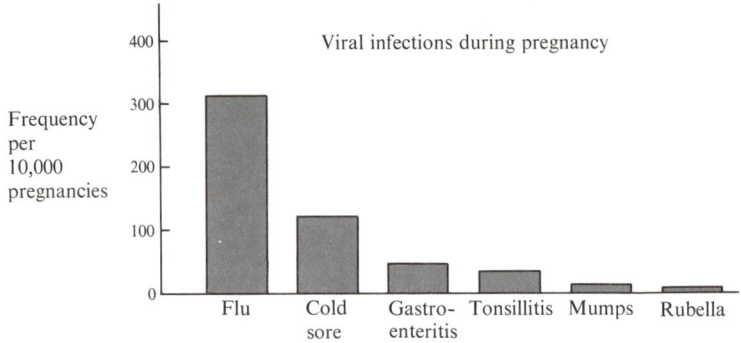

FIGURE 2.10

Question 2.5.5. In this example, does the *order* in which the bars are arranged, from left to right, matter?

Question 2.5.6. In 1967, there were approximately 3,521,000 live births in the United States. During about how many of those pregnancies did the mother have tonsillitis?

2.6
DESCRIPTIVE STATISTICS FOR INTERVAL DATA

With nominal and ordinal data, the possible outcomes (as they might appear on the horizontal axis of a bar graph) are essentially predetermined by the nature of the observations. The same is not true for interval data. For example, if the data collected are blood pressures recorded as low, normal, or high, then these three outcomes automatically become the scale values. But if these same blood pressures were measured on an interval scale, as mm of Hg, the data would be a set of numbers (102, 135, 110, etc.), and the resulting frequency distribution (using the integers from, say, 90 to 200 as possible outcomes) might be nothing more than a series of 0's and 1's (unless the sample size was very large):

Blood pressure (mm of Hg)	Frequency
90	0
91	1
.	.
.	.
.	.
199	0
200	1

From a descriptive standpoint, a listing like this would not be very enlightening. It would be far better to combine (or group) consecutive blood pressures into classes and then record the number of times each class was represented. That way it would be possible to get a much clearer picture of the overall shape of the data.

Blood pressure (mm of Hg)	Frequency
90–99	3
100–109	5
.	.
.	.
200–209	1

Of course, it is not obvious how these classes are to be defined. Why, for example, was the first class chosen to be "90–99" and not "90–95"? Like so many other questions in descriptive statistics, this one has no clearcut answer. But there are three rules of thumb that can provide at least some guidance. First, each of the classes should have the same width. Second, the width selected should divide the range of the sample measurements into a reasonable *number of classes*. ("Reasonable" often means between 5 and 15.) And third, the lower limit of each class should be kept simple — a multiple of 5, if possible. (More will be said about the construction of classes in some of the examples.)

Three basic formats are used with interval data: frequency distributions (Example 2.6.1), histograms (Examples 2.6.2 and 2.6.3), and frequency polygons (Examples 2.6.4 and 2.6.5). A *histogram* is like a bar graph except that the bars are adjacent, in deference to the nature of the scale. In some situations it is more convenient to represent the frequency of a given class by a point rather than by a bar. If consecutive points are then connected with straight lines the resultant figure is known as a *frequency polygon*. This is a particularly useful format when several sets of data are to be displayed on the same graph.

EXAMPLE 2.6.1. Traffic Mortality

In 1971, over 55,000 Americans died in traffic accidents. Connecticut had the safest highways, with a fatality rate of 2.8 deaths per 100 million motor vehicle miles, while Alaska had the most dangerous, 8.8 deaths per 100 million mvm.

Contrary to what we might think, the nationwide fatality rate, 4.7 deaths per 100 million mvm, was the lowest on record. By way of contrast, the nationwide traffic mortality rate in the 1920s and '30s was more than twice as high as the 1971 figure ("Medical News," 1972).

Traffic deaths per 100,000 mvm					
Ala	6.4	La	7.1	Ohio	4.5
Alaska	8.8	Maine	4.6	Okla	5.0
Ariz	6.2	Mass	3.5	Ore	5.3
Ark	5.6	Md	3.9	Pa	4.1
Cal	4.4	Mich	4.2	RI	3.0
Color	5.3	Minn	4.6	SC	6.5
Conn	2.8	Miss	5.6	SD	5.4
Del	5.2	Mo	5.6	Tenn	7.1
Fla	5.5	Mont	7.0	Tex	5.2
Ga	6.1	NC	6.2	Utah	5.5
Hawaii	4.7	ND	4.8	Va	4.5
Idaho	7.1	Nebr	4.4	Vt	4.7
Ill	4.3	Nev	8.0	WVa	6.2
Ind	5.1	NH	4.6	Wash	4.3
Iowa	5.9	NJ	3.2	Wisc	4.7
Kans	5.0	NM	8.0	Wy	6.5
Ky	5.6	NY	4.7		

To form classes for any set of data, we first locate the smallest and largest observations (in this case, 2.8 and 8.8) and then choose limits that satisfy the three criteria cited earlier. Here, a reasonable set of classes would be "2.0–2.9," "3.0–3.9," ..., "8.0–8.9."

Traffic death rate per 100 million mvm	Number of states
2.0–2.9	1
3.0–3.9	4
4.0–4.9	16
5.0–5.9	15
6.0–6.9	7
7.0–7.9	4
8.0–8.9	3
	50

Question 2.6.1. Look again at the state-specific traffic death rates. What are some of the factors that might "explain" the observed variation among the states? Why should Alaska have the highest death rate? Why are the rates along the heavily-populated Eastern seaboard so low?

The next two examples illustrate the construction of histograms. Like the bar graphs of Section 2.5, histograms supply the visual dimension that frequency distributions lack.

EXAMPLE 2.6.2. Tuberculosis in the United States

In the early years of the nineteenth century, almost one-quarter of all deaths in the United States were due to tuberculosis. Today antibiotics have brought it under control but there is still a sizeable fraction of the U.S. population with inapparent TB infections. It was estimated, for example, that in 1960 almost 40,000,000 people in the United States (about 1 in every 5) would have given a positive reaction to a tuberculin test (Lowell, Edwards, and Palmer, 1969).

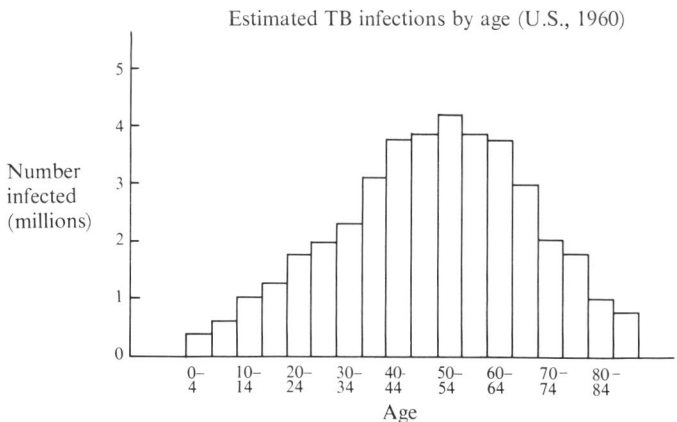

FIGURE 2.11

Comment

Graphically, the only difference between a histogram and a bar graph is the adjacency of the bars. All the other conventions mentioned in Example 2.5.3, such as leaving a space between the vertical axis and the leftmost bar, also apply to histograms.

Question 2.6.2. In 1960 there were 41,738,000 people in the United States fifty years or older. Approximately what percentage were infected with the tubercle bacillus? Is this percentage more likely to be higher or lower in 1970?

EXAMPLE 2.6.3. Etruscan Skulls

In the eighth century B.C., the Etruscan civilization was the most advanced in all of Italy but, militarily, it proved to be no match for the Roman legions. By the dawn of Christianity it was all but gone. Unfortunately, no chronicles of the Etruscan empire were ever written and to this day it remains shrouded in mystery. Much of what *is* known has come from anthropometric studies — the use of body measurements to determine racial characteristics. These data were adapted from one such study (Barnicot and Brothwell, 1959).

Model One — Descriptive Statistics

Maximum head breadths (in mm)
of 84 Etruscan males

141	148	132	138	154	142	150
146	155	158	150	140	147	148
144	150	149	145	149	158	143
141	144	144	126	140	144	142
141	140	145	135	147	146	141
136	140	146	142	137	148	154
137	139	143	140	131	143	141
149	148	135	148	152	143	144
141	143	147	146	150	132	142
142	143	153	149	146	149	138
142	149	142	137	134	144	146
147	140	142	140	137	152	145

Here the smallest observation is 126 and the largest, 158. A suitable set of classes would be "125–129," "130–134," "135–139," etc.

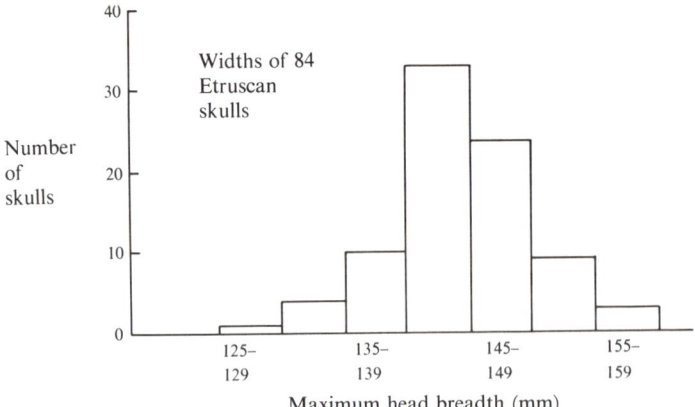

FIGURE 2.12

Comment

Another way to label a class is by designating its center (or *midpoint*) rather than its upper and lower limits. (See Figure 2.13.) For example, the midpoint of the "125–129" class is given by

$$\frac{125 + 129}{2} = 127$$

Question 2.6.3. Why are the bars of the histograms in Figure 2.13 adjacent even though the intervals defined by the class limits are not?

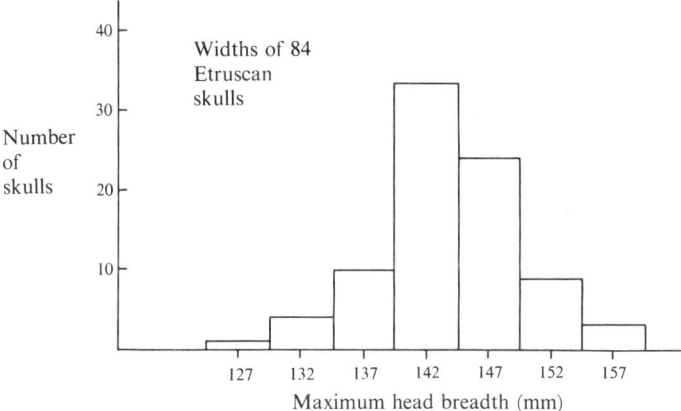

FIGURE 2.13

Another way of representing the number of observations that belong to a certain class is by plotting a point above each class midpoint at a height equal to the class frequency. If consecutive points are then connected with straight lines the resulting figure is known as a *frequency polygon*.

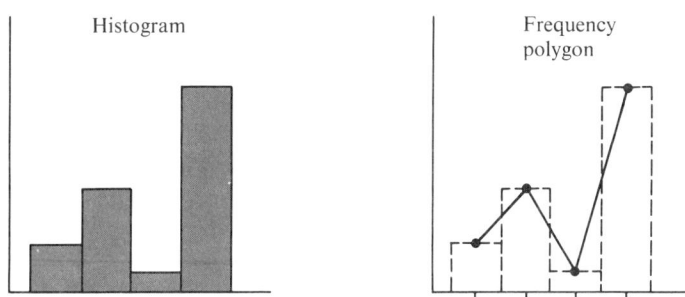

FIGURE 2.14

In many instances, histograms and frequency polygons can be used interchangeably, but the latter are especially effective when several sets of data are to be shown on the same graph. (See Example 2.6.5.)

EXAMPLE 2.6.4. Prothrombin Times

Blood coagulates only after a very complex series of chemical reactions has taken place. The final step is the transformation of fibrinogen, a protein found in the plasma, into fibrin, which forms the clot. The fibrinogen–fibrin reaction is triggered by another protein called thrombin, which itself is formed under the influence of still other proteins, including one called prothrombin.

One procedure for measuring clotting ability is the one-stage Quick test. This consists of adding to a blood sample a substance (thromboplastin) that initiates the prothrombin–thrombin reaction, and, thereby, the clotting process.

Model One — Descriptive Statistics

The interval between the addition of thromboplastin and the formation of a clot is called the prothrombin time. Shown below are prothrombin times found for ten samples of normal blood (Biggs, 1951).

Sample	Prothrombin time (seconds)
1	17.0
2	20.0
3	25.0
4	18.5
5	13.0
6	17.0
7	8.5
8	16.0
9	27.5
10	12.0

If "6.0–9.9," "10.0–13.9," ..., "26.0–29.9" are used as classes, the midpoints along the horizontal axis of the frequency polygon will be 7.95, 11.95, ..., 27.95.

Prothrombin time (sec)	Midpoint	Frequency
6.0– 9.9	7.95	1
10.0–13.9	11.95	2
14.0–17.9	15.95	3
18.0–21.9	19.95	2
22.0–25.9	23.95	1
26.0–29.9	27.95	1
		10

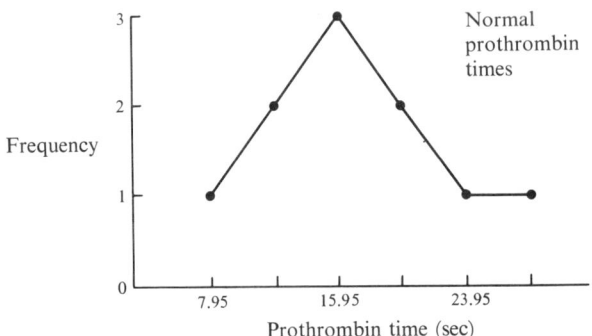

FIGURE 2.15

Question 2.6.4. With the frequency polygon format, why is the frequency of, say, the "6.0–9.9" class represented by the height of a point located above the number 7.95 on the horizontal scale and not above the number 6.0 or 9.9?

Question 2.6.5. To which sample-population model do these data belong?

EXAMPLE 2.6.5. Politics and Academia

Until recently, very little was known about the political leanings of university faculties. It was tacitly assumed that a teacher would vote according to the patterns established by his or her ethnic group, religious affiliation, or socioeconomic level. But that does not seem to be the case. In 1969, an extensive survey of American college and university professors revealed that their political preferences were closely tied to their fields of interest. A "typical" physicist, for example, will react to public issues quite differently than a "typical" engineer, even though the two might be next-door neighbors and identical with respect to all the usual political indices.

Shown below are the political philosophies of faculty members from four different academic disciplines — agriculture, medicine, law, and social science (Ludd and Lipsit, 1972).

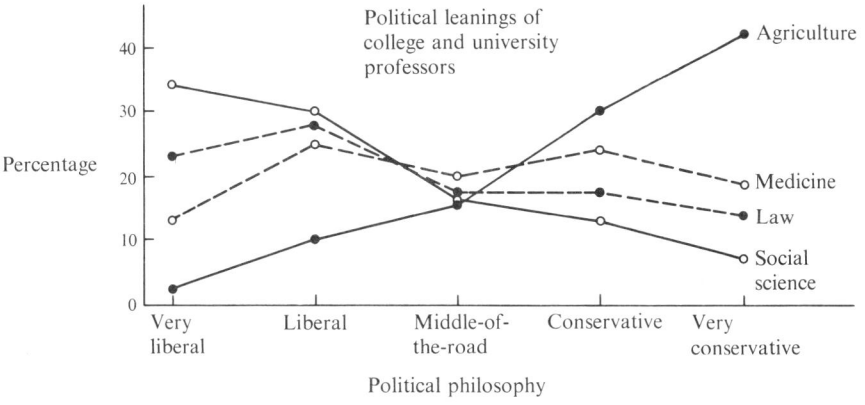

FIGURE 2.16

Question 2.6.6. How might this same information be displayed on a single graph using the histogram format?

Often more than one attribute of a sample member is measured. In Example 1.9.1, for instance, each patient was rated according to (1) the seriousness of his illness and (2) the amount of recent change in his lifestyle. In cases like these, the *relationship* between the two sets of measurements is what is important, and one very effective way of picturing that relationship is by drawing a *scatterdiagram*. This is simply a graph of points where the x and y coordinates of a given point are the two measurements recorded for some particular sample member.

EXAMPLE 2.6.6. **Dental Caries and Fluoridation**

Many water supplies throughout the United States contain sizeable amounts of naturally occurring fluorides. This suggests that by determining the frequency of dental problems from place to place, it should be possible to measure the effectiveness of fluoride as a decay preventative. The scatterdiagram in Figure 2.18 shows how this has actually been done (World Health Organization, 1970); the data points refer to dental surveys done in 21 cities throughout Ohio, Indiana, and Illinois.

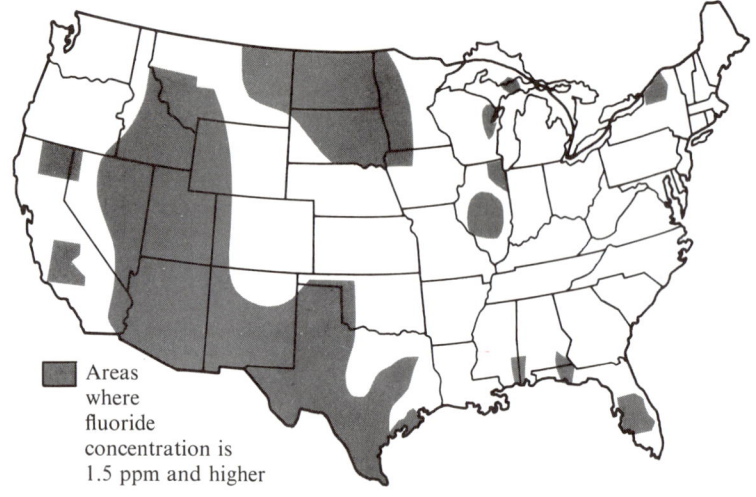

FIGURE 2.17

Here the beneficial effects of fluoride are unmistakable: children living in cities with higher fluoride concentrations tend to have fewer caries. (It was this sort of evidence that provided the impetus for artificially raising the fluoride concentrations of water supplies in certain parts of the country.)

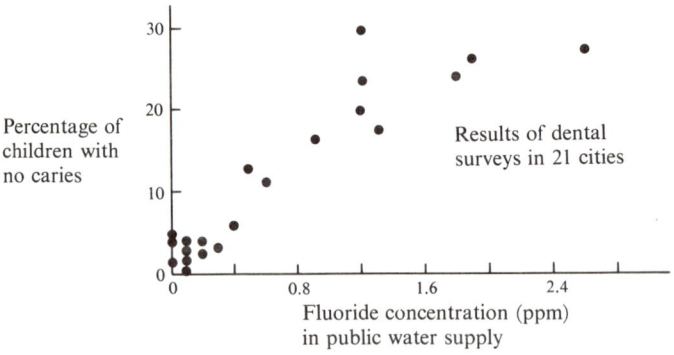

FIGURE 2.18

Question 2.6.7. What are the 21 sample members referred to in this problem?

Question 2.6.8. What other factors (besides fluoride content) might have influenced these results?

Question 2.6.9. Comparisons of medical histories of the sort described above are known as *retrospective* studies. They draw on information and conditions already present (for example, the fact that fluoride concentrations vary from place to place). What are some other medical problems whose solutions might depend on data gathered from retrospective studies?

2.7 SPECIAL TECHNIQUES

Bar graphs, histograms, frequency polygons, and scatterdiagrams are, unquestionably, the most popular ways of displaying data, but sometimes they can be improved upon. Don't let your ingenuity be stifled by convention. Approach each set of data with the basics firmly in mind but, at the same time, try to think of modifications that might be even more effective.

Probably the most typical reason for embellishing any of the basic formats is the need to display two or more kinds of information on the same graph. Example 2.7.1 falls into this category.

EXAMPLE 2.7.1. Mode of Childbirth in the United States

In 1935 almost two-thirds of the mothers in the United States had their babies at home. Today that figure has shrunk to less than 2%. The modified histogram below gives by five-year intervals (1) the total number of births and (2) the number and percentage of births that were delivered by either a "physician in a hospital," "a physician not in a hospital," or a "midwife" (Anderson, 1969).

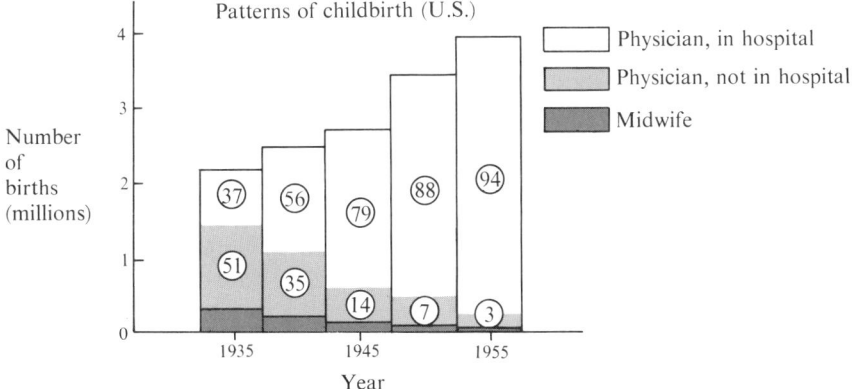

FIGURE 2.19

Question 2.7.1. Records kept during the 30s and 40s showed that mothers having their babies in hospitals had a higher mortality rate (from the childbirth) than mothers delivering their babies at home. What would account for this?

Sometimes the best approach to take when graphing a set of data is to abandon the standard formats and look for something new.

EXAMPLE 2.7.2. Fetal Heart Rates

Traditionally, obstetricians have used the stethoscope to listen to fetal heart rates (FHR) just prior to delivery. This technique, however, is far from satisfactory, with the main problem being the difficulty in isolating the FHR from all the other sounds picked up by the stethoscope. The magnitude of these measurement errors was brought out very clearly in a study where fifteen obstetricians were asked to "count" a series of simulated fetal heart beats (Hon, 1970).

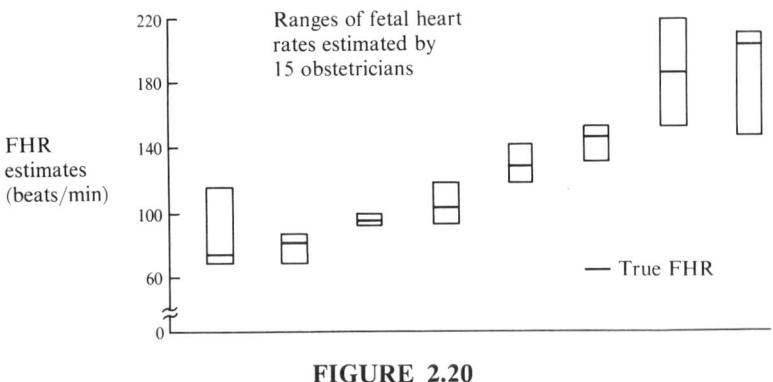

FIGURE 2.20

Question 2.7.2. Is there any indication in these data that, in counting fetal heart beats, obstetricians are influenced by what they think the rate *should* be?

The last two examples in this section are variations of histograms. The first is commonly used in epidemiology; the second, in demography.

Epidemiology is the study of epidemics, where they start and how they are transmitted. In everyday language, the word has grandiose connotations. We think of cholera epidemics or flu epidemics affecting thousands, maybe even hundreds of thousands, of people. To an epidemiologist, though, twenty people coming down with food poisoning after attending a church supper also constitutes an epidemic.

Regardless of its size, the first step taken in describing an epidemic, statistically, is the construction of a histogram showing the number of new cases diagnosed each day (or whatever time period is appropriate). These graphs are called *epidemic curves*.

EXAMPLE 2.7.3. Vaccine Contamination

The search for a polio vaccine was a major medical research effort during the 1940s and '50s, ending, temporarily, with the discovery of the Salk vaccine. Tested in 1954 on almost 500,000 children, the vaccine was found to be safe and effective.

But in the spring of 1955, shortly after a second immunization campaign had begun, a disturbingly large number of polio cases were reported among children recently inoculated. An investigation revealed that some of the vaccine produced by one of the suppliers contained live virus. Ultimately, a total of 61 cases of paralytic polio were linked to the contaminated vaccine (Langmuir, 1963).

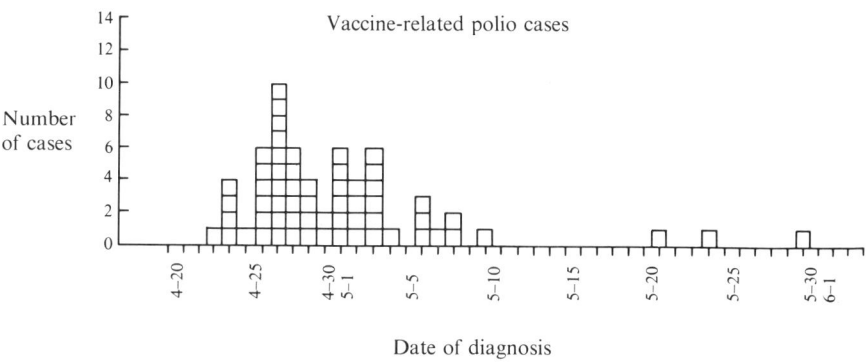

FIGURE 2.21

Comment

A widely-accepted convention in drawing epidemic curves is to subdivide the bars into blocks, letting each block represent one case. The blocks make it easy to add another variable to the graph. For example, an x might be put in each block corresponding to a case living in a certain area. Any obvious nonrandomness in the locations of the x-blocks might suggest a previously undetected pattern in the spread of the disease.

Question 2.7.3. What other information, besides residence, might it be helpful to incorporate into an epidemic curve?

Whereas epidemiology focuses on events affecting only highly selected groups within a population, the science of demography looks at characteristics shared by the *entire* population. Example 2.7.4 shows how some of this information — namely, the age and sex distribution of a population — is typically presented. The format used here is a histogram known as a *population pyramid*.

EXAMPLE 2.7.4. Population Pyramids

The age and sex distribution of a country's population reflects its position on the socioeconomic continuum (Benjamin, 1969). Underdeveloped nations have high birth rates and high death rates which combine to produce a very young population (see, for example, Brazil in 1960). Conversely, countries that are highly developed have lower birth rates and lower death rates, so much larger proportions of their populations are in older age brackets (see England and Wales in 1967).

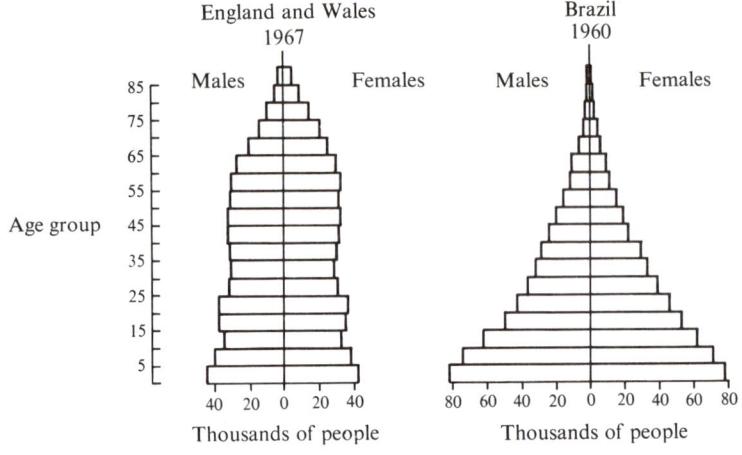

FIGURE 2.22

Question 2.7.4. Major events in the history of a country are sometimes mirrored in the shape of its population pyramid. Figure 2.23 shows the age and sex distribution of Russia in 1959 (Hollingsworth, 1969). Why are the percentages of men and women in the 10–19 age group so disproportionately small?

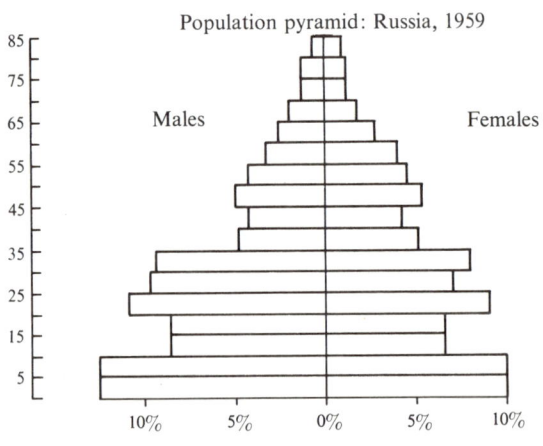

FIGURE 2.23

2.8
LOGARITHMIC SCALING

So far, all the frequency scales (vertical axes) we have encountered have been *arithmetic*. The "distance" between any two frequencies on such a scale is determined by their numerical difference. For example, the scale distance between 2 and 8 is three times as great as the distance between 12 and 14.

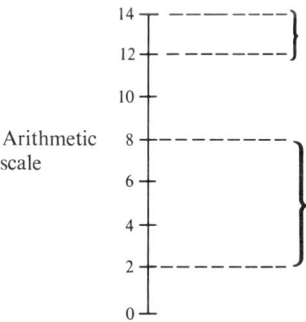

FIGURE 2.24

But frequency scales can also be constructed so that the distance between two numbers is determined from their ratio rather than by their difference; scales of this kind are called *logarithmic* (or *log*). Consider the mortality associated with two hypothetical diseases, A and B. Suppose Disease A accounted for 20,000 deaths in 1900 and 4000 in 1970, while the numbers of deaths attributed to Disease B were 500 and 100 during the same two periods. For each disease the number of fatalities declined by 80% [(20,000 − 4000)/20,000 = 0.80 = (500 − 100)/500]. On a log scale the distance between 4000 and 20,000 would be the same as the distance between 100 and 500.

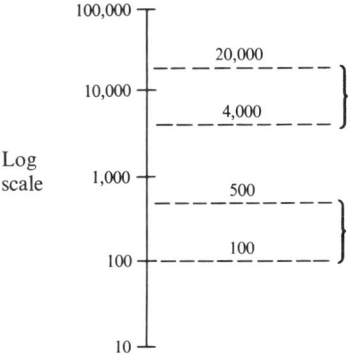

FIGURE 2.25

In medical statistics, graphs with log scales are often used to compare, over time, the *proportional* changes in either (1) the mortality or morbidity due to several diseases (Example 2.8.1) or (2) various aspects, such as cases and deaths, of a single disease (Example 2.8.2). The graphical format used with a log scale is always the frequency polygon.

EXAMPLE 2.8.1.   Mortality Trends in the United States

Figure 2.26 shows the trends in mortality rates from (1) all causes, (2) malignant neoplasms, (3) measles, and (4) automobile accidents for the period 1900–1959

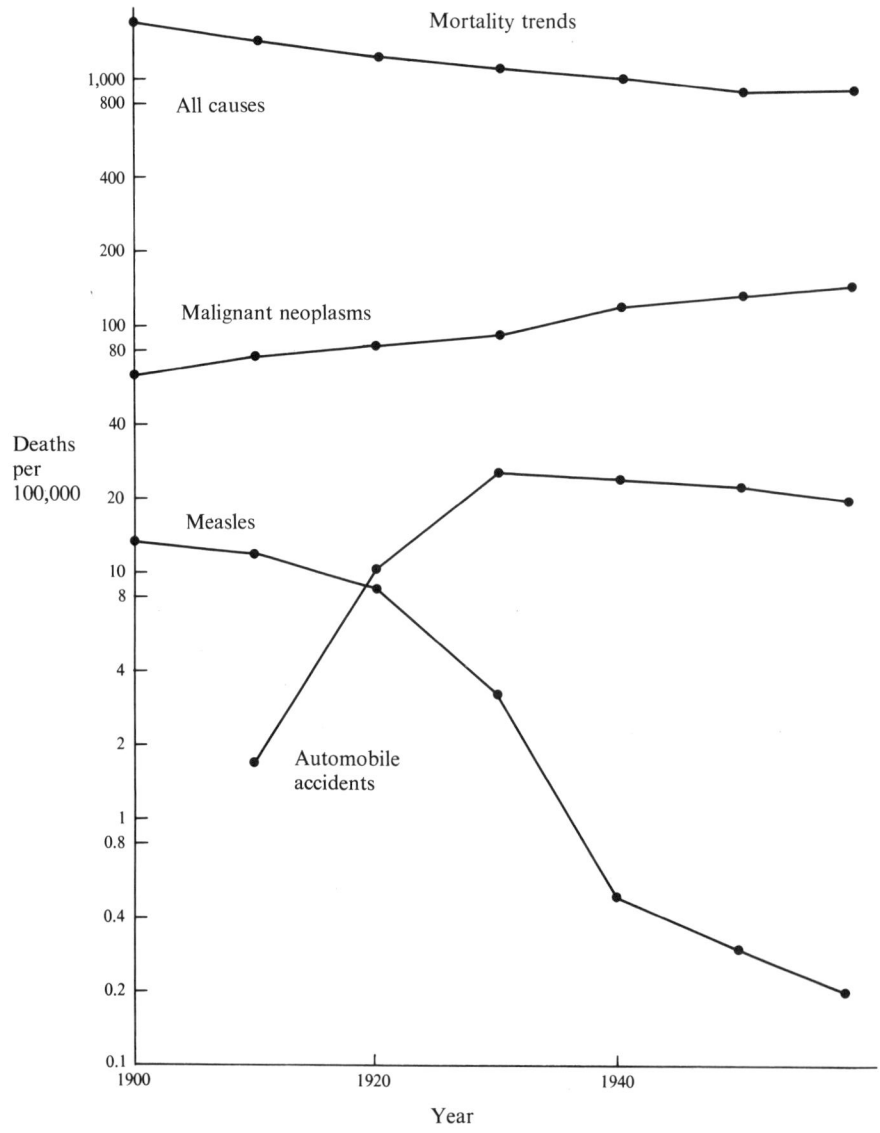

FIGURE 2.26

(Graham, 1963). The rates are plotted on a log scale to facilitate the comparison of their percentage changes over time. Mortality rates from all causes and measles, for example, both declined during this period, but the rate for measles declined much faster.

Question 2.8.1. When were measles and automobiles equally lethal in terms of the number of fatalities each was responsible for?

EXAMPLE 2.8.2. Malaria in the United States

Surveys taken during the 1930s indicated that malaria was a major health problem in certain parts of the United States. The disease was endemic along the southern Atlantic coast and in the Mississippi delta region; the number of

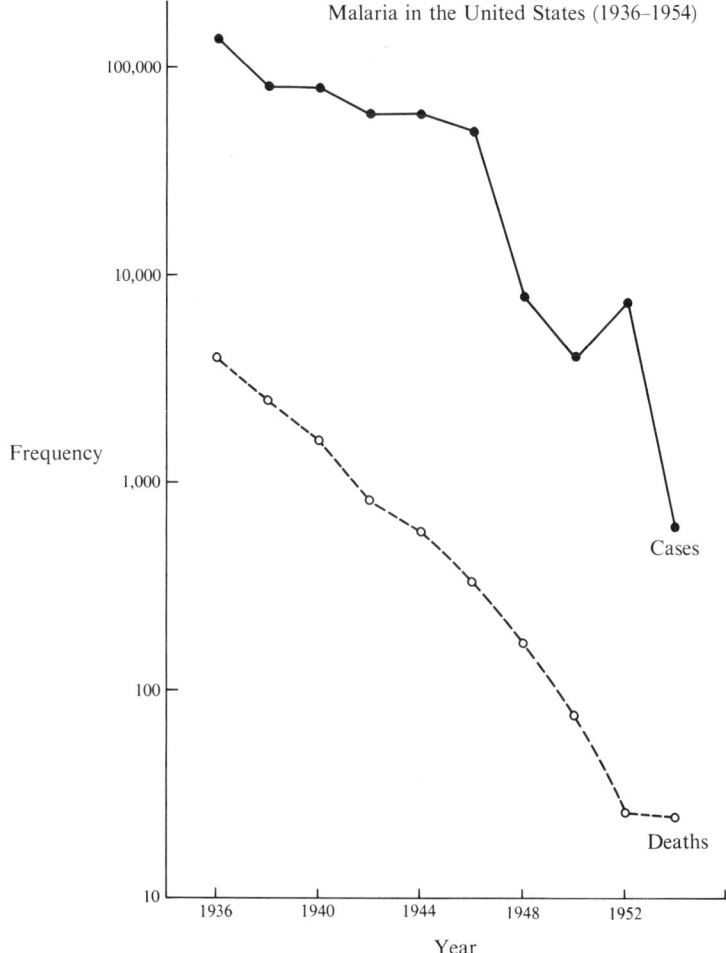

FIGURE 2.27

reported cases was averaging close to 100,000 a year. Extensive public health programs directed at the many aspects of the problem were eventually implemented and by the early 1950s malaria was virtually eliminated from the United States (Langmuir, 1963).

Malaria in the United States*

Year	Cases	Deaths
1936	140,000	4000
1938	81,000	2500
1940	80,000	1600
1942	60,000	840
1944	60,000	590
1946	50,000	340
1948	8,100	170
1950	4,100	79
1952	7,600	26
1954	630	25

*See Figure 2.27.

Question 2.8.2. What would explain the sharp increase in the number of cases reported for 1952?

2.9
SUMMARY

Chapter 2 has focused on the mechanics of summarizing and presenting data. Among the more standard formats discussed are *frequency distributions, bar graphs, histograms, frequency polygons,* and *scatterdiagrams.* In Section 2.7 some nonstandard methods are introduced — graphs specially designed to fit particular situations. Included here are *epidemic curves* and *population pyramids.*

All these many methods for going from raw data to a final table or graph are called *descriptive statistics.* Although there is no single right way to present any given set of data, there are, nevertheless, some well-established conventions that help narrow down the options. Bar graphs, for example, are preferred for either nominal or ordinal data whereas histograms and frequency polygons are used for interval data.

An important concept in medical statistics is the notion of a *rate.* In principle, a rate is an attempt to quantify the likelihood that a certain event will happen to an individual belonging to a certain class. There are three basic kinds of rates — *crude, specific,* and *adjusted.* The first two differ in refinement. Crude rates apply to broad, largely unrestricted populations (e.g., total U.S. deaths in 1970 divided by total U.S. population in 1970). Specific rates involve more particular numerator and denominator populations (e.g., all female suicides in Ohio, ages 25–29, divided by all females in Ohio, ages 25–29). The third kind of rate is fundamentally different. An adjusted rate is computed by applying a set of specific rates to a standard population. Its objective is to compensate for biases in the composition of the population at risk. All three of these rates are discussed in Sections 2.3 and 2.4.

Concluding this chapter is an introduction to the use of logarithmic scaling. This is a technique often used in medical statistics to characterize individual trends — in, say, the morbidity of a disease — or to compare one trend with another.

Definitions

Adjusted rate. A rate corrected for certain biases (age, race, sex, etc.) in the composition of the population at risk.

Arithmetic scale. A vertical axis marked off so that the physical distance between any two numbers on the scale is proportional to their numerical difference.

Bar graph. A graph that summarizes a set of data by using the heights of bars to denote the number of times each possible outcome occurred; suitable for nominal and ordinal data.

Class. A group of possible outcomes treated as a single entity; often an interval.

Crude rate. A rate whose numerator and denominator refer to a very general population.

Descriptive statistics. Methods for summarizing and displaying data.

Epidemic curve. A modified histogram that shows the accumulation, over time, of all cases making up an epidemic.

Frequency distribution. A listing of the possible outcomes of an experiment together with the number of times each actually occurred; typically the first step taken in summarizing data.

Frequency polygon. A line graph related to the histogram; class frequencies are represented by points and consecutive points are connected with straight lines; used for interval data.

Histogram. A graph used for interval (and sometimes ordinal) data; the height of a bar denotes the frequency of a class.

Interval scale. An ordinal scale with the added property that the physical distance between any two points has numerical meaning.

Logarithmic scale. A vertical axis marked off in such a way that the physical distance between any two numbers is proportional to their quotient.

Midpoint. The center of a class interval; used in drawing frequency polygons.

Morbidity rates. Rates referring to the occurrences of diseases.

Mortality rates. Rates referring to deaths.

Natality rates. Rates referring to births.

Nominal scale. A scale where the possible outcomes are unordered and mathematically unrelated.

Ordinal scale. A scale whose possible outcomes satisfy a "less than" relationship.

Population pyramid. A modified histogram showing the age and sex distribution of a country's population.

Rate. The quotient formed by dividing the annual number of events of a certain kind by a specified population "at risk."

Retrospective study. A study making use of what has already happened (as opposed to a *prospective study*, where the experimental conditions are established in advance).

Scale. A listing of the possible outcomes of an experiment or survey; the properties of that listing determine whether the scale is nominal, ordinal, or interval.

Scatterdiagram. A graph of points on a rectangular grid; the x- and y-coordinates of each point correspond to the two measurements made on some particular sample member.

Specific rate. A rate referring to a population at risk which has been intentionally restricted (often by some combination of age, sex, race, or state of residence).

Review Exercises

2.1 One of the mysteries surrounding the Etruscans, referred to in Example 2.6.3, is their origin. Were they native Italians or were they immigrants? And if they were immigrants, where did they come from? Listed below (adapted from Barnicot and Brothwell, 1959) are the maximum head breadths (in mm) of 70 "modern" Italians.

133	138	130	138	134	127	128
138	136	131	126	120	124	132
132	125	139	127	133	136	121
131	125	130	129	125	136	131
132	127	129	132	116	134	125
128	139	132	130	132	128	139
135	133	128	130	130	143	144
137	140	136	135	126	139	131
133	138	133	137	140	130	137
134	130	148	135	138	135	138

Construct a frequency distribution for this sample using the same classes given in Example 2.6.3. Then superimpose the corresponding histogram over the graph shown on page 56. Does it appear that these data support the hypothesis that the Etruscans were native Italians?

2.2 Towards the end of the nineteenth century, one of the worst slums in the United States was the tenement district in New York City's lower East Side. Mortality rates for residents of this area, particularly for young children, were extremely high. In 1888, of the 944 children under five years of age who lived in the heart of this ghetto, along Baxter and Mulberry streets, a total of 132 died (Riis, 1971). Compute the corresponding mortality rate.

72   Model One — Descriptive Statistics

2.3 Graph the annual cigarette consumptions for the 21 countries referred to in Example 1.2.3. (Divide the "outcomes" into classes and use the histogram format.)

2.4 Surveys have indicated that the nature as well as the frequency of mental illness is related to social class. The results of one such study, showing the prevalence of neurotics and psychotics in New Haven, Connecticut, are given in Figure 2.28 (Lindgren, Byrne, and Petrinovich, 1966). Graph this same information using some other format.

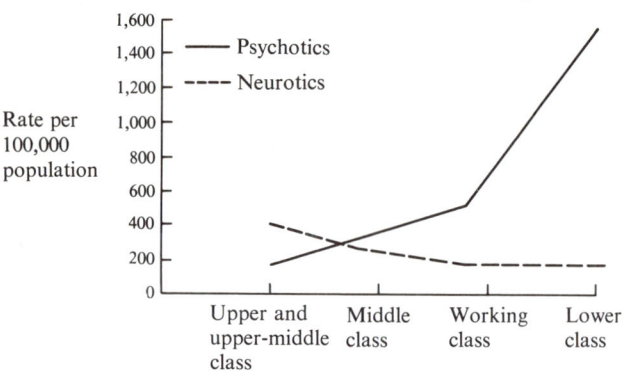

FIGURE 2.28

2.5 In North Dakota in 1960, there were 2,194 deaths due to diseases of the circulatory system. Of that number, 1,410 were males and 784 were females. The total population of North Dakota that year was 632,446, including 323,208 males.

(a) Compute the state-specific mortality rate for diseases of the circulatory system.

(b) Compute the corresponding sex-specific mortality rates.

The total U.S. population in 1960 was 179,323,175. There were 88,331,494 males and 90,991,681 females.

(c) Compute North Dakota's sex-adjusted mortality rate for diseases of the circulatory system.

2.6 Draw a histogram for the air-flow rates (FEV_1/VC) of the nineteen workers described in Review Exercise 1.9.

2.7 The following table gives the numbers and percentages of men and women physicians receiving various specialty certifications in 1966 (Holton, 1969).

Specialty board	Women		Men	
	Number	Percent	Number	Percent
Pediatrics	152	33.6	79	10.6
Psychiatry and neurology	62	13.7	55	7.4
Internal medicine	45	10.0	127	17.0
Anesthesiology	41	9.1	30	4.0
Pathology	39	8.6	34	4.6
General surgery	7	1.6	116	15.5
Other	106	23.4	305	40.9

(a) What kind of scale is involved here?

(b) Display this information graphically.

2.8 Listed below are the 1960 age breakdowns for (1) the United States, (2) Kentucky, and (3) 267,566 deaths due to malignant neoplasms (in the U.S.).

Age	United States	Kentucky	Number of U.S. deaths from malignant neoplasms
<5	20,320,901	342,496	2,060
5–14	35,465,272	637,261	2,415
15–29	34,889,128	622,342	3,600
30–44	36,030,538	561,366	17,215
45–64	36,057,756	582,368	98,059
65+	16,559,580	292,323	144,217

(a) Compute the crude mortality rate in the United States for this condition.
(b) How many deaths due to malignant neoplasms could have been "expected" in Kentucky during 1960?
(c) Estimate Kentucky's state-specific mortality rate for malignant neoplasms.
(d) What would a comparison of the answers to parts (a) and (c) reveal about the relative age of the Kentucky population?

2.9 An epidemic of aseptic meningitis involving Echovirus type 30 occurred in Metropolitan Seattle during the latter half of 1968. The case listing is given below. Draw the epidemic curve. (Data adapted from Hall, Cooney, and Fox, 1970).

Patient	Onset (week ending)	Patient	Onset (week ending)
J.C.	Sept. 5	C.K.	Aug. 8
A.B.	Aug. 1	G.J.	July 11
F.B.	Sept. 12	S.B.	Aug. 15
N.S.	Oct. 24	K.W.	Oct. 3
S.T.	Sept. 5	T.T.	Sept. 12
M.C.	Sept. 26	W.B.	Oct. 31
R.R.	Aug. 15	S.R.	Oct. 3
H.C.	Aug. 8	B.O.	Aug. 8
A.O.	Aug. 8	J.C.	Sept. 5
H.M.	Sept. 12	C.C.	Oct. 24
J.M.	Oct. 3	P.M.	Oct. 3
E.F.	Aug. 8	I.R.	Sept. 5
T.K.	Aug. 22	L.J.	Aug. 1
N.G.	Sept. 26	D.P.	Aug. 8
B.C.	Aug. 8	L.Y.	Aug. 8
K.K.	Sept. 12	Y.D.	Aug. 8
A.F.	Sept. 12	M.T.	Sept. 5
L.T.	Oct. 17	A.C.	Oct. 3
S.P.	Nov. 21	H.W.	Oct. 13
P.B.	Aug. 8	E.P.	Aug. 1
D.M.	Aug. 1	D.R.	Aug. 15
M.P.	Aug. 15	A.D.	Aug. 8
S.L.	Oct. 3	K.G.	Aug. 15

2.10 Graph the energy expenditures listed in Review Exercise 1.12.

2.11 According to their stereotypes, artists are both introverted and neurotic — in degrees proportional to their abilities. If the following study is any indication, the stereotype is probably true. One hundred students enrolled in a leading art conservatory were rated by their teachers as being either (1) highly gifted, (2) less gifted, or (3) ungifted. Each student was then given the Maudsley Personality Inventory (MPI). On the basis of the test, each was assigned an extroversion score (E) and a neuroticism score (N). Subjects with E scores less than 25 would be considered introverts; those with N scores greater than 20 would be considered neurotics. Listed below are the individual E and N scores for the 15 highly gifted students, the average E and N scores for the 35 less gifted and the 50 ungifted students, and the established British and American "norms" (Gotz and Gotz, 1973).

Highly gifted:	E	N
	22	36
	21	35
	20	31
	20	34
	18	40
	13	33
	18	30
	10	38
	12	31
	20	36
	18	34
	10	44
	15	30
	14	31
	16	37

Less gifted: Average E Score = 21
Average N Score = 26

Ungifted: Average E Score = 27
Average N Score = 22

Normal British: Average E Score = 25
Average N Score = 20

Normal American: Average E Score = 28
Average N Score = 22

Display all this information on a single graph.

2.12 A variation of the histogram that is sometimes used in medical statistics is the *cumulative frequency polygon*. Suppose the following pulse rates were recorded for a group of twenty blood donors:

Pulse rate	Number of persons
50–69	6
70–89	8
90–109	5
110–129	1
	20

These data could be described by saying that 6 persons had pulse rates less than or equal to 69, 14 (= 6 + 8) had rates less than or equal to 89, etc. Or, since pulse rates are recorded only to the nearest integer, it could be said that 6 persons had pulse rates less than 69.5; 14, less than 89.5, etc. The numbers 69.5, 89.5, 109.5, and 129.5 are called *class boundaries;* the numbers 6, 14, 19, and 20 are called *cumulative frequencies*.

Pulse rate	Cumulative frequency
< 69.5	6
< 89.5	14
<109.5	19
<129.5	20

The graph that is obtained by plotting cumulative frequencies against class boundaries and then connecting consecutive points with straight lines is called a *cumulative frequency polygon*.

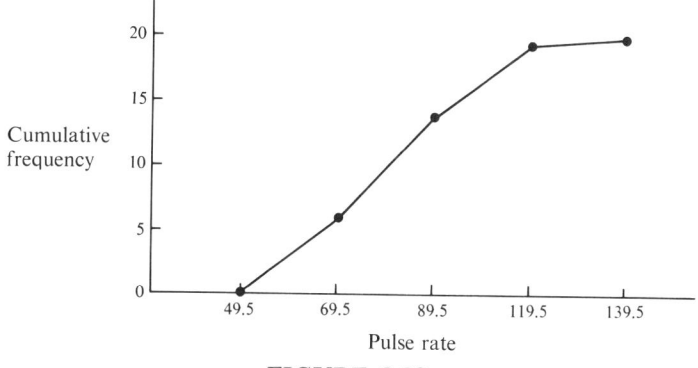

FIGURE 2.29

Draw a cumulative frequency polygon for the traffic mortality rates given in Example 2.6.1.

3

Principles of Inference

*We sail within a vast sphere,
ever drifting in uncertainty,
driven from end to end.*
                              Pascal

3.1
INTRODUCTION

It was pointed out in Chapter 1 that the six different sample-population models can be put into two broad groupings: descriptive (Model One) and inferential (Models Two through Six). In the first model, our knowledge of the population distribution is complete, since the sample includes every individual in the population. But in the remaining five models, the sample contains only a fraction of the total number in the population, meaning that any statement made about the population distribution (or distribution*s*) is only a guess. We call these guesses *inferences*.

Suppose, for example, a group of pharmacologists is working on an oral substitute for insulin. What they ultimately would like to know is whether or not their product is effective enough medically to be successful financially. Yet they cannot possibly test their product on every single diabetic. The best they can hope to do is test it on 50, or maybe 100, diabetics and on the basis of those results decide whether to pursue it any further.

78 Principles of Inference

The inference that is drawn from this sample is obviously extremely important. If they decide the drug is not good enough — when, in fact, it really is — they will have passed up an opportunity to make a nice profit. But if they conclude the drug *is* marketable — when it isn't — they will begin investing time and money into what, inevitably, will be a failure.

Unfortunately, there is no way the pharmacologists can be guaranteed of drawing the right inference. Making generalizations on the basis of limited information is always risky. But with the proper application of the principles of statistical inference, much of that uncertainty can be removed.

We begin this chapter by defining the *sample mean and* the *sample standard deviation*. These are two numbers that prove to be useful in summarizing data to an even greater degree than was possible with the graphical methods of Chapter 2. Then the very important concept of a *sampling distribution* is discussed, followed by a first look at the principles of *hypothesis testing* as they relate to the one-sample problem. Chapter 3 concludes with an introduction to probability and the normal curve.

3.2
THE SAMPLE MEAN

Histograms summarize data to the extent that each of the original sample measurements is put into one of several classes, with the frequency of each class being represented by the height of a bar. In many cases, though, data can be "reduced" even further without sacrificing any significant information. In particular, we can often condense what needs to be known about a histogram into just two numbers. One of these numbers, the *sample mean*, is discussed in this section; the other, the *sample standard deviation*, is developed in Section 3.5.

Recall the ten prothrombin times of Example 2.6.4. For later reference, the observations are denoted here by the symbols $x_1, x_2, \ldots, x_{10}$.

Blood sample	Prothrombin time (seconds)
1	$x_1 = 17.0$
2	$x_2 = 20.0$
3	$x_3 = 25.0$
4	$x_4 = 18.5$
5	$x_5 = 13.0$
6	$x_6 = 17.0$
7	$x_7 = 8.5$
8	$x_8 = 16.0$
9	$x_9 = 27.5$
10	$x_{10} = 12.0$

Using "6.0–9.9," "10.0–13.9," ..., "26.0–29.9" as classes, these observations can be reduced to the histogram shown in Figure 3.1.

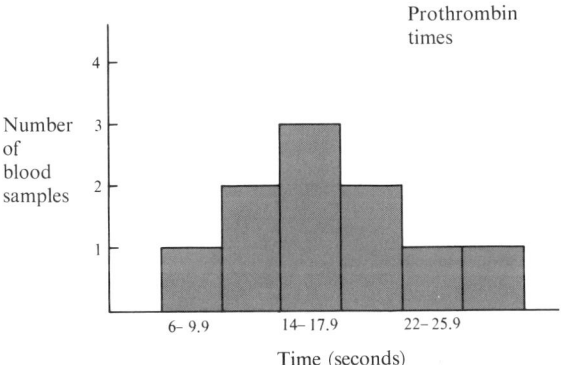

FIGURE 3.1

Note that two characteristics of this (or any) histogram are immediately apparent: (1) its *location* with respect to the horizontal scale and (2) its *shape*. A case in point is the set of histograms in Figure 3.2 showing systolic blood pressures for women of different ages (Pickering, 1960). As the ages of the sample subjects increase, the histograms not only shift in location to the right but also change in shape by becoming more dispersed. A blood pressure of 150 mm of Hg, for example, is abnormally high for a 15-year-old but is relatively low for a 60-year-old. Likewise, while most of the blood pressures for the youngest group were fairly similar (falling between 90 and 130), those for the oldest group were much more scattered, ranging from a low of less than 120 to a high of over 240.

Comment

The population distributions (and sample distributions) of many numerical measurements, regardless of their source, have a *bell shape:* the most frequently observed values are intermediate ones while extremely small or extremely large values occur only sparingly.

Both the prothrombin times and the systolic blood pressures belong to this type. For reasons that will be brought out in the next chapter, this particular shape plays a key role in almost every inference procedure.

Ignoring shape for the moment, how might we describe, numerically, the *location* of a histogram (or, equivalently, the location of a set of n measurements)? One solution would be simply to list the smallest and largest observations, thus "locating" the others in between. A better answer, though — for mathematical reasons — can be obtained by computing a single number that corresponds to the "center" of the sample distribution.

To be more precise, imagine the horizontal axis to be a bar and the observations to be weights attached at various points along its length. That is, x_1 is a weight attached at the point marked "17.0," x_2 is an equal weight attached at "20.0," and so on. If a fulcrum is placed at just the right point under the bar (which is assumed to be weightless), the system will be in balance. In physics,

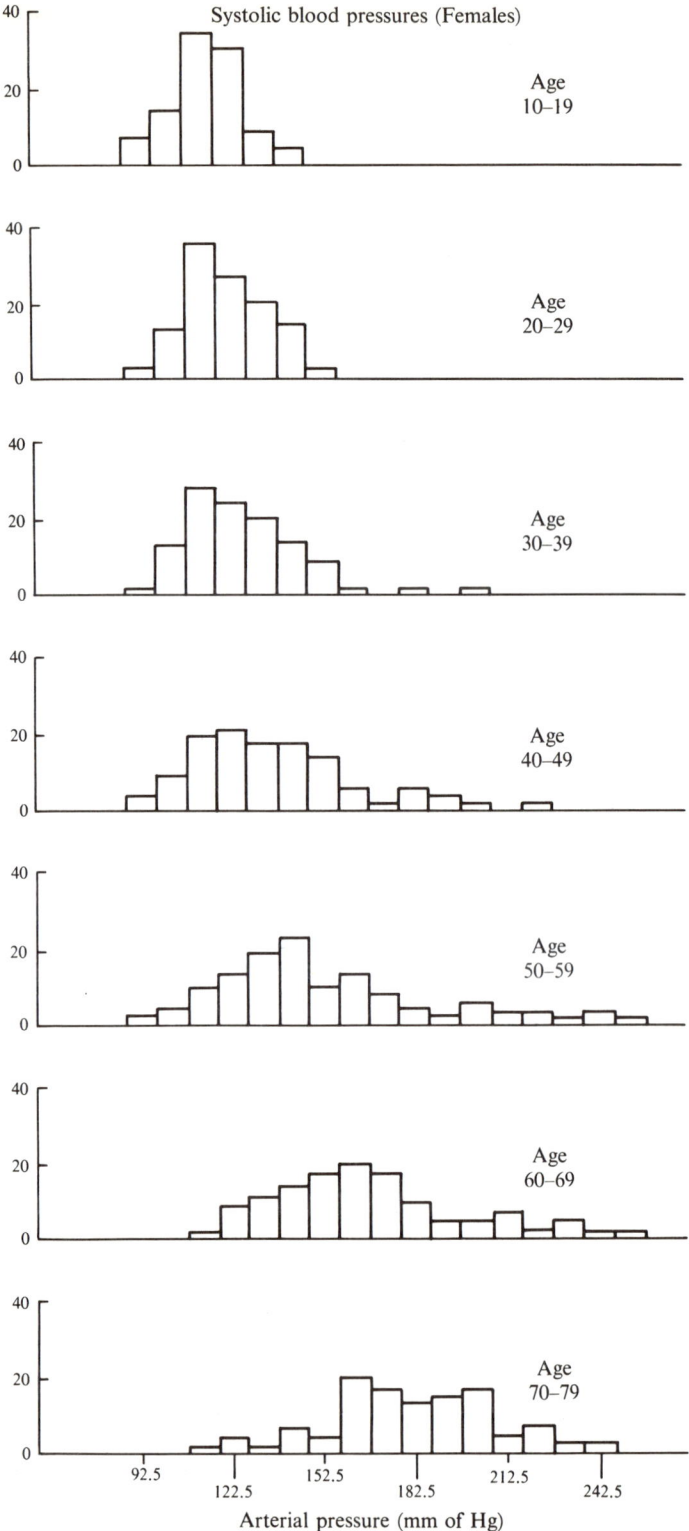

FIGURE 3.2

the point having this property is called the center of gravity. In statistics, we call it the *sample mean* and denote it by the symbol $\bar{x}$.

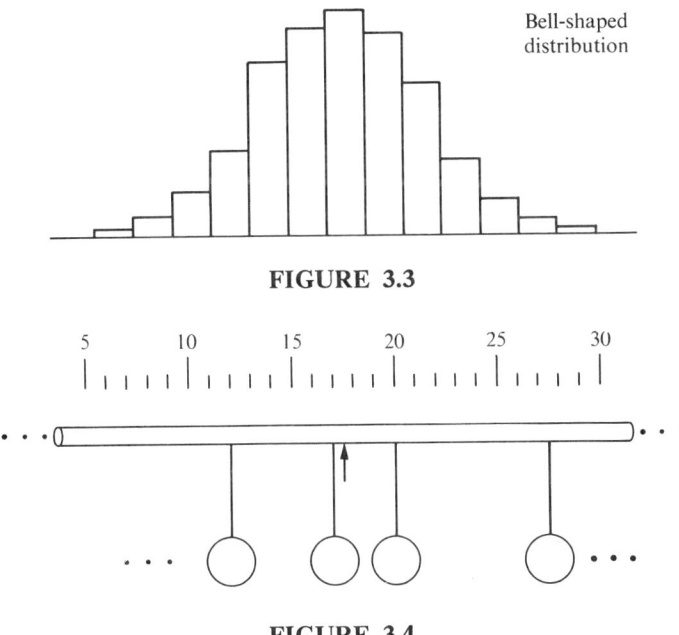

FIGURE 3.3

FIGURE 3.4

Computationally, $\bar{x}$ is just the *average* of the sample measurements,

$$\bar{x} = \frac{17.0 + 20.0 + \cdots + 12.0}{10} = 17.4 \text{ seconds}$$

The next section introduces sigma notation, a mathematical shorthand for expressing quantities such as the sample mean in a more general way.

3.3 SIGMA NOTATION

It is often necessary when working with data to add together a set of observations, as in the case of $\bar{x}$, or a set of quantities computed from those observations. The writing of these sums can be greatly facilitated by a mathematical shorthand known as *sigma notation*. Consider the sum of the first three prothrombin times: $17.0 + 20.0 + 25.0 = 62.0$ (or, $x_1 + x_2 + x_3$). In sigma notation, this same sum would be written $\sum_{i=1}^{3} x_i$. The expression appearing after the sigma sign (in this case, x_i) denotes the *type* of quantity to be added. All terms of that type having subscripts equal to or "between" the ones appearing at the bottom and top of the sigma sign are to be included in the sum.

EXAMPLE 3.3.1. Summation Examples

Let $x_1, x_2, \ldots, x_{10}$ denote the ten prothrombin times.

(a) $$\sum_{i=1}^{4} x_i = x_1 + x_2 + x_3 + x_4$$
$$= 17.0 + 20.0 + 25.0 + 18.5$$
$$= 80.5$$

(b) $$\sum_{i=1}^{3} x_i^2 = x_1^2 + x_2^2 + x_3^2$$
$$= (17.0)^2 + (20.0)^2 + (25.0)^2$$
$$= 289.0 + 400.0 + 625.0$$
$$= 1314.0$$

(c) $$\sum_{i=7}^{8} 3x_i = 3x_7 + 3x_8$$
$$= 3(8.5) + 3(16.0)$$
$$= 25.5 + 48.0$$
$$= 73.5$$

(d) $$\sum_{i=1}^{5} (2x_i + 1) = (2x_1 + 1) + (2x_2 + 1) + (2x_3 + 1)$$
$$+ (2x_4 + 1) + (2x_5 + 1)$$
$$= (34.0 + 1) + (40.0 + 1) + (50.0 + 1)$$
$$+ (37.0 + 1) + (26.0 + 1)$$
$$= 192.0$$

(e) $$\sum_{i=9}^{10} (x_i - 0.5)^2 = (x_9 - 0.5)^2 + (x_{10} - 0.5)^2$$
$$= (27.5 - 0.5)^2 + (12.0 - 0.5)^2$$
$$= (27.0)^2 + (11.5)^2$$
$$= 861.25$$

Further applications of sigma notation are presented in Examples 3.5.1* and 3.5.3*.

Question 3.3.1. Let $x_1 = 2.0$, $x_2 = 1.0$, $x_3 = 4.0$, and $x_4 = 6.0$. Express the following two sums in sigma notation and evaluate each one numerically:
(a) $x_1^3 + x_2^3 + x_3^3 + x_4^3$
(b) $(x_1 + x_2 + x_3 + x_4)^3$

Question 3.3.2. Refer to the data of Example 1.2.2. Let $x_1 = 32$, $x_2 = 36$, etc. Evaluate the following sums:

(a) $\sum_{i=3}^{4} x_i^2$

(b) $\sum_{i=1}^{3} (x_i - 36)^2$

(c) $\left[\sum_{i=1}^{3} (x_i - 36) \right]^2$

(d) $\dfrac{1}{4} \sum\limits_{i=1}^{4} x_i$

(e) $\sum\limits_{i=1}^{4} \left(\dfrac{x_i}{4}\right)$

Definition 3.3.1 gives the general formula for the sample mean in sigma notation.

> **Definition 3.3.1.** The sample mean, $\bar{x}$, of n numerical measurements, $x_1, x_2, \ldots x_n$, is given by
>
> $$\bar{x} = \dfrac{\sum\limits_{i=1}^{n} x_i}{n} = \dfrac{1}{n} \sum\limits_{i=1}^{n} x_i$$

EXAMPLE 3.3.2. Platelet Counts

What effects, if any, does age have on a person's blood? Do clotting times change? Is the hemoglobin content altered? Are immunological functions diminished? Questions of this sort prompted a hematologic study (Szalontai and Timaffy, 1964) involving 24 female rest home patients. One of the several variables measured were their platelet counts; that is, the number of platelets in a cubic millimeter of blood. (In a normal population, platelet counts tend to range from 140,000 to 440,000 per mm^3).

Platelet counts (per mm^3)

Subject	Count	Subject	Count
1	125,000	13	180,000
2	170,000	14	180,000
3	250,000	15	280,000
4	270,000	16	240,000
5	144,000	17	270,000
6	184,000	18	220,000
7	176,000	19	110,000
8	100,000	20	176,000
9	220,000	21	280,000
10	200,000	22	176,000
11	170,000	23	188,000
12	160,000	24	176,000

Letting $x_1 = 125,000$, $x_2 = 170,000, \ldots, x_{24} = 176,000$, it follows that

$$\bar{x} = \dfrac{1}{24} \sum_{i=1}^{24} x_i = \dfrac{125,000 + \cdots + 176,000}{24}$$

$$= \dfrac{4,645,000}{24} = 193,500/\text{mm}^3$$

84 Principles of Inference [3.3]

These data point strongly to the conclusion that platelet counts *are* reduced in elderly women. None of the 24 counts was near the normal upper limit but three fell less than the lower limit and another 12 were fairly close. The sample mean itself was far to the left of the center of the normal range (290,000/mm^3).

Comment

By convention, sample means are recorded to either the same number of significant digits as the observations, or to one more.

In this case, the counts are given to the nearest thousand and $\bar{x}$ is expressed to the nearest hundred — that is, $4,645,000/24 = 193,541.7$ is rounded off to 193,500. On the other hand, the average prothrombin time of Section 3.2 was given to *one* decimal place, the same as the observations.

Question 3.3.3. Draw a histogram for these data. Indicate the location of the sample mean along the horizontal axis.

Comment

For distributions that are bell-shaped, or nearly so, $\bar{x}$ is numerically similar to the most frequently occurring values; in that sense, it represents a "typical" observation. However, for certain other shapes, the sample mean may be nowhere near the value of a typical observation.

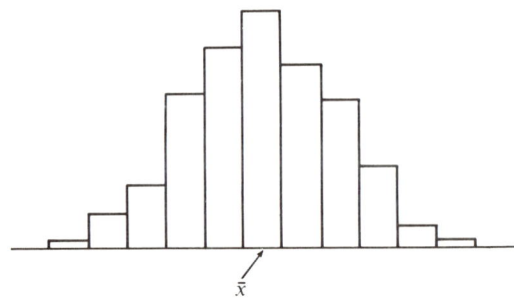

FIGURE 3.5

EXAMPLE 3.3.3. Number of Births per Woman — U.S. and Mexico

Data collected in 1950 revealed that, in the United States, women who were then in their fifties had had an average of 2.8 children; in Mexico, the average for a similar group was 5.1 children. The two bar graphs in Figure 3.6 give the percentages of women in the 50 to 59 age group according to the number of children they had (Barclay, 1958).

In contrast to distributions having a bell shape, the Mexican data show the extremes, "zero" children and "eight or more" children, occurring more often than any of the intermediate values. When this is the case, the distribution is said to be *U-shaped*.

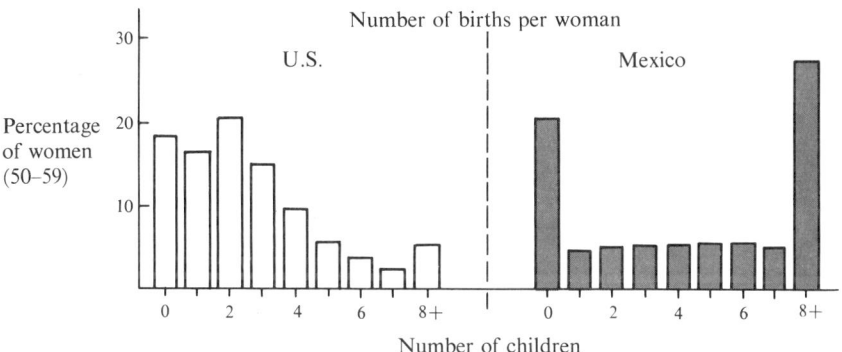

FIGURE 3.6

It should be clear that the average of 5.1 is a poor indicator of the number of children borne by a typical Mexican woman. In general, the more a histogram deviates from a bell shape, the less reliance should be put on $\bar{x}$ as a descriptive measure. The most relevant information in these instances is often the shape of the histogram itself, and that information should not be oversummarized.

Question 3.3.4. What are some other histogram shapes for which $\bar{x}$ would not be similar to a typical observation?

The next section introduces some alternatives to the sample mean. These are to be used when the shape of the data is such that computing $\bar{x}$ would be inappropriate.

3.4
ALTERNATIVES TO THE SAMPLE MEAN

Without question, the most frequently used number for summarizing the location of a set of measurements is the sample mean. Nevertheless, we have seen (Example 3.3.3) that $\bar{x}$ can be misleading when the sample distribution has a shape other than a bell shape. Fortunately, there are other ways of describing location. One of these, the *sample median*, will be discussed in this section. Another, the *geometric mean*, will be deferred until Chapter 6.

Given a set of n measurements, where n is an odd number, the sample median is defined to be the "middle" value, in terms of magnitude. If the sample observations were $x_1 = 12$, $x_2 = 8$, $x_3 = 26$, $x_4 = 32$, and $x_5 = 7$, the sample median would be 12, since

$$7 < 8 < 12 < 26 < 32$$

The symbol for the sample median is $\tilde{x}$.

If the number of measurements is even, the sample median is taken to be the average of the middle two (after the data have been arranged from smallest to largest). For example, the numbers $x_1 = 260$, $x_2 = 108$, $x_3 = 135$, $x_4 = 137$, $x_5 = 208$, and $x_6 = 198$, when ordered, become

$$108 < 135 < 137 < 198 < 208 < 260$$

so that

$$\tilde{x} = \frac{137 + 198}{2} = 167.5$$

Note that the sample median represents the "center" of a set of measurements in the sense that the number of observations that are *less than* $\tilde{x}$ is the same as the number that are *greater*. This is not the same definition of center that was used for the sample mean but for data that are more-or-less bell-shaped, $\bar{x}$ and $\tilde{x}$ will be quite similar anyway. Where the median is most often used — and where it may be quite different from the mean — is for samples having one or two observations either much smaller or much larger than all the others. The sample mean would be unduly influenced (and distorted) by these extreme values; the sample median would not be.

For example, suppose the following data were recorded:

Subject	Response
1	$x_1 = 91$
2	$x_2 = 78$
3	$x_3 = 87$
4	$x_4 = 79$
5	$x_5 = 2$

The sample mean is

$$\bar{x} = \frac{\sum_{i=1}^{5} x_i}{5} = 67.4$$

and the sample median is

$$\tilde{x} = 79$$

since $2 < 78 < 79 < 87 < 91$. Here, 79 is clearly more indicative than 67.4 of the values the observations tend to have. So, in this case, $\tilde{x}$ would be preferred over $\bar{x}$ as a measure of location.

EXAMPLE 3.4.1. Bone Marrow Transplants and Leukemia

Listed below are the survival times of eleven acute leukemia patients after having received bone marrow transplants (Graw and Santos, 1971).

Patient	Post-transplant survival time (days)
J.B.	131
Y.O.	451+
S.A.	90
L.P.	332
J.J.	33
M.P.	66
D.V.	92
J.T.	47
W.E.	32
T.W.	215
P.W.	75

The sample median is the only way to describe the location of these data because one of the subjects, Y.O., was still alive when the study ended, making it impossible to compute an average. Arranging the observations from shortest to longest gives

$$32 < 33 < 47 < 66 < 75 < 90 < 92 < 131 < 215 < 332 < 451+$$

so that

$$\tilde{x} = 90 \text{ days}$$

is the median survival time.

Question 3.4.1. Find $\bar{x}$ and $\tilde{x}$ for the bacteria counts listed in Review Exercise 1.2.

3.5
THE SAMPLE STANDARD DEVIATION

Describing the *shape* of a histogram is not as easy as describing its *location*. One problem is the lack of a physical analog, like the center of gravity, to suggest an answer. Another is that "shape" is too general a concept to be easily handled mathematically. A better approach is to focus on a more workable, but related, property — in this case, *dispersion*. By definition, the dispersion of a set of observations is the extent to which those observations are scattered away from a central value.

But just defining a new term does not solve the original problem. The *concept* of dispersion still needs to be translated into a mathematical formula. Unfortunately, as the next two paragraphs show, what seems to be the "obvious" formula turns out to be completely useless.

Suppose $\bar{x}$ is chosen to be the central value referred to in the dispersion definition. The amount of scatter associated with an arbitrary observation, x_i, could be set equal to the algebraic "distance" of x_i from $\bar{x}$: namely, $x_i - \bar{x}$.

This would make the dispersion of, say, the first prothrombin time equal to $x_1 - \bar{x} = 17.0 - 17.4 = -.4$; of the second prothrombin time, $2.6 (= x_2 - \bar{x} = 20.0 - 17.4)$; and so on.

Then, given a sample of size n, it might seem reasonable to add up the n deviations from $\bar{x}$, divide the sum by n, and let the quotient, $1/n \sum_{i=1}^{n} (x_i - \bar{x})$, be our measure of dispersion. But this does not work. It can be shown (see Example 3.5.1*) that this expression will *always* equal 0, regardless of the values of $x_1, x_2, \ldots, x_n$.

EXAMPLE 3.5.1.* A Proof that $(1/n)\sum_{i=1}^{n}(x_i - \bar{x}) = 0$

(Note: This example and Example 3.5.3* are optional. The results are important and should be understood, but the proofs may be omitted.)

Derivations involving sigma notation are simplified when the following three rules of summation are used.

Rule 1 Let $x_1, x_2, \ldots, x_n$ and $y_1, y_2, \ldots, y_n$ be any two sets of numbers. Then

$$\sum_{i=1}^{n}(x_i + y_i) = (x_1 + y_1) + (x_2 + y_2) + \cdots + (x_n + y_n)$$
$$= \sum_{i=1}^{n} x_i + \sum_{i=1}^{n} y_i$$

In words, the summation of a sum is equal to the sum of the summations.

Rule 2 The summation of a constant, k, times a set of numbers is equal to the constant times the summation of the numbers.

$$\sum_{i=1}^{n} kx_i = kx_1 + kx_2 + \cdots + kx_n = k \sum_{i=1}^{n} x_i$$

Rule 3 The summation of a constant, k, is equal to the number of terms in the summation times k.

$$\sum_{i=1}^{n} k = \underbrace{k + k + \cdots + k}_{n \text{ terms}} = nk$$

Now, using the principle of Rule 1,

$$\sum_{i=1}^{n}(x_i - \bar{x}) = \sum_{i=1}^{n} x_i - \sum_{i=1}^{n} \bar{x}$$

Note that $\bar{x}$ is a constant (given $x_1, x_2, \ldots, x_n$) so that from Rule 3,

$$\sum_{i=1}^{n} x_i - \sum_{i=1}^{n} \bar{x} = \sum_{i=1}^{n} x_i - n\bar{x}$$

But

$$\bar{x} = \frac{1}{n}\sum_{i=1}^{n} x_i,$$

making
$$n\bar{x} = \sum_{i=1}^{n} x_i$$

Therefore,
$$\sum_{i=1}^{n}(x_i - \bar{x}) = \sum_{i=1}^{n} x_i - \sum_{i=1}^{n} x_i = 0$$

which means that
$$\frac{1}{n}\sum_{i=1}^{n}(x_i - \bar{x}) = 0$$

Question 3.5.1. Make up a set of four numbers and verify that
$$\sum_{i=1}^{4}(x_i - \bar{x}) = 0$$

The reason that $1/n \sum_{i=1}^{n}(x_i - \bar{x})$ is always 0 (and, consequently, of no value as a measure of dispersion) is that, for any sample, the negative deviations from $\bar{x}$ are exactly equal to the positive deviations. But suppose the scatter of the ith observation were to be equated to its *squared* deviation from $\bar{x}$, $(x_i - \bar{x})^2$. Since $(x_i - \bar{x})^2$ is always nonnegative, the expression

$$\frac{1}{n}\sum_{i=1}^{n}(x_i - \bar{x})^2$$

would be a valid measure of dispersion. A more workable formula, though, is the slightly different *sample standard deviation*, as given in Definition 3.5.1.

Definition 3.5.1. The dispersion of a set of n numerical measurements, $x_1, x_2, \ldots, x_n$ is described by the *sample standard deviation*, s, where

$$s = \sqrt{\frac{1}{n-1}\sum_{i=1}^{n}(x_i - \bar{x})^2}$$

An equivalent formula for s that simplifies the computations is

$$s = \sqrt{\frac{n\sum_{i=1}^{n} x_i^2 - \left(\sum_{i=1}^{n} x_i\right)^2}{n(n-1)}}$$

Comment

The square root was introduced in the formula for s to make its units compatible with those of the data. Had the observations been recorded, say, in seconds, then the units of any quantity such as

$$\frac{1}{n}\sum_{i=1}^{n}(x_i - \bar{x})^2$$

would be seconds squared. The reason for replacing n with $n-1$ in the denominator was a mathematical one; numerically, the change makes very little difference.

Comment

Not much has been said about the *interpretation* of s except that it represents a measure of dispersion. Later that statement will be made more precise.

Comment

The square of the sample standard deviation is known as the *sample variance*. That is,

$$s^2 = \text{sample variance} = \frac{1}{n-1} \sum_{i=1}^{n} (x_i - \bar{x})^2$$

In textbooks on *mathematical* statistics, the sample variance, rather than the sample standard deviation, is the quantity most often used to describe dispersion.

Comment

The equivalence of the two formulas for s given in Definition 3.5.1 will be established in Example 3.5.3*.

EXAMPLE 3.5.2. Calculation of s

Let $x_1, x_2, \ldots, x_{10}$ be the ten prothrombin times referred to in Section 3.2. The calculations below indicate the steps required to evaluate s using the first formula of Definition 3.5.1. (Recall that $\bar{x} = 17.4$.)

Prothrombin time: x_i	Deviation: $x_i - \bar{x}$	$(x_i - \bar{x})^2$
17.0	−0.4	.16
20.0	2.6	6.76
25.0	7.6	57.76
18.5	1.1	1.21
13.0	−4.4	19.36
17.0	−0.4	.16
8.5	−8.9	79.21
16.0	−1.4	1.96
27.5	10.1	102.01
12.0	−5.4	29.16
		297.75

$$\sum_{i=1}^{10} (x_i - \bar{x})^2 = 297.75$$

$$s = \sqrt{\frac{297.75}{10-1}} = \sqrt{33.08} = 5.8 \text{ seconds}$$

The second formula for s is much easier to use than the first, particularly when the computations are being done on a desk calculator. Also, it leads to fewer rounding errors.

Prothrombin time: x_i	x_i^2
17.0	289.00
20.0	400.00
25.0	625.00
18.5	342.25
13.0	169.00
17.0	289.00
8.5	72.25
16.0	256.00
27.5	756.25
12.0	144.00
174.5 $(= \sum_{i=1}^{n} x_i)$	3342.75 $(= \sum_{i=1}^{10} x_i^2)$

$$s = \sqrt{\frac{10(3342.75) - (174.5)^2}{10(9)}} = \sqrt{\frac{2977.25}{90}}$$

$$= \sqrt{33.08} = 5.8 \text{ seconds}$$

Comment

In practice, we *always* use the computing formula

$$\sqrt{\frac{n \sum_{i=1}^{n} x_i^2 - \left(\sum_{i=1}^{n} x_i \right)^2}{n(n-1)}}$$

when finding s. The first formula was introduced solely for the purpose of showing *how* the sample standard deviation measures dispersion.

Question 3.5.2. Use the computing formula to find the sample standard deviation for the marihuana data given in Example 1.2.2.

EXAMPLE 3.5.3.* A Proof that

$$\sqrt{\frac{\sum_{i=1}^{n} (x_i - \bar{x})^2}{n-1}} = \sqrt{\frac{n \sum_{i=1}^{n} x_i^2 - \left(\sum_{i=1}^{n} x_i \right)^2}{n(n-1)}}$$

Note, first of all, that to establish the equivalence of the two formulas for s, it is sufficient to show that

$$\sum_{i=1}^{n} (x_i - \bar{x})^2 = \frac{n \sum_{i=1}^{n} x_i^2 - \left(\sum_{i=1}^{n} x_i \right)^2}{n}$$

Consider the left-hand term. Since $(x_i - \bar{x})^2 = x_i^2 - 2x_i \bar{x} + \bar{x}^2$, it follows from Rule 1 (Example 3.5.1*) that

$$\sum_{i=1}^{n} (x_i - \bar{x})^2 = \sum_{i=1}^{n} x_i^2 - \sum_{i=1}^{n} 2x_i \bar{x} + \sum_{i=1}^{n} \bar{x}^2$$

Recognizing that $\bar{x}$ is a constant and using Rules 2 and 3,

$$\sum_{i=1}^{n}(x_i - \bar{x})^2 = \sum_{i=1}^{n} x_i^2 - 2\bar{x}\sum_{i=1}^{n} x_i + n\bar{x}^2$$

But
$$n\bar{x} = \sum_{i=1}^{n} x_i$$

which, when substituted into the above equation, gives

$$\sum_{i=1}^{n}(x_i - \bar{x})^2 = \sum_{i=1}^{n} x_i^2 - 2n\bar{x}^2 + n\bar{x}^2$$

$$= \sum_{i=1}^{n} x_i^2 - n\bar{x}^2$$

$$= \sum_{i=1}^{n} x_i^2 - \frac{\left(\sum_{i=1}^{n} x_i\right)^2}{n}$$

$$= \frac{n\sum_{i=1}^{n} x_i^2 - \left(\sum_{i=1}^{n} x_i\right)^2}{n}$$

proving the equality of the two formulas.

Question 3.5.3. What is another expression, besides $(x_i - \bar{x})^2$, that would measure the scatter of the ith observation, and whose sum over i would not be zero?

Question 3.5.4. Find $\bar{x}$ and s for the Etruscan data of Example 2.6.3. Note that

$$\sum_{i=1}^{84} x_i = 12{,}077$$

and

$$\sum_{i=1}^{84} x_i^2 = 1{,}739{,}315$$

3.6
THE SAMPLING DISTRIBUTION OF $\bar{X}$

Variability is a statistical fact of life. No matter how well an experiment is planned, or how elaborate a lab procedure might be, what is measured will still vary from trial to trial. The reason, of course, is that to control, or even to be aware of, *every* factor influencing the outcome of an experiment is impossible.

Suppose, for example, an antismoking therapy is being clinically tested on five adults, each of whom smokes, at the outset, two packs a day. The measured response will be the number (x_i) of cigarettes a subject smokes each day after being on the program for, say, 10 weeks. Now if the only factor involved was the therapy itself, all the x_i's would be the same, since each person received the same treatment. But that would not happen. Many other factors would enter in — the subject's perseverance, his desire to stop smoking, how much encouragement he gets from his family and friends, and so on.

The implication of this is that the $\bar{x}$ computed from any sample distribution should be considered a variable, in the sense that if the experiment was repeated, both the new sample and the new sample mean would be different. It seems reasonable, then, to hypothesize a distribution of $\bar{x}$ values, even though the result of any particular series of trials will be a single $\bar{x}$. The properties of this distribution — that is, its shape, location, and dispersion — would reflect the "behavior" of the sample mean if the same experiment were repeated over and over again under presumably identical conditions. We call this imaginary set of $\bar{x}$ values the *sampling distribution of $\bar{X}$*. It plays a vital role in the theory of statistical inference.

Comment

In the future, it will be necessary to make the distinction between a variable and a particular realization of that variable. The former will be denoted by a capital letter and the latter by a small letter. In the experiment just described, X_1 would be used to denote the (unknown) number of cigarettes Subject #1 will smoke daily, after the study is over. But when the study actually *is* over and Subject #1 still smokes, say, 10 cigarettes a day, we would write $x_1 = 10$. Likewise, the sample mean, *before* the data are taken, is denoted by the symbol $\bar{X}$; *after* the data are taken, by the symbol $\bar{x}$.

In more mathematical developments of statistical theory, expressions such as X_1 and $\bar{X}$ are called *random variables*. The numbers x_1 and $\bar{x}$ are simply values taken on by the random variables.

EXAMPLE 3.6.1. Sampling Distribution of Prothrombin Time Averages

Based on the definition in Chapter 1, the population distribution of prothrombin times is the totality of measurements that would result after repeating

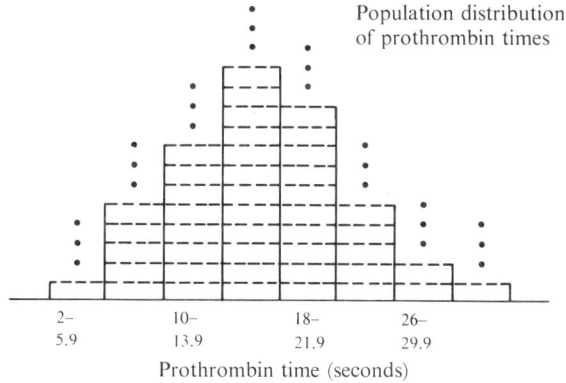

FIGURE 3.7

the procedure over and over again (in fact, after repeating the procedure an *infinite* number of times).

For the purposes of this example, the bars have been divided into blocks to represent individual measurements. The broken lines are intended to reinforce the fact that the number of blocks shown here is only an infinitesimal fraction of the total number that would comprise the population distribution.

According to Example 2.6.4, the prothrombin times actually found were 17.0, 20.0, 25.0, 18.5, 13.0, 17.0, 8.5, 16.0, 27.5, and 12.0, giving a sample mean of $\bar{x} = 17.4$ seconds. For the purposes of this example, we will denote 17.4 by the symbol $\bar{x}_1$. In Figure 3.8, the 1's are meant to indicate where in the population distribution the *first* sample came from. Of course, their locations along a particular bar are arbitrary.

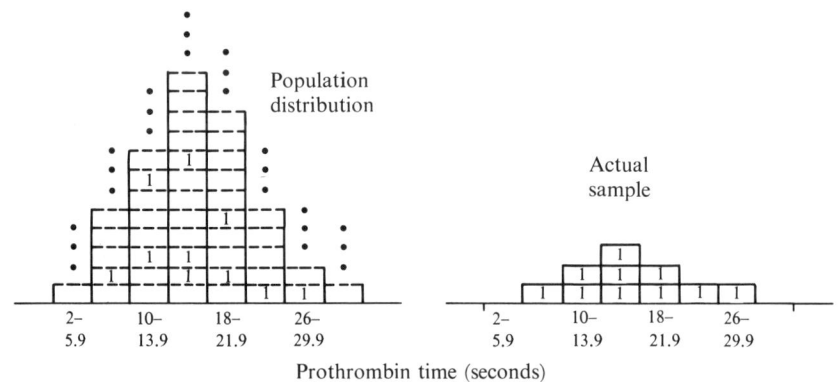

FIGURE 3.8

Now, suppose the test was done ten more times. The results *might* be 8.0, 15.5, 10.0, 10.0, 23.5, 5.5, 14.0, 11.5, 19.5, and 28.5, in which case the sample mean would be $\bar{x}_2 = 14.6$.

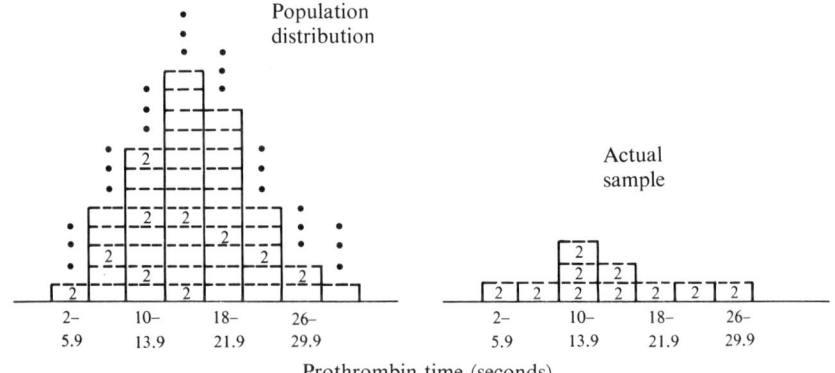

FIGURE 3.9

Still a third sample of size ten might give $\bar{x}_3 = 19.5$, and so on. Averages computed from many such samples could, themselves, be displayed with a histogram.

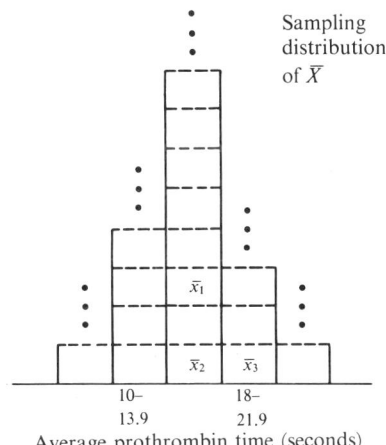

FIGURE 3.10

If all possible samples of size ten had been recorded, the collection of $\bar{x}$ values, together with their frequencies, would be called the *sampling distribution of $\bar{X}$*.

Question 3.6.1. Suppose an entire population consists of only six individuals, on each of whom a single response has been measured. Construct a histogram of the sampling distribution of $\bar{X}$ based on samples of size two drawn from this particular population.

Subject	Response, x_i
1	16
2	4
3	10
4	12
5	8
6	8

The properties of the sampling distribution of $\bar{X}$ that make it so important in statistical inference will be the topic of Section 4.2. For the present, it is sufficient to understand what the sampling distribution of $\bar{X}$ is and how it relates to the population distribution. Also, it should be clear how this same concept could be applied to *any* quantity computed from sample data. We could define, for example, the sampling distribution of s, of $\bar{X}/s$, of the largest observation minus the smallest observation, and so on.

Question 3.6.2. For the six responses referred to in Question 3.6.1, find the sampling distribution of the median, $\tilde{X}$, based on samples of size three. Construct the corresponding histogram.

3.7 INTRODUCTION TO HYPOTHESIS TESTING

For samples whose histograms are essentially bell-shaped, $\bar{x}$ and s provide very useful measures of location and dispersion. But what about population distributions? Can the same sort of numerical descriptions be applied to them? The answer is yes, with one qualification — quantities computed from entire populations, unlike their sample counterparts, exhibit *no* variability. To emphasize this distinction, the *population mean* and the *population standard deviation* are given their own set of symbols — the Greek letters μ and σ.

Comment

As we will see later, the exact form of a population distribution is typically described in terms of certain constants called *parameters*. For bell-shaped distributions, the two parameters are μ and σ. In contrast to a parameter, whose numerical value is derived from an entire population distribution, any quantity that is computed solely from the information contained in a sample is called a *statistic*. The sample mean, for instance, is a statistic, as is the sample standard deviation.

Much of what we do from this point on centers around methods for estimating the numerical values of the parameters of a population distribution on the basis of certain statistics computed from samples representing that distribution. Consider, for example, the data of Review Exercise 1.9, showing air-flow rates found for persons involved in the manufacture of enzyme detergents.

Subject	FEV_1/VC	Subject	FEV_1/VC
R.H.	.61	W.S.	.78
R.B.	.70	R.V.	.84
M.B.	.63	E.N.	.83
D.M.	.76	W.D.	.82
W.B.	.67	F.R.	.74
R.B.	.72	P.D.	.85
B.F.	.64	E.B.	.73
J.T.	.82	P.C.	.85
P.S.	.88	R.W.	.87
R.B.	.82		

As administrators, or perhaps as health officials, we would like to decide on the basis of these nineteen observations whether manufacturing detergents (1) *is* or (2) *is not* hazardous to the respiratory system.

Introduction to Hypothesis Testing

To begin, note that from a conceptual standpoint there are *two* population distributions to be considered here. The first is the population distribution of air-flow rates for all persons *not* involved in the production of enzyme detergents. The second is the distribution of air-flow rates of all persons who now work, or who will work, under conditions similar to those experienced by the nineteen subjects.

There are certain things that are known about the first distribution simply because, over the years, many non-detergent workers have been tested for this particular respiratory function. For example, as mentioned in Review Exercise 1.9, the *average* air flow rate for healthy persons is 0.80. Conceivably, the standard deviation and shape of this first distribution might also be known.

But the second distribution is a different matter. These nineteen persons may be among the first detergent workers whose air-flow rates have ever been measured so we can only speculate about the "properties" of the distribution that *their* responses represent. Compared to the first distribution, this second one may have a different mean, a different standard deviation, or a different shape; it may differ in several of these respects, or in none. Some of these situations are pictured in Figure 3.11.

Unless a very large number of observations is taken (considerably more than nineteen), there is no way to investigate all these possibilities. In Model Two, it is usually assumed that *if this second distribution has "changed," it has done so only with respect to location*. Bear in mind that for any given problem there is likely to be little or no a priori justification for making such an assumption. However, experience with many different phenomena from many different areas of applied science suggests that shifts in location are often the dominant effects elicited by different "treatments."

Let μ denote the mean of the population distribution of air-flow rates for detergent workers. Our assumption gives rise to two hypotheses regarding its value. One, representing the status quo, states that the location of the distribution of air-flow rates for detergent workers has *not* shifted (that is, it still equals 0.80). This is called the *null hypothesis* and is denoted H. The second, or *alternative hypothesis*, denoted A, states that the mean *has* shifted, to some unspecified lower value. In formal notation, we would write

$$H: \quad \mu = 0.80 \quad \text{versus} \quad A: \quad \mu < 0.80$$

Our decision to believe either the null hypothesis or the alternative hypothesis must come, ultimately, from the sample data. In particular, since the problem has been narrowed down to a decision involving the *population mean* (μ), it seems reasonable that the decision should be based on the *sample mean* ($\bar{x}$).

For these data,

$$\bar{x} = \frac{1}{19}\sum_{i=1}^{19} x_i = \frac{0.61 + 0.70 + \cdots + 0.87}{19} = \frac{14.56}{19} = 0.77$$

At this point, the choice between H and A might seem obvious: accept A as the true hypothesis; after all, 0.77 is *not* equal to 0.80. But remember that $\bar{x}$ varies from sample to sample *naturally* so that even if the population mean were 0.80,

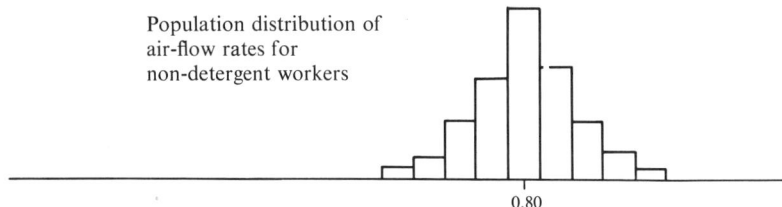

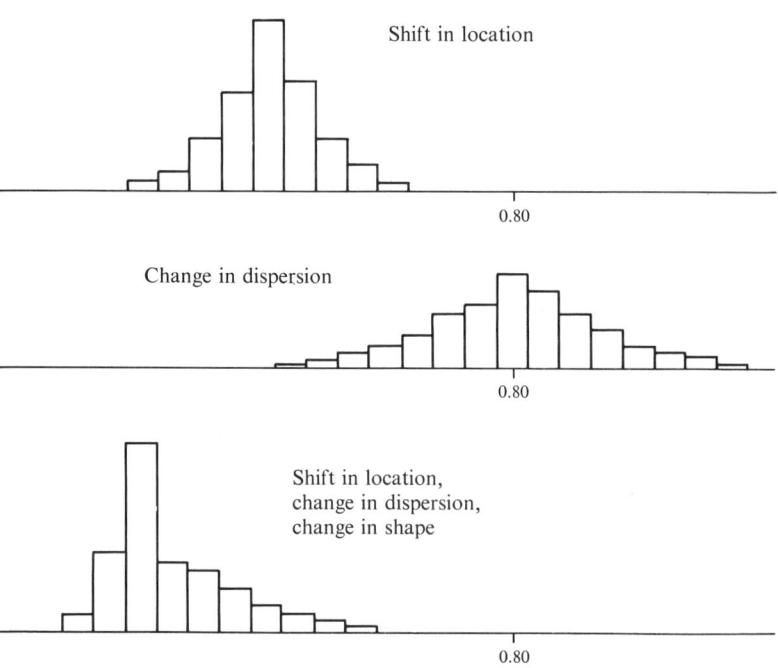

FIGURE 3.11

$\bar{x}$ would not always equal that value. In fact, usually it wouldn't! There are always two conflicting reasons to explain why an observed $\bar{x}$ does not equal the value of μ specified in the null hypothesis:

(1) The null hypothesis is true, and the difference between the observed mean and the hypothesized value for μ is simply due to the sampling variability of $\bar{X}$.

(2) The null hypothesis is false.

Methods for deciding between (1) and (2) make up the important branch of statistical inference known as *hypothesis testing*. At least some of the conclusions of almost all statistical studies are expressed in the language of hypothesis testing.

But whatever the setting, decision making of this sort is a highly structured procedure. The null hypothesis always states some *particular* value of the parameter in question (for example, H: $\mu = 0.80$). The alternative hypothesis includes some or all of the other possible values for μ. More precisely, A is said to be *two-sided* if it includes *all* the other possibilities (like A: $\mu \neq 0.80$) and *one-sided* if it includes values of μ in only one "direction" (for example A: $\mu < 0.80$).

Within the hypothesis testing framework, there are two ways to make correct decisions and two ways to make incorrect decisions. A correct decision results if either (1) H is accepted when H is true or (2) H is rejected when H is false. On the other hand, H might be rejected when true (this is called a *Type I error*) or accepted when false (this is called a *Type II error*). The next two examples show what Type I and Type II errors represent in real problems.

		True hypothesis	
		H	A
Our decision	Accept H	Correct decision	Type II error
	Reject H	Type I error	Correct decision

EXAMPLE 3.7.1. Polygraphs

Polygraphs are used in criminal investigations as a means of establishing the guilt or innocence of a suspect. They typically measure five functions: (1) thoracic respiration, (2) abdominal respiration, (3) blood pressure and pulse rate, (4) muscular movement and pressure, and (5) galvanic skin response. In principle, the magnitudes of these responses, when the subject is asked a relevant question ("Did you murder John Smith?"), indicate whether he is lying or telling the truth.

Of course, the procedure is not infallible. The purpose of the experiment described below (Horvath and Reid, 1971) was to determine how accurate polygraphs really are, under actual test conditions.

Seven experienced polygraph examiners were given a set of 40 records — 20 from innocent suspects and 20 from guilty suspects. The subjects had been asked 11 questions, on the basis of which each examiner was to make an overall judgment: innocent or guilty. The resulting 280 decisions were categorized according to what was actually true and what the examiner thought was true.

		Suspect's true status	
		Innocent	Guilty
Examiner's decision	Innocent	131	15
	Guilty	9	125
		140	140

If the null hypothesis is taken to be the legal standard that a person is innocent until proven guilty, then each of the 280 decisions reduces to a choice between

H: Suspect is innocent   versus   A: Suspect is guilty

As the table shows, correct decisions were made 91.4% of the time

$$\left[= \frac{131 + 125}{280} \times 100 \right]$$

Type I errors (rejecting H when H is true) were made 3.2% of the time $[= (9/280) \times 100]$; and Type II errors (accepting H when H is false) were made 5.4% of the time $[= 15/280 \times 100]$.

Question 3.7.1. In this particular setting, are Type I and Type II errors of equal consequence?

EXAMPLE 3.7.2. Alcohol and Writing Speed

To measure the effects on coordination associated with mild intoxication, thirteen subjects were each given 15.7 ml of ethyl alcohol per square meter of body surface area and asked to write a certain phrase as many times as they could in the space of one minute (Nash, 1972). The number of correct letters written was scaled, and each subject was assigned the score shown. (Negative scores indicate *decreased* writing speeds; positive scores, *increased* writing speeds.) Assuming the scale was defined so that subjects *not* under the influence achieve, on the average, a score of 0, can it be concluded that the amount of alcohol given in this study has any effect?

Subject	Score	Subject	Score
1	−6	8	0
2	10	9	−7
3	9	10	5
4	−8	11	−9
5	−6	12	−10
6	−2	13	−2
7	20		

Here the two distributions of interest are:

(1) The distribution of writing scores that would be achieved by persons not intoxicated.

(2) The distribution of writing scores that would be achieved by persons mildly intoxicated.

If μ denotes the mean of the second distribution, the initial question can be rephrased to read

H: $\mu = 0$ (Alcohol *does not* have an effect)

versus

A: $\mu \neq 0$ (Alcohol *does* have an effect)

If H is true, but the analysis of the data leads us to conclude that alcohol *does* have an effect, then we have committed a Type I error. On the other hand, if A is really true but we conclude that $\mu = 0$, then we have committed a Type II error. Of course, we might also make a correct decision, by accepting H when H is true or rejecting H when H is false.

Question 3.7.2. In Question 3.7.1, it was possible to determine after a decision had been made whether that judgment had been correct or not. Will this be possible for any decision made regarding the data in Example 3.7.2?

Comment

Type I and Type II errors are important concepts in hypothesis testing. If it were possible to choose between H and A and never make either kind of error, there would be no need for statistics. But Type I and Type II errors *are* made, and, as Chapter 4 will show, the reason is the sampling variability of $\bar{X}$.

The last two sections in this chapter develop some basic ideas about probability models and normal curves. This material, together with certain properties of the sampling distribution of $\bar{X}$, will be used in Chapter 4 to make formal the tests of H versus A.

3.8
PROBABILITY AND AREA

When histograms were discussed in Chapter 2, no restrictions were put on how the vertical axis could be scaled. For some of the examples, the vertical axis denoted a frequency; for others, a rate. In this section, two other kinds of vertical scales are introduced, *relative frequency* and *modified relative frequency*.

A relative frequency is simply a proportion. For example, suppose that a set of data consists of 50 observations grouped into three classes: "10–19," "20–29," and "30–39," denoted A, B, and C; and that these three classes occurred 10, 25, and 15 times, respectively. It follows that the relative frequency (or proportion of the time) that class A occurred was 10/50, or 0.20. Similarly, the relative frequencies of B and C were (25/50) = 0.50 and (15/50) = 0.30, respectively.

(1) Class	(2) Frequency	(3) Relative frequency
10–19 (A)	10	10/50 = .20
20–29 (B)	25	25/50 = .50
30–39 (C)	15	15/50 = .30
	50	1.00

According to the definition given in Chapter 2, Columns (1) and (2) of the table constitute a frequency distribution. For reasons soon to be explained, Columns (1) and (3) are called a *probability distribution*.

To see the implications of Column (3), it is necessary to picture the meaning of relative frequency in a sampling context. Imagine writing the class (A, B, or C) of each of these 50 observations on a separate slip of paper, putting all the slips into a box, and drawing one out without looking. We define the *probability* of the event "A will be drawn" to be the number of slips favorable to A (10) divided by the total number of slips that may be selected (50). In symbols, we abbreviate the word probability to P and write

$$P\{A \text{ is drawn}\} = 10/50 = 0.20$$

But note that this is just another way of representing the relative frequency of A. Similarly,

$$P\{A \text{ or } B \text{ is drawn}\} = (10 + 25)/50 = 0.70$$
$$= \text{relative frequency of A} + \text{relative frequency of B}$$

Comment

Since probabilities are proportions, it follows that the probability of any event must be a number between 0 and 1, inclusive. If an event *cannot* happen it has probability equal to 0 — for example, drawing a slip bearing the letter D. If an event is *sure* to happen it has probability equal to 1 — for example, drawing a slip with either the letter A, B, or C. This latter property implies that the *sum* of the probabilities associated with each of the classes must add to 1. In this case, $0.20 + 0.50 + 0.30 = 1.00$.

Expressions such as "$P\{A \text{ is drawn}\}$" can also be interpreted in a more operational way. Suppose that instead of drawing just *one* slip of paper, we drew many, but only one at a time. After choosing a slip we record whether or not it had written on it the letter A, then mix it back with the others, draw another slip, etc. The "data," after making nine such drawings, might look like this:

Draw number	Outcome	Proportion of A's
1	A	1/1 = 1.00
2	not A	1/2 = .50
3	not A	1/3 = .33
4	not A	1/4 = .25
5	not A	1/5 = .20
6	not A	1/6 = .17
7	A	2/7 = .28
8	not A	2/8 = .25
9	not A	2/9 = .22

If n selections are made, during which time m A's are recorded, the fraction m/n can be thought of as an empirical estimate of the probability that the event "A is drawn" occurs. Figure 3.12 shows how this estimate evolves and becomes better as sample information accumulates.

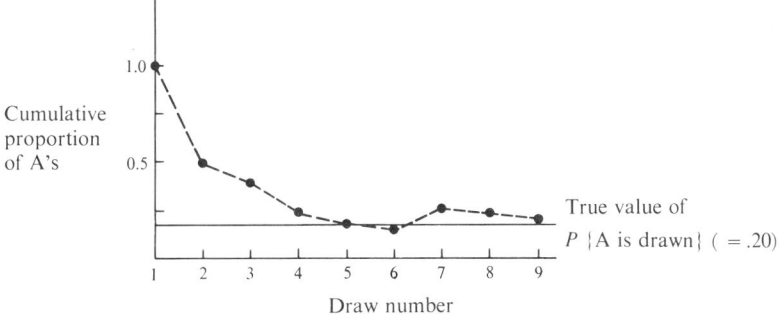

FIGURE 3.12

In the discussion that follows, it will always be helpful to think of probabilities in this way; that is, as limiting values of relative frequencies.

Question 3.8.1. Refer to the data described in Example 3.3.2. Estimate the probability that the platelet count of a new patient admitted to the rest home will be less than 150,000/mm³.

The last part of this section relates the concepts of probability and relative frequency to the interpretation of a histogram. Recall that in previous discussions, the location and dispersion of a histogram were singled out as being very important characteristics. *Area* is a third property that needs to be considered. From geometry, the area of a histogram can be calculated by adding together the products formed by multiplying the height of each bar by its width. Consider the histogram in Figure 3.13 which describes the occurrences of classes A (10–19), B (20–29), and C (30–39). Here the width of each class is 10, so the total area of the histogram is

Area = base × height for A + base × height for B + base × height for C
= 10(10) + 10(25) + 10(15)
= 500

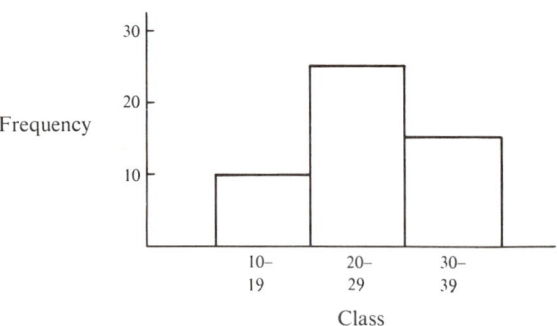

FIGURE 3.13

Comment

Remember that the 10–19 class actually extends from 9.5 to 19.5 so the class width is, indeed 10 (= 19.5 − 9.5) and not 9 (= 19−10).

Note that neither the location nor the shape of any histogram will be changed if every number on the vertical scale is multiplied or divided by the same positive constant. That is, whether the heights of the 10–19 and 20–29 bars are labeled as 10 and 25 or as $10c$ and $25c$, where c is any positive constant, is irrelevant as far as location and shape are concerned. Of course, by including the factor c the total area of the histogram is changed from 500 to $500c$:

$$\text{Area} = 10(10c) + 10(25c) + 10(15c)$$
$$= 500c$$

This implies that by choosing c properly, we can make the histogram area equal to any number desired. In particular, there are advantages, which will be discussed shortly, in having the area equal to 1. Here this can be accomplished by letting

$$c = \frac{1}{500} = \frac{1}{\text{Total number of observations} \times \text{class width}} = \frac{1}{50 \times 10}$$

In general, to force the area of a histogram to equal 1 we need simply make the height of, say, the A bar equal to

$$\frac{\text{Frequency of class A}}{\text{Total number of observations} \times \text{class width}} = \frac{10}{50 \times 10} = 0.02$$

Scale units of this sort are called *modified relative frequencies*.

[3.8] Probability and Area

Class	Frequency	Modified relative frequency
10–19 (A)	10	$\frac{10}{50 \times 10} = .02$
20–29 (B)	25	$\frac{25}{50 \times 10} = .05$
30–39 (C)	$\frac{15}{50}$	$\frac{15}{50 \times 10} = .03$

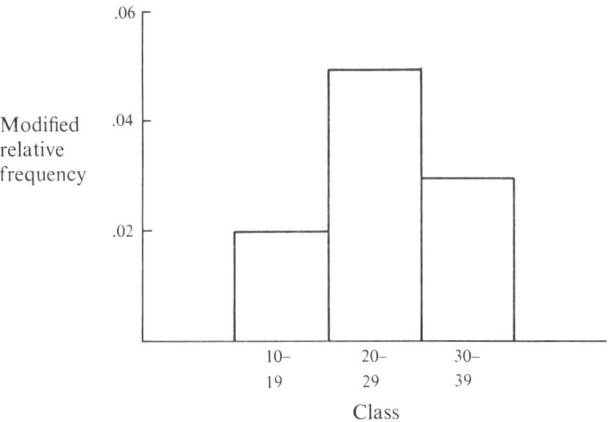

FIGURE 3.14

Since neither location nor shape is affected by scale changes along the vertical axis, it may seem that modified relative frequencies serve no purpose, but they do. By making the total area of a histogram equal to 1, it is possible to associate the area of a bar (or group of bars) with the probability that a sample observation will belong to a particular class (or group of classes). For example, the area of the bar corresponding to class C is equal to

$$\text{Base} \times \text{Height} = 10 \times 0.03 = 0.30$$

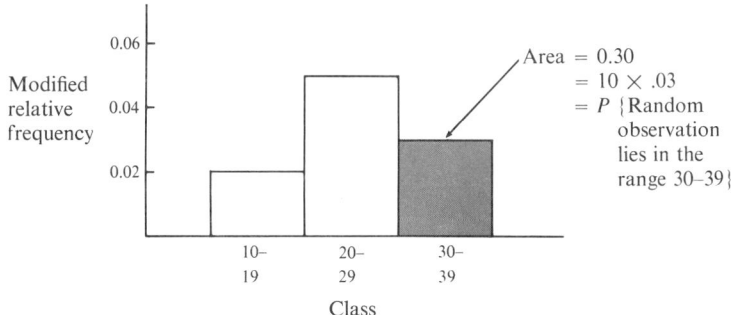

FIGURE 3.15

which, as seen earlier, is the probability that an observation chosen at random will lie in the range 30–39.

EXAMPLE 3.8.1. Area Computations

The maximum head breadths of 84 Etruscan skulls were listed in Example 2.6.3, along with Figure 3.16. To convert this histogram to one whose total area equals 1, it is necessary to rescale the vertical axis by replacing "Frequency" with

$$\frac{\text{Frequency}}{84 \times 5}$$

since there is a total of 84 observations and the class width is 5.

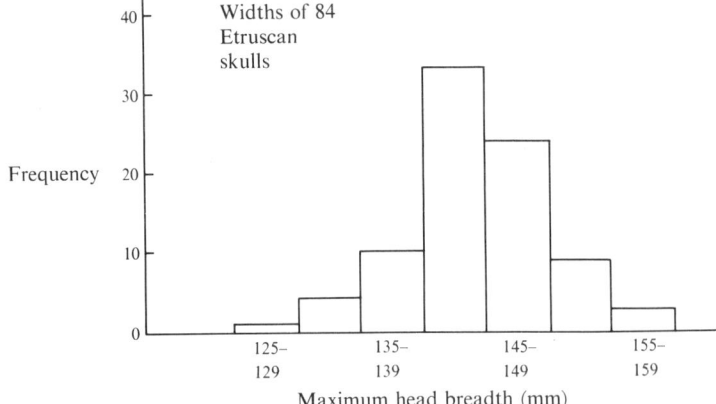

FIGURE 3.16

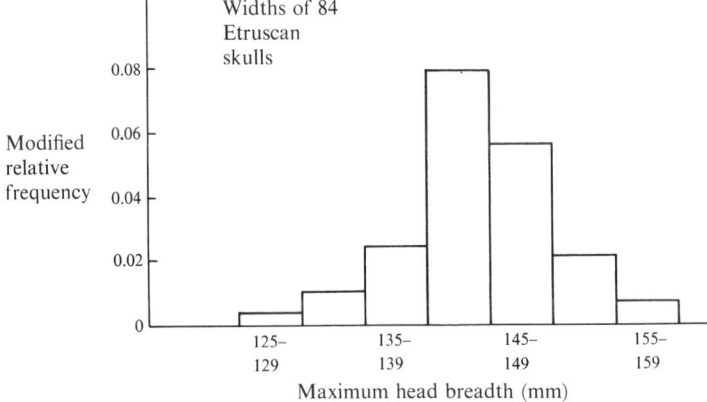

FIGURE 3.17

Let X denote the value of an observation selected at random from this distribution. As an example of the relationship between probability and area, note that

$$P\{130 < X < 144\} = \text{Relative frequency of} \\ \text{130–134 class} + \text{relative frequency of} \\ \text{135–139 class} + \text{relative frequency of} \\ \text{140–144 class}$$

$$= \frac{4}{84} + \frac{10}{84} + \frac{33}{84} = \frac{47}{84}$$

$$= 0.56$$

Also,

$$P\{130 < X < 144\} = \text{Sum of the areas of the} \\ \text{130–134, 135–139, and 140–144 bars}$$

$$= 5\left(\frac{4}{84 \times 5}\right) + 5\left(\frac{10}{84 \times 5}\right) + 5\left(\frac{33}{84 \times 5}\right) = \frac{235}{420}$$

$$= 0.56$$

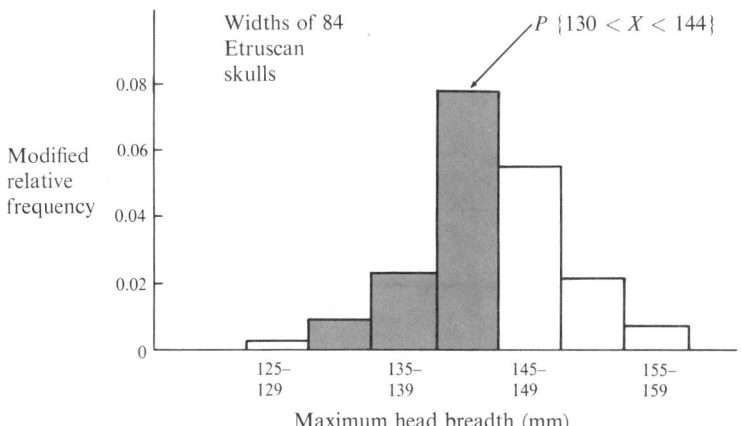

FIGURE 3.18

Comment

Probability expressions like the ones above refer to the likelihood that a measurement *will* be in a particular interval so that measurement (that is, the random variable) is denoted by a capital letter, in this case, X. It would be incorrect to write $P\{130 < x < 144\}$.

Question 3.8.2. Compute $P\{X < 135\}$ two ways: (1) by using relative frequencies and (2) by finding the corresponding area on the appropriately scaled histogram.

Question 3.8.3. Define a set of classes for the bacterial counts of Review Exercise 1.2. Then:
(1) Draw a histogram of the corresponding frequency distribution.
(2) Scale the histogram so its total area is 1.

3.9 AREAS UNDER NORMAL CURVES

Certain histogram shapes reappear in a variety of experimental settings. The bell shape, for example, has already described prothrombin times, blood pressures, traffic death rates, and skull widths. Some of the other patterns that frequently occur are shown in Figures 3.19 and 3.20.

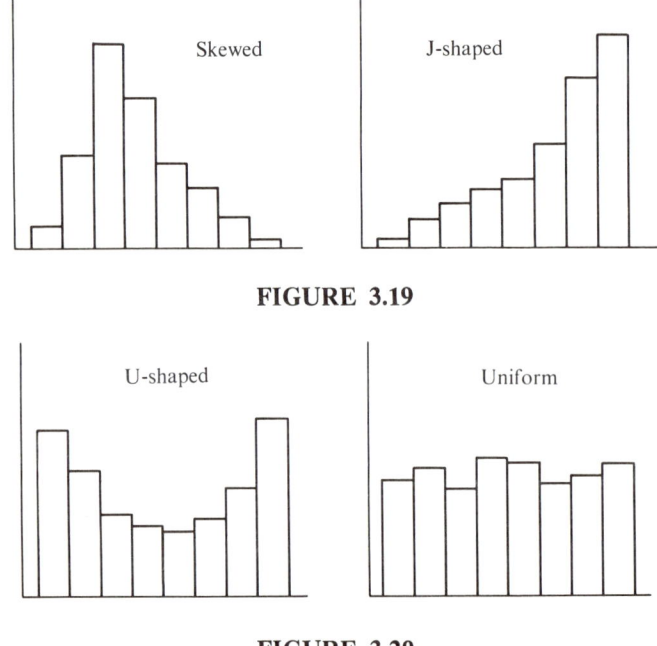

FIGURE 3.19

FIGURE 3.20

It often proves helpful to approximate a histogram having a certain shape with a *mathematical model;* that is, with a probability distribution whose basic properties are determined by a formula rather than from the sample data. By far the most important mathematical model in statistics is the *normal curve*. This is the one that approximates bell-shaped histograms.

The equation of a normal curve will not be given, but it depends on the two parameters mentioned in Section 3.7, μ and σ. Furthermore, each distinct set of parameter values generates a different normal curve.

Areas Under Normal Curves

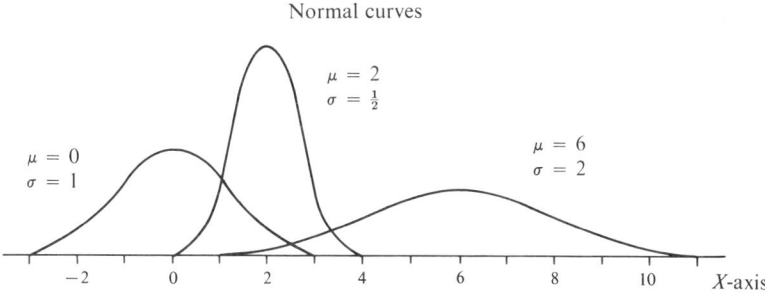

FIGURE 3.21

Comment

All normal curves have certain characteristics in common. First, they all have areas equal to 1. Second, each is symmetric around μ. That is, the heights of the curve at $\mu - k$ and $\mu + k$ are the same, for any particular value of k. And, finally, the curve itself never touches the horizontal axis; the defining equation is such that the left-hand tail extends to "minus infinity" and the right-hand tail to "plus infinity." Nevertheless, about 95% of the area under any normal curve is concentrated above the interval ranging from $\mu - 2\sigma$ to $\mu + 2\sigma$. In the normal curve having $\mu = 6$ and $\sigma = 2$, for example, almost all the area lies above the interval from 2 to 10.

EXAMPLE 3.9.1. A Normal Curve Approximation

Figure 3.22 shows the Etruscan skull histogram of Example 3.8.1 and a normal curve that approximates it. The parameters μ and σ for the normal curve have been set equal to the values found for $\bar{x}$ and s in the sample data — 143.8 and 6.0, respectively (see Question 3.5.4).

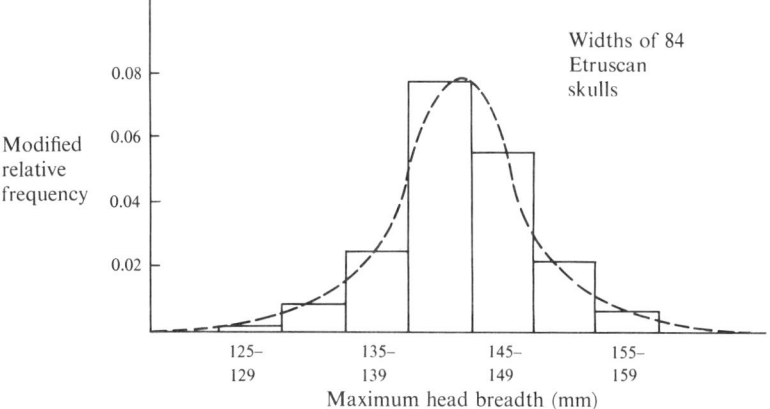

FIGURE 3.22

Of the infinite number of normal curves, the one having $\mu = 0$ and $\sigma = 1$ is of special interest. This is called the *standard normal curve* and any variable whose "behavior" it describes is denoted by the letter Z. Two properties make the standard normal curve so important:

(1) Tables have been constructed for finding the area under this particular curve between any two points, a and b, on the horizontal axis.

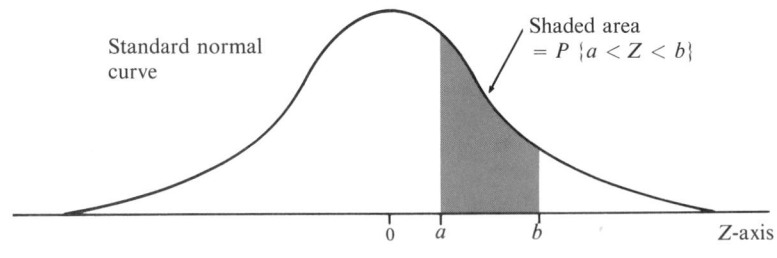

FIGURE 3.23

(2) Suppose X is a variable whose distribution is approximated by an arbitrary normal curve, having mean μ and standard deviation σ; if c and d are any two points on the horizontal axis, then the area under the curve between c and d — that is, $P\{c < X < d\}$ — can be determined by first transforming X into a standard normal variable (see Theorem 3.9.1) and then using the tables referred to in (1).

The remainder of this section explains how to find areas under both standard normal curves and arbitrary normal curves.

First, let Z denote a standard normal variable. The table in Appendix I allows us to find, in one step, the numerical value of expressions such as "$P\{Z < 1.13\}$" — namely, the probability that a randomly selected observation, Z, from a standard normal distribution will equal some number less than 1.13. The numbers listed in the body of Appendix I are the areas under the standard normal distribution *to the left* of the numbers listed along the left-hand margin. A second decimal point for the margin numbers defines the columns going across the table. In particular, the area to the left of a Z-value of 1.13 is 0.8708; that is, $P\{Z < 1.13\} = 0.8708$.

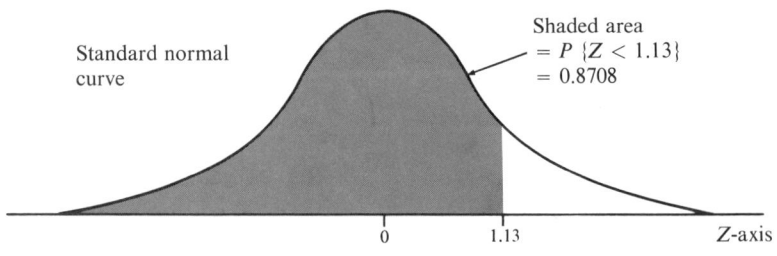

FIGURE 3.24

Sometimes more than one step is required to find a particular area. Suppose, for example, that we wanted to know the area under a standard normal curve between -1.02 and $+0.57$.

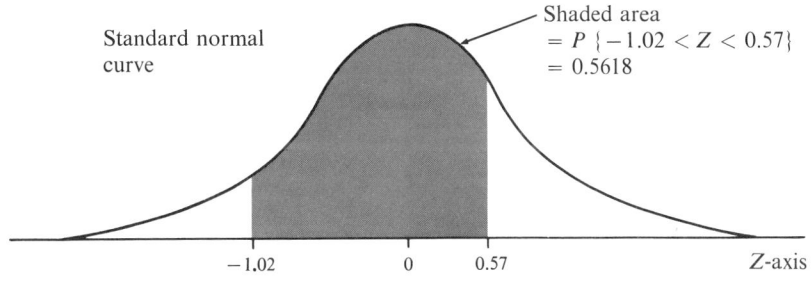

FIGURE 3.25

Here there is no direct way to look up the answer but note that

Area between -1.02 and 0.57
$\quad=$ (Area to the left of 0.57) $-$ (area to the left of -1.02)

or

$$P\{-1.02 < Z < 0.57\} = P\{Z < 0.57\} - P\{Z < -1.02\}$$

Since the two probabilities on the right-hand side *can* be found in the table (they equal 0.7157 and 0.1539, respectively), it follows that

$$P\{-1.02 < Z < 0.57\} = 0.7157 - 0.1539$$
$$= 0.5618$$

EXAMPLE 3.9.2. Areas Under the Standard Normal Curve

Let Z denote a standard normal variable.
(a) Find $P\{Z \geq 0.65\}$

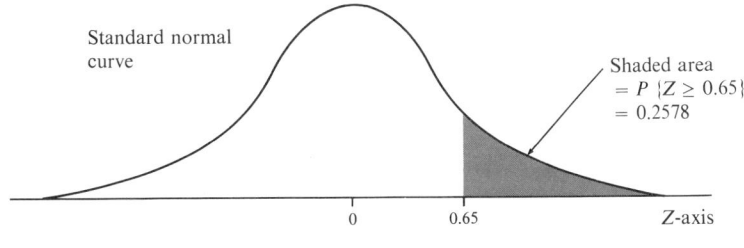

FIGURE 3.26

Since the total area under the curve is equal to 1,

$$P\{Z < 0.65\} + P\{Z \geq 0.65\} = 1$$

in which case

$$P\{Z \geq 0.65\} = 1 - P\{Z < 0.65\}$$
$$= 1 - 0.7422$$
$$= 0.2578$$

Comment

The continuous nature of the normal curve makes it necessary to assign a probability of 0 to the occurrence of any particular number. That is, $P\{Z = 1.16\} = 0$, $P\{Z = -0.46\} = 0$, etc. This means that the numerical value of expressions such as $P\{Z \geq 0.65\}$ is the same with or without the equal sign:

$$P\{Z \geq 0.65\} = P\{Z > 0.65\}$$

(b) Find $P\{-0.60 < Z < -0.12\}$

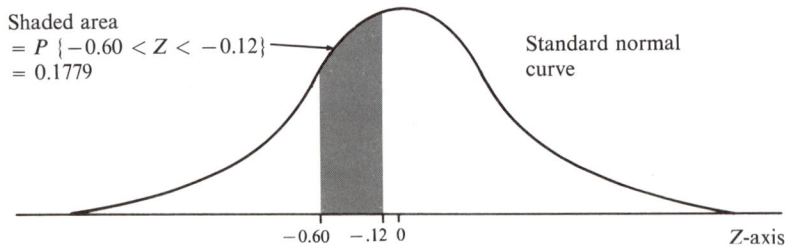

FIGURE 3.27

From Figure 3.27,

$$P\{-0.60 < Z < -0.12\} = P\{Z < -0.12\} - P\{Z < -0.60\}$$
$$= 0.4522 - 0.2743$$
$$= 0.1779$$

(c) Find $P\{Z > 0\}$

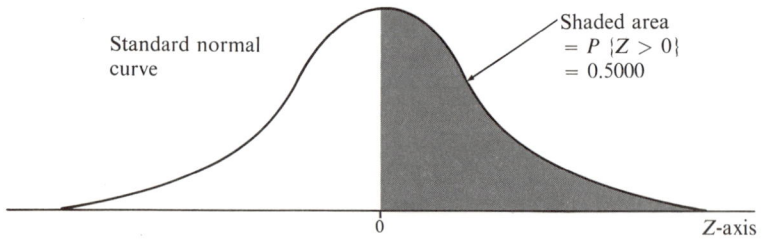

FIGURE 3.28

Here Appendix I is not needed. From the symmetry of the standard normal curve, it follows that

$$P\{Z > 0\} = P\{Z < 0\}$$
$$= 0.5000$$

Question 3.9.1. Find the following probabilities associated with areas under a standard normal curve. In each instance, draw a diagram showing the area in question.
(1) $P\{Z > -0.17\}$
(2) $P\{-1.69 < Z < 0.98\}$
(3) $P\{Z < 4.82\}$

Question 3.9.2. In a previous comment it was noted that about 95% of the area under any normal curve lies between $\mu - 2\sigma$ and $\mu + 2\sigma$. *Exactly* what percentage of the area under a standard normal curve lies between these limits? How much of the area is contained within *one* standard deviation of the mean?

The following theorem relates the first property that makes the standard normal so important to the second (see page 110).

Theorem 3.9.1. Suppose that X denotes a measurement, or variable, whose probability distribution is described by a normal curve with mean and standard deviation equal to μ and σ, respectively. Then the probability distribution of

$$\frac{X - \mu}{\sigma}$$

will be described by the *standard* normal curve.

Figure 3.29 on p. 114 illustrates the meaning of Theorem 3.9.1. It compares for two special cases, the properties of an X distribution with those of the corresponding $(X - \mu)/\sigma \, (= Z)$ distribution.

Theorem 3.9.1 is easy to apply. Suppose we want to find the area under a normal curve between the points 40 and 65 — that is, $P\{40 < X < 65\}$ — and suppose the curve can be assumed to have mean 50 and standard deviation 10. Recall that one of the properties of inequalities (such as $40 < X < 65$) is that their meaning remains unchanged if the same positive number multiplies (or divides) each term, or if the same positive or negative number is added to (or subtracted from) each term. Therefore,

$$40 < X < 65$$

is equivalent to

$$\frac{40 - 50}{10} < \frac{X - 50}{10} < \frac{65 - 50}{10}$$

or

$$-1.00 < \frac{X - 50}{10} < 1.50$$

Transforming an arbitrary normal distribution into a standard normal distribution

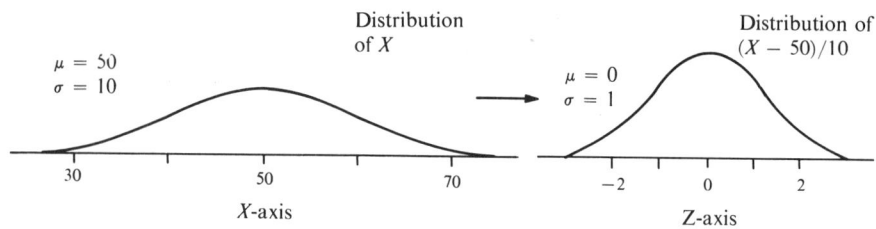

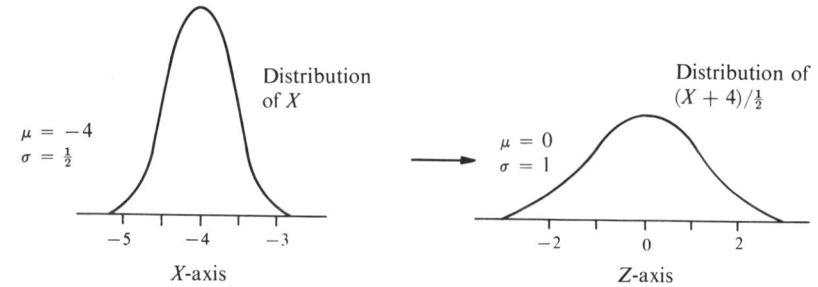

FIGURE 3.29

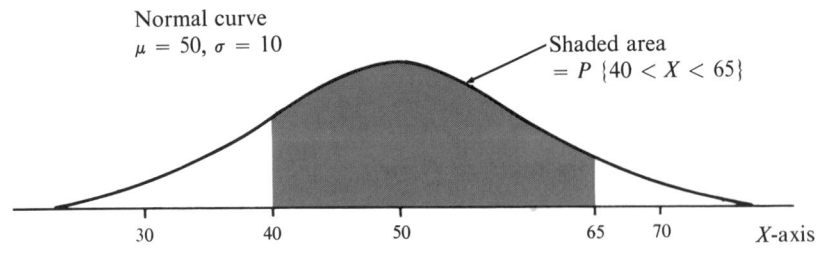

FIGURE 3.30

But since 50 and 10 are the values of μ and σ for the distribution of X, Theorem 3.9.1 implies that the distribution of

$$\frac{X - 50}{10} \quad (= Z)$$

is described by a standard normal curve. Therefore,

$$\begin{aligned} P\{40 < X < 65\} &= P\{-1.00 < Z < 1.50\} \\ &= P\{Z < 1.50\} - P\{Z < -1.00\} \\ &= 0.9332 - 0.1587 \\ &= 0.7745 \end{aligned}$$

The next example shows how this type of calculation is used to approximate areas under histograms.

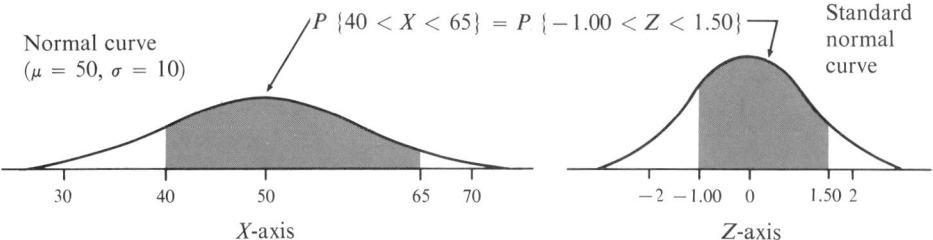

FIGURE 3.31

EXAMPLE 3.9.3. IQs and the Normal Curve

The revised Stanford-Binet test is a battery of examinations designed to measure various mental capacities, from simple manipulative skills to abstract verbal aptitude. Individual results are combined to form an "intelligence quotient," which is defined to be 100 times the ratio of a child's mental and chronological ages:

$$\text{IQ} = \frac{\text{Mental age}}{\text{Chronological age}} \times 100$$

The grading of the Stanford-Binet test is scaled so that the probability distribution of IQ scores is bell-shaped with a mean (μ) of 100 and a standard deviation (σ) of 16.

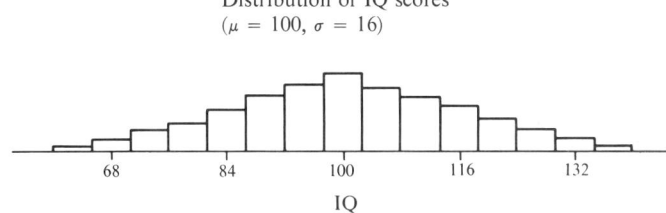

FIGURE 3.32

Suppose a child is selected at random. What is the probability that his or her IQ will be between 90 and 115?

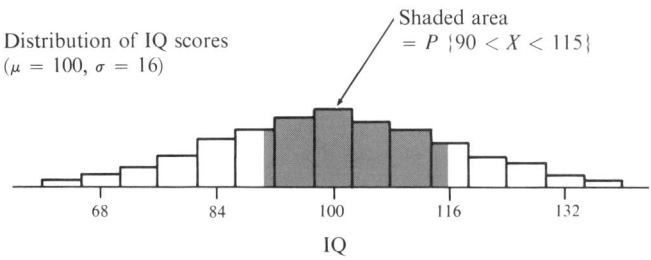

FIGURE 3.33

Using Theorem 3.9.1,

$$P\{90 < X < 115\} = P\left\{\frac{90-100}{16} < \frac{X-100}{16} < \frac{115-100}{16}\right\}$$
$$= P\{-0.62 < Z < 0.94\}$$
$$= P\{Z < 0.94\} - P\{Z < -0.62\}$$
$$= 0.8264 - 0.2676$$
$$\approx 0.56$$

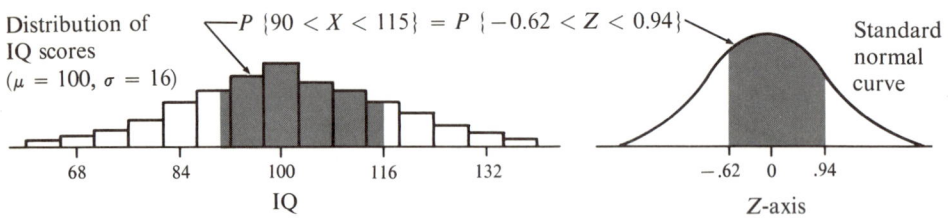

FIGURE 3.34

One more example should clarify these ideas. What would be the chances of selecting a child with an IQ greater than 140? Using the Z transformation,

$$P\{X > 140\} = P\left\{\frac{X-100}{16} > \frac{140-100}{16}\right\}$$
$$= P\{Z > 2.50\}$$
$$= 1 - P\{Z \le 2.50\}$$
$$= 1 - 0.9938$$
$$\approx 0.01$$

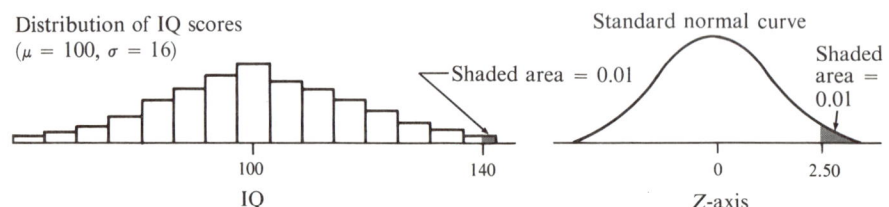

FIGURE 3.35

Question 3.9.3. What is the probability of selecting a child with an IQ in the range 104 to 122? In the range 99 to 101? Less than 60? Either less than 75 or greater than 125? Draw diagrams for both the original distribution and the transformed standard normal curve, shading the areas in question.

Question 3.9.4. Mensa is an international society whose only requirement for membership is to have an IQ in the upper 2% of the population. Assuming that $\mu = 100$ and $\sigma = 16$, what is the *lowest* IQ that will qualify a person to belong to Mensa?

Question 3.9.5. Draw a histogram of the prothrombin times listed in Section 3.2, using modified relative frequencies on the vertical axis. Superimpose a freehand sketch of a normal curve approximating that histogram. Assume that the parameters of the normal curve are numerically equal to the corresponding statistics computed from the sample data; that is, assume that $\mu = 17.4$ and $\sigma = 5.8$. Let X denote a random prothrombin time. Use normal curve calculations to estimate the probability that X will be in the interval from 13.6 to 20.5.

Question 3.9.6. In women, the hemoglobin (Hb) content of venous blood is normally distributed with a mean of 14.0 grams per 100 ml and a standard deviation of 2.0 grams per 100 ml (Diem, 1962). Let X denote the hemoglobin content of a randomly selected woman. Find $P\{X > 18.1\}$.

3.10
SUMMARY

The first five sections of Chapter 3 extended the tabular and graphical forms of descriptive statistics to include two numerical measures, the *sample mean* and the *sample standard deviation*. At the same time, *sigma notation* was introduced to simplify the writing of formulas like the ones that define $\bar{x}$ and s. Then Sections 3.6 and 3.7 presented some of the fundamentals of statistical inference. More specifically, Section 3.6 developed the notion of the *sampling distribution of* $\bar{X}$, while Section 3.7 drew the very important distinctions between a *statistic* and a *parameter*, between the *null hypothesis* and the *alternative hypothesis*, and between a *Type I error* and a *Type II error*.

The final two sections covered *probability distributions* and *normal curves*. In principle, probability distributions are listings of the possible outcomes of an experiment together with the relative likelihoods that each will occur. In a graphical format, they look very much like the histograms of Chapter 2 except that the vertical axes are scaled with *modified relative frequencies*.

Certain types of probability distributions — that is, certain shapes — tend to occur over and over again in a variety of experimental settings. We find it convenient to approximate these distributions with families of theoretical distributions known as *mathematical models*. The most important of these mathematical models is the *normal curve*.

For reasons that will become obvious in the next chapter, it is necessary to be able to compute areas under normal curves. This would be a formidable task if it were not for the fact that any area involving an arbitrary normal variable, X, with mean μ and standard deviation σ, can always be expressed in terms of an area involving a *standard normal* variable, Z, whose mean equals 0 and whose standard deviation equals 1. In particular,

$$P\{a < X < b\} = P\{(a - \mu)/\sigma < Z < (b - \mu)/\sigma\}$$

Written in this way, the area indicated by the right hand side of the equation can be found using the table in Appendix I.

Definitions

Alternative hypothesis (A). What is accepted as being true when the data fail to support the null hypothesis; can be either one-sided or two-sided.

Bell shape. A term loosely describing a common data pattern: the most frequently occurring values are near the mean, with extreme deviations on either side of $\bar{x}$ occurring much less often.

Hypothesis testing. The procedure for choosing between two conflicting statements concerning the numerical value of a parameter.

Mathematical model. A theoretical probability distribution used to approximate the behavior of a particular variable; for example, the normal curve.

Modified relative frequency. A particular scale used on the vertical axis of a histogram for the purpose of making the total area of the histogram equal to 1.

Normal curve. A mathematical model for approximating bell-shaped histograms.

Null hypothesis (H). The hypothesis that gives the "status quo" (or "no effect") value for the parameter being tested.

One-sided alternative. An alternative hypothesis having either the form A: $\mu < \mu_0$ or A: $\mu > \mu_0$, where μ_0 is some specified constant.

Parameter. A constant characterizing some aspect of a population distribution; the problem of numerically estimating parameters on the basis of information contained in samples is central to much of statistics.

Population mean (μ). A parameter; a number denoting the "location" of the distribution of all possible measurements of a certain kind; the population analog of $\bar{x}$.

Population standard deviation (σ). A parameter; a number describing the "dispersion" of the distribution of all possible measurements of a certain kind; the population analog of s.

Probability. A number between 0 and 1, inclusive; quantifies the likelihood with which a certain event will occur.

Probability distribution. For discrete data, a listing of all the possible outcomes of an experiment together with the relative frequencies with which they can be expected to occur; for continuous data, a curve describing the behavior of a variable X in the sense that for any two points a and b, $P\{a < X < b\}$ is the area under the curve between a and b.

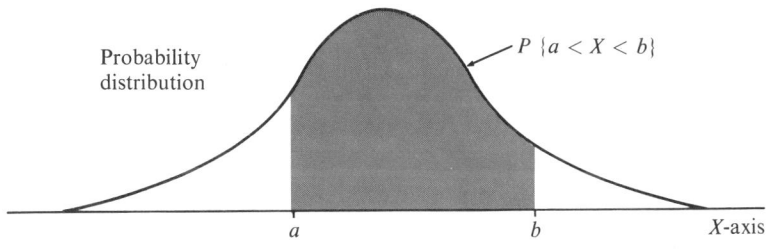

FIGURE 3.36

Relative frequency. The proportion of times a certain event occurs.

Sample mean ($\bar{x}$). A statistic; the most frequently used way of quantifying the center (or location) of a set of measurements; given $x_1, x_2, \ldots, x_n$,

$$\bar{x} = \frac{1}{n} \sum_{i=1}^{n} x_i$$

Sample median ($\tilde{x}$). The "middle" observation, in terms of magnitude; a way of characterizing the location of a set of measurements; used in place of the sample mean when the data contain one or more extreme values that would unduly influence (and distort) the value of $\bar{x}$.

Sample standard deviation (s). A statistic; measures the amount of dispersion in a set of measurements; given $x_1, x_2, \ldots, x_n$,

$$s = \sqrt{\frac{n \sum_{i=1}^{n} x_i^2 - \left(\sum_{i=1}^{n} x_i\right)^2}{n(n-1)}}$$

Sample variance (s^2). The square of the sample standard deviation; a measure of dispersion.

Sampling distribution of $\bar{X}$. A probability distribution describing the behavior of averages; the properties of the sampling distribution of $\bar{X}$ figure prominently in the procedures for testing hypotheses about μ.

Sigma notation. Certain conventions related to the use of the symbol Σ; simplifies the writing of formulas involving sums of subscripted variables.

Standard normal curve. The particular normal curve having $\mu = 0$ and $\sigma = 1$; areas under this curve are tabulated in Appendix I; the letter Z is used to denote any variable whose distribution is described by the standard normal curve.

Statistic. Any number computed solely on the basis of information contained in the sample data; for example, $\bar{x}$ and s.

Two-sided alternative. An alternative hypothesis of the form A: $\mu \neq \mu_0$, where μ_0 is a specified constant.

Type I error. In hypothesis testing, concluding that H is false when, in fact, H is true.

Type II error. In hypothesis testing, concluding that H is true when, in fact, H is false.

Review Exercises

3.1 The average gestation time for humans is 266 days, with a standard deviation of 16 days. If the distribution of gestation times is assumed to be normal, what is the probability that a pregnancy will exceed 310 days? In 1967, there were an estimated 318,000 illegitimate births in the United States. How many of those pregnancies might have been expected to exceed 310 days?

3.2 Four groups of subjects were recruited to participate in a psychological study involving self-esteem. Group 1 were recently admitted inmates of a Montana prison; Group 2 were maximum security prisoners confined for extended sentences; Group 3 were college students taking an introductory psychology course; and Group 4 were white, Anglo-Saxon members of a small, rural Protestant church. Each subject was given a verbal test that measured his or her self-esteem by contrasting the subject's opinions of his *actual* self and his *ideal* self. Higher scores denoted greater differences between the actual and the ideal, and, consequently, a lower self-esteem. The four test score distributions are shown in Figure 3.37 (Fichtler, Zimmerman, and Moore, 1973). What "principle" of statistical inference do these data violate?

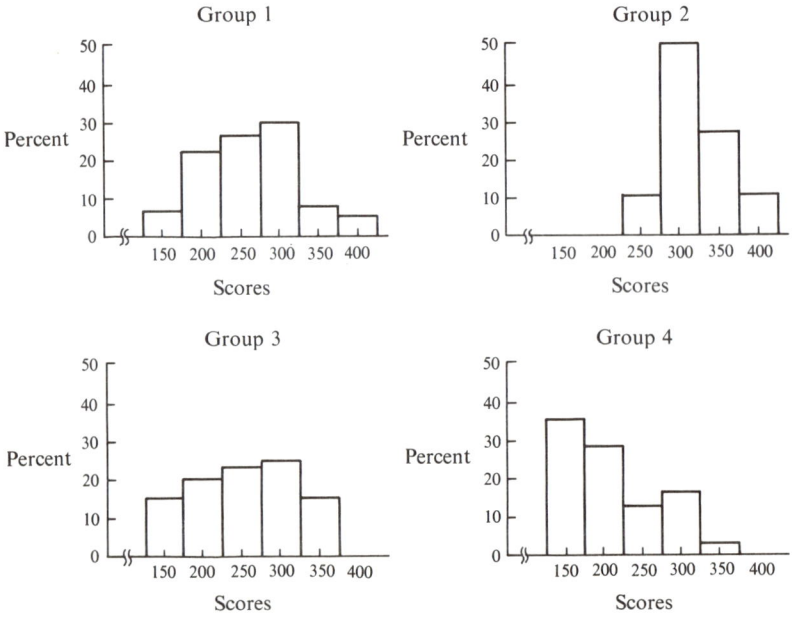

FIGURE 3.37

3.3 The systolic blood pressure of 18-year-old women is normally distributed with a mean of 120 mm of Hg and a standard deviation of 12 mm of Hg (Diem, 1962). What is the probability that the blood pressure of a randomly selected 18-year-old woman will be greater than 150? Less than 115? Between 110 and 130?

3.4 The pth percentile, x_p, of any distribution is the value of the variable that is exceeded $(100 - p)\%$ of the time. Compute the 90th percentile, x_{90}, for the blood pressure distribution referred to in Exercise 3.3. What is another name for x_{50}?

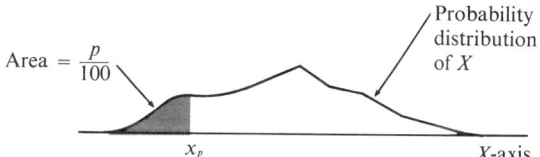

FIGURE 3.38

3.5 For any distribution, the interquartile range, Q, is defined to be the difference between the 75th and 25th percentile — that is, $Q = x_{75} - x_{25}$. Find the interquartile range for the IQ distribution of Example 3.9.3. Is Q a measure of location or dispersion?

3.6 In Example 1.6.1, a graph was shown of the radiation levels measured in 10 department stores selling color televisions. The actual numbers that were recorded are listed below.

Location	Net mr/hour
1	.40
2	.48
3	.60
4	.15
5	.50
6	.80
7	.50
8	.36
9	.16
10	.89

Find the sample mean and the sample standard deviation.

3.7 Given that $x_1 = -2$, $x_2 = 1$, $x_3 = 0$, and $y_1 = 4$, $y_2 = 3$, $y_3 = 1$, compute:

(a) $\sum_{i=1}^{3} (x_i + y_i)$

(b) $\sum_{i=1}^{3} x_i y_i$

(c) $\left(\sum_{i=1}^{3} x_i \right) \left(\sum_{i=1}^{3} y_i \right)$

(d) $\sqrt{\sum_{i=1}^{3} x_i + \sum_{i=1}^{3} y_i}$

(e) $\dfrac{\left[3 \sum_{i=1}^{3} (x_i - 3)^3 \right]^3}{3} - 3$

3.8 Dental structure provides an effective criterion for classifying certain fossils. Listed below are the third molar lengths of nine baboons belonging to the genus *Papio* (Minkoff, 1972). Find $\bar{x}$ and s. Not long ago, a baboon skull of unknown origin was discovered in a cave in Angola; its third molar length was 9.0 mm. Is that value "compatible" with the nine listed below? Be as quantitative as possible.

Specimen	Third molar length (mm)
MCZ 8466	8.3
MCZ 29790	8.5
MCZ 10570	8.6
MCZ 11395	7.8
MCZ 29791	8.1
MCZ 29792	8.1
MCZ 26472	7.2
MCZ 29789	8.2
MCZ 22752	8.8

3.9 Compute the sample mean and the sample standard deviation for the thirteen writing scores described in Example 3.7.2.

3.10 Sometimes it is necessary to compute the sample mean and/or the sample standard deviation from data presented in histogram form. That is, the *numbers* of observations belonging to each class are known, but the exact values of the x_i's are not. In these cases, $\bar{x}$ and s can be estimated by making the assumption that each observation has a value equal to the midpoint of the class to which it belongs. For example, in the following data:

Class	Frequency, f_i	Midpoint, m_i
10–19	5	14.5
20–29	6	24.5
30–39	4	34.5

the *grouped mean* ($\bar{x}_g$) and the *grouped standard deviation* (s_g) — by analogy with the formulas for $\bar{x}$ and s — are given by

$$\bar{x}_g = \frac{\Sigma f_i m_i}{n} = \frac{5(14.5) + 6(24.5) + 4(34.5)}{15}$$

$$= \frac{357.5}{15}$$

$$= 23.8$$

$$s_g = \sqrt{\frac{n \Sigma f_i m_i^2 - (\Sigma f_i m_i)^2}{n(n-1)}}$$

$$= \sqrt{\frac{15[5(14.5)^2 + 6(24.5)^2 + 4(34.5)^2] - (357.5)^2}{15(14)}}$$

$$= \sqrt{\frac{13{,}400.00}{210}} = \sqrt{63.81}$$

$$= 8.0$$

Suppose the exact values of $x_1, x_2, \ldots, x_n$ *were* known, in addition to their histogram. Would $\bar{x}$ equal $\bar{x}_g$, in general? If not, would $\bar{x}_g$ tend to be larger or smaller?

3.11 In normal adults, the average diameter of red blood cells is 7.5 microns, with a standard deviation of 0.3 microns (Diem, 1962). Assume the distribution of diameters is bell-shaped. Let X denote the diameter of a randomly chosen red blood cell.

(a) Find $P\{7.1 < X < 7.6\}$
(b) Find $P\{X < 7.0 \quad \text{or} \quad 7.4 < X < 7.6\}$
(c) What would be the "standardized" diameter of a red blood cell whose length was 7.4 microns?

3.12 It is estimated that 80% of all 18-year-old girls have weights ranging from 103.5 to 144.5 pounds (Diem, 1962). Assuming the weight distribution can be adequately approximated by a normal curve, and assuming that 103.5 and 144.5 are equal distances from the average weight, μ, calculate σ.

4

MODEL TWO
The One-Sample Problem

*A reasonable probability is the
only certainty.*
      E. G. Bulwer-Lytton

4.1
INTRODUCTION

In this chapter, the principles of sampling distributions, finding areas under normal curves, and hypothesis testing are all brought together for the first time. The result is a "philosophy" of statistical inference — that is, a formalized way of generalizing, quantitatively, from the known to the unknown.

More than anything else, making inferences is what statistics is all about. For example, suppose the drug "of choice" for a certain disease has been found, over the years, to be effective 80% of the time. But now a new drug is being developed, and it has been credited with 170 cures among an initial sample of 200 patients, giving it a cure rate of 85% ($= (170/200) \times 100$). Should this second treatment be considered superior to the first? Or must we defer judgment, pointing to the fact that the sample size is probably too small for the results to be definitive? Questions of this sort arise quite often in experimental research. For their solution, they require the methods presented in this chapter.

Almost all applications of statistical inference fall into two broad categories: *hypothesis tests* and *confidence intervals*. The former are taken up in Sections

4.2, 4.3, 4.5, and 4.6; the latter, in Sections 4.4 and 4.5. Although both approaches are very similar mathematically, hypothesis tests are used much more often in practice.

In most cases, hypothesis tests and confidence intervals for one-sample problems involve a location parameter. For the first part of this chapter we deal with continuous data, where the location parameter is μ. Here there are two variations on the basic inference procedures, with the critical factor being the sample size, n. When n is fairly large (meaning greater than 30), hypothesis tests and confidence intervals for μ involve the normal curve; but when n is less than or equal to 30, another mathematical model, the *Student t curve*, is usually more appropriate.

These same two techniques — hypothesis tests and confidence intervals — can also be applied to *binomial data* (Section 4.5). These are measurements recorded on a nominal scale that has only two possible outcomes ("yes" or "no", "lived" or "died", "normal" or "abnormal", etc.). Data of this sort are very common in medical research.

The last section in this chapter looks at the structure of hypothesis testing from a more theoretical perspective. Among the topics covered are the computation of Type II error probabilities and the interpretation of *operating characteristic curves*.

4.2
LARGE SAMPLE HYPOTHESIS TESTS FOR μ

In Section 3.6, the sampling distribution of $\bar{X}$ was defined to be the hypothetical collection of $\bar{X}$ values that would result from selecting all possible sets of n measurements from some given population distribution. For the present, it will be helpful to think of the sampling distribution of $\bar{X}$ as a histogram (whose total area is 1).

Comment

If the variable X can take on many different values and if n is fairly large, the sampling distribution of $\bar{X}$ can be thought of as a continuous curve, as in Figure 4.1(a) rather than a histogram as in Figure 4.1(b).

However, to emphasize the distinction between the exact sampling distribution and the mathematical model that will be used to approximate it, we will almost always picture the former as a histogram and the latter as a smooth curve.

There is a very important relationship between the sampling distribution of $\bar{X}$ and the normal curve. The nature of that relationship is the subject of the *Central Limit Theorem*, which is one of the most far-reaching results in all of mathematics. Without it, the principles of hypothesis testing — and statistical inference, in general — would be extremely difficult to put into practice.

[4.2]   Large Sample Hypothesis Tests For μ 127

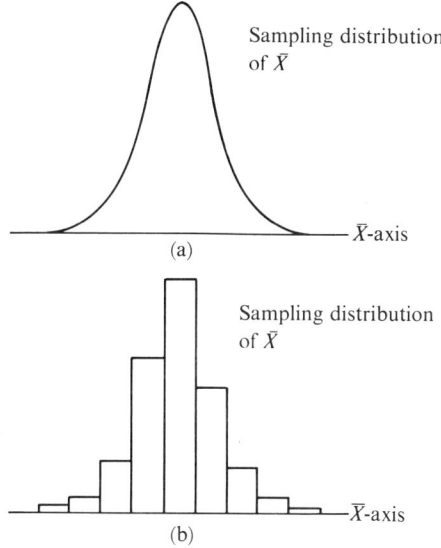

FIGURE 4.1

Central Limit Theorem. Suppose a variable X has a probability distribution with mean μ and standard deviation σ. Imagine random samples of size n being drawn and their means computed. Regardless of the shape of the probability distribution of X, the sampling distribution of $\bar{X}$ will be approximated by a normal curve having mean equal to μ and standard deviation equal to $\sigma/\sqrt{n}$.

Comment

For a given probability distribution, the larger the sample size, the better the approximation; in many cases, though, sample sizes as small as four or five will give values for $\bar{X}$ that are very nearly "normal."

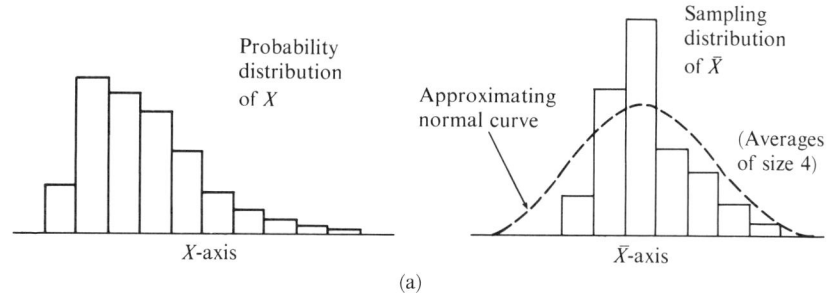

FIGURE 4.2

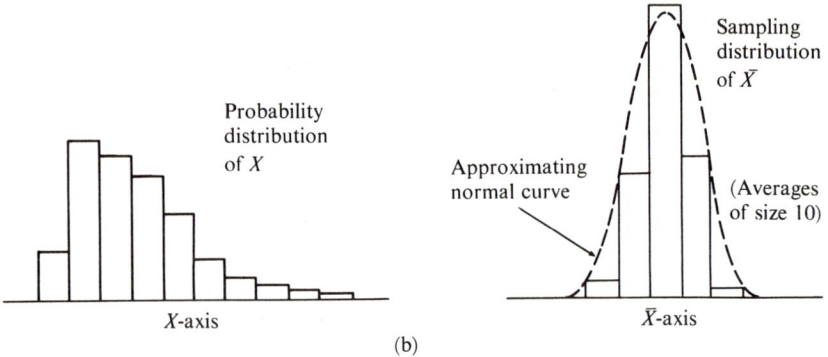

(b)

FIGURE 4.2 Continued

Comment

As n increases, $\sigma/\sqrt{n}$ decreases so the sampling distribution of $\bar{X}$ becomes more and more concentrated around μ.

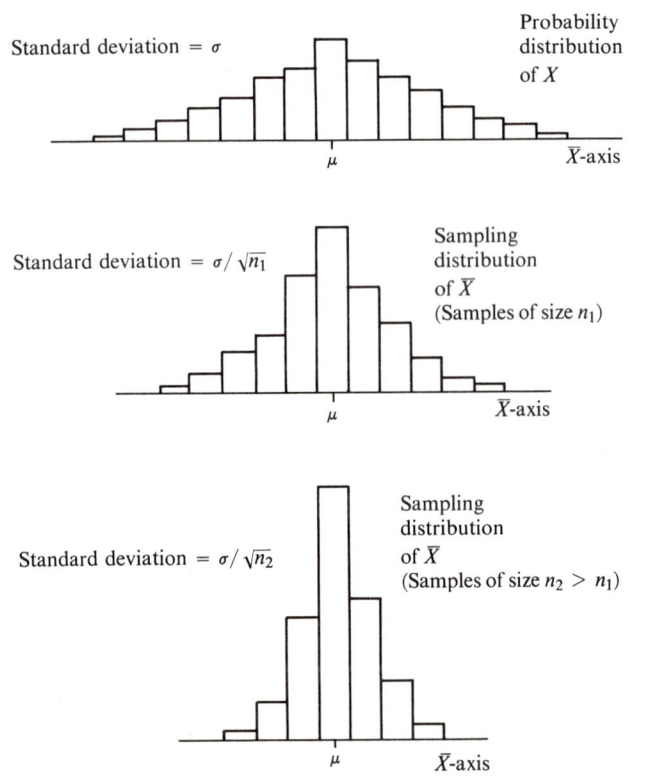

FIGURE 4.3

Comment

If σ is unknown but $n > 30$, then s, the sample standard deviation, is likely to be numerically close to σ and the sampling distribution of $\bar{X}$ will be approximated by a normal curve with mean μ and standard deviation $s/\sqrt{n}$.

The next example shows how the Central Limit Theorem is used to approximate areas under the sampling distribution of $\bar{X}$. Notice the difference between finding areas under an $\bar{X}$ distribution and areas under an X distribution (recall Theorem 3.9.1).

EXAMPLE 4.2.1. Fingerprints

There are many features of a fingerprint that can be measured. One that is particularly useful for identification purposes is the *ridge count*. This is determined by counting, for each finger, the number of ridges separating the triradius and the point of core. Then the sum of these numbers for the ten fingers is computed. That sum is defined to be a person's "ridge count" (Carter, 1970). For males, the ridge count has a distribution that is more or less bell-shaped with an average (μ) of 145 and a standard deviation (σ) of about 55.

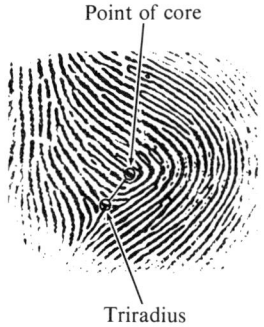

FIGURE 4.4

Suppose the ridge counts $x_1, x_2, \ldots, x_9$ for nine males selected at random were recorded and the corresponding sample average, $\bar{x}$, computed. According

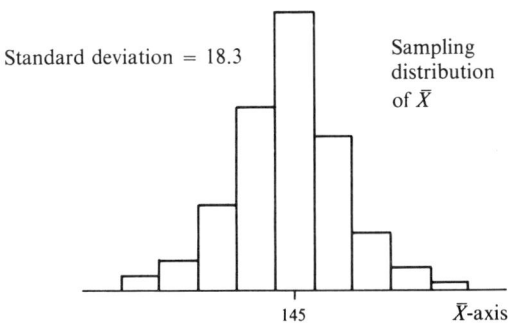

FIGURE 4.5

to the Central Limit Theorem, the sampling distribution that would describe the behavior of $\bar{X}$ would be similar in shape to a normal curve; it would have a mean equal to 145 and a standard deviation equal to $55/\sqrt{9} = 18.3$.

Areas under the $\bar{X}$ distribution can be approximated with a method similar to that used in Section 3.9. For example, suppose we wanted to find the area to the left of 140. Since the distribution of

$$\frac{\bar{X} - \mu}{\frac{\sigma}{\sqrt{n}}} = \frac{\bar{X} - 145}{18.3}$$

will be approximated by a standard normal curve,

$$P\{\bar{X} < 140\} = P\left\{\frac{\bar{X} - 145}{18.3} < \frac{140 - 145}{18.3}\right\}$$
$$\approx P\{Z < -0.27\}$$
$$= 0.3936$$

That is, the shaded area under the original histogram shown in Figure 4.7 is similar to the shaded area under the approximating normal curve in Figure 4.8, which, in turn, is equal to a corresponding area under a standard normal curve (Figure 4.9).

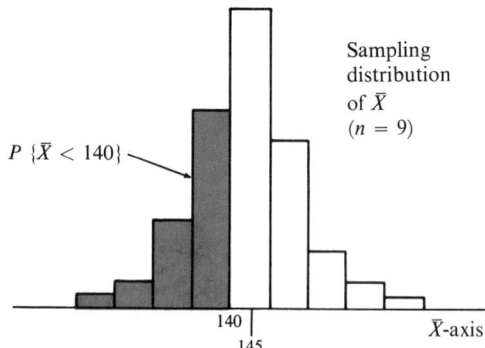

FIGURE 4.6

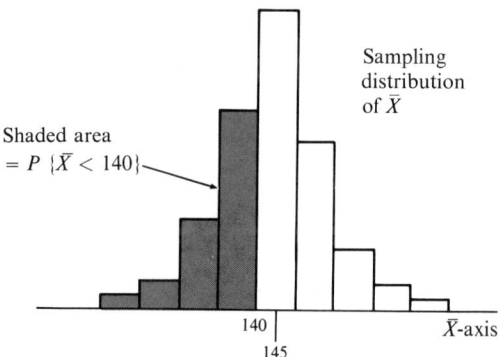

FIGURE 4.7

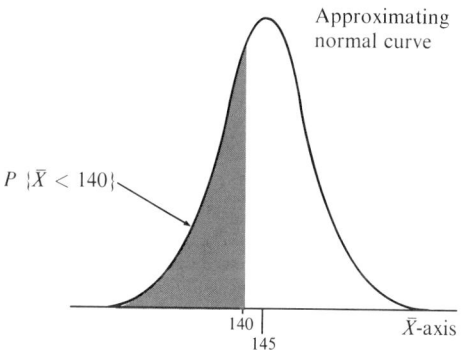

FIGURE 4.8

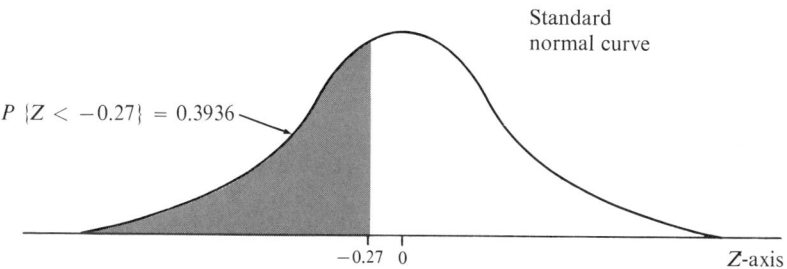

FIGURE 4.9

Note that if samples of size 25, rather than 9, had been considered, the distribution of $\bar{X}$ would still have a mean of 145, but the standard deviation would be reduced to $55/\sqrt{25} = 11.0$. More of the distribution would then be concentrated around the mean and the probability of the average count being less than, say, 140 would be smaller. Specifically,

$$P\{\bar{X} < 140\} = \left\{\frac{\bar{X} - 145}{11.0} < \frac{140 - 145}{11.0}\right\}$$
$$\approx P\{Z < -0.45\}$$
$$= 0.3264$$

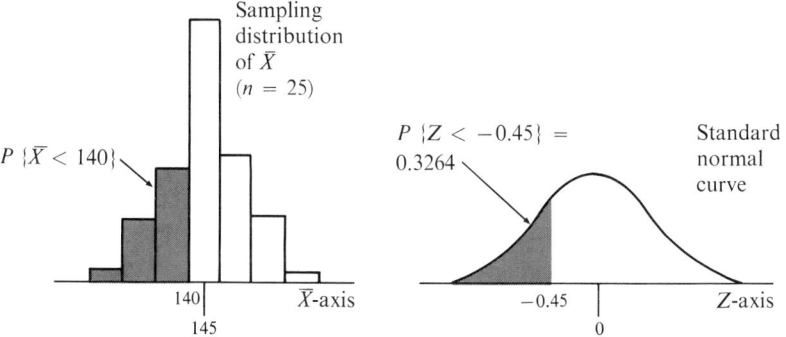

FIGURE 4.10

Comment

To avoid confusing the parameters of an X distribution with those of an $\bar{X}$ distribution, we need to introduce a second set of symbols. As analogs of μ and σ, the mean and standard deviation of the sampling distribution of $\bar{X}$ will be denoted by $\mu_{\bar{X}}$ and $\sigma_{\bar{X}}$. It follows, then, from the Central Limit Theorem that for samples of size n,

$$\mu_{\bar{X}} = \mu \quad \text{and} \quad \sigma_{\bar{X}} = \frac{\sigma}{\sqrt{n}}$$

This latter expression is often called the *standard error of the mean*, and written S.E.M. In words, the standard error of the mean is the standard deviation of the sampling distribution of $\bar{X}$.

Comment

The symbol $s_{\bar{X}}$ will be used to denote the sample estimate of $\sigma_{\bar{X}}$. Since s estimates σ, $s_{\bar{X}} = s/\sqrt{n}$.

Question 4.2.1. The standard deviation of the $\bar{X}$ distribution decreases as n increases. What does this imply about the effect the sample size has when $\bar{x}$ is used to estimate the unknown value of the population mean?

The next three examples show how the properties of the sampling distribution of $\bar{X}$ are applied to the problem of hypothesis testing (when $n > 30$).

EXAMPLE 4.2.2. Educating the Deaf

At the New York School for the Deaf a study was done to determine the effect, if any, of psychological adjustment on achievement (Getz, 1953). The performances in vocational training classes of 35 "maladjusted" students were carefully monitored and evaluated. Teachers rated each student on the basis of conduct, attitude, and general skill; the highest possible score was 10.

Performance scores						
4.7	5.0	8.0	3.5	5.0	4.3	7.0
5.6	8.1	8.0	10.0	4.0	7.8	6.0
6.8	2.0	5.9	7.3	5.8	4.7	6.1
3.9	8.0	5.0	8.0	8.0	6.4	7.0
6.8	4.4	7.0	5.5	6.4	5.0	4.2

(For these data, $\bar{x} = 6.0$ and $s = 1.7$.)

Suppose it is known from past experience with large numbers of "adjusted" students that *their* average score on a similar rating scale is 6.8. Since the sample mean (6.0) for these particular maladjusted students is less than the "established" mean for adjusted students, can we conclude that maladjusted students, *on the average*, perform less capably than adjusted students?

Let μ denote the (population) mean of the vocational training grades that would be achieved, under similar circumstances, by *all* maladjusted students — past, present, and future. Put in the language of hypothesis testing, the question posed above reduces to choosing between the null hypothesis H: $\mu = 6.8$ (the maladjusted students *do* perform as well as the adjusted students) and the one-sided alternative A: $\mu < 6.8$ (the maladjusted students *don't* perform as well as the adjusted students).

Comment

As explained here, this problem belongs to Model Two and not Model Three because all the sample observations have come from *one* population, the maladjusted group. What has been assumed about the adjusted student population — namely, the fact that its mean score is 6.8 — is information presumably accumulated *prior* to this particular study.

The decision to believe either H or A is based on what the sampling distribution of $\bar{X}$ would be like if H were, in fact, true. More precisely, if H were true, then $\mu = 6.8$ and σ would be approximately 1.7 (since $\sigma \approx s$ when $n > 30$), and the $\bar{X}$ distribution would be closely approximated by a normal curve with a mean of 6.8 ($= \mu_{\bar{x}}$) and a standard deviation of $1.7/\sqrt{35} = 0.29$ ($= s_{\bar{x}}$). Since the interval $\mu_{\bar{x}} - 2s_{\bar{x}}$ to $\mu_{\bar{x}} + 2s_{\bar{x}}$ (or, 6.2 to 7.4) corresponds to approximately 95% of the area under the $\bar{X}$ distribution (see Question 3.9.2), it follows that the observed sample mean of 6.0 is well out in the left-hand tail.

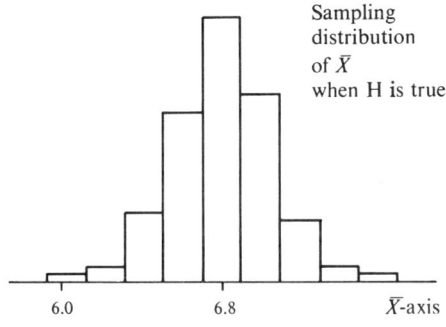

FIGURE 4.11

It seems clear that a sample mean this small would have to be considered a rather extraordinary event if we held to the null hypothesis that $\mu = 6.8$. In fact, the area under the sampling distribution to the left of 6.0 is:

$$P\{\bar{X} \leq 6.0\} = P\left\{\frac{\bar{X} - 6.8}{0.29} \leq \frac{6.0 - 6.8}{0.29}\right\}$$
$$\approx P\{Z \leq -2.76\}$$
$$= 0.0029$$

In other words, less than 0.3% of the time would a sample mean this small, or smaller, be observed if, in fact, H were true. While this does not totally refute the null hypothesis, it diminishes its credibility to the extent that the only "reasonable" decision is to reject H and accept A.

As another example of these calculations, suppose the sample mean had equaled 6.6. Then what would our decision have been? Note that the area to the left of 6.6 is

$$P\{\bar{X} \leq 6.6\} = P\left\{\frac{\bar{X} - 6.8}{0.29} \leq \frac{6.6 - 6.8}{0.29}\right\}$$
$$\approx P\{Z \leq -0.69\}$$
$$= 0.2451$$

meaning that almost one out of four sample averages will be less than 6.6 *by chance* even if $\mu = 6.8$. As a standard procedure, the null hypothesis will be accepted unless, as in the previous calculation, the data establish, *beyond a reasonable doubt*, that H is false. Therefore, in this second case, H would be accepted; knowing that, if H were true, 25% of all sample means would be even further away from the null hypothesis value for μ (6.8) than what was actually observed ($\bar{x} = 6.6$), we could hardly claim that the evidence is overwhelming that H is false.

For both these examples ($\bar{x} = 6.0$ and $\bar{x} = 6.6$), the appropriate decision was clearcut. But what if the observed sample mean was somewhere *between* 6.0 and 6.6? Would we reject H if $\bar{x}$ equaled 6.2? Or 6.5? Clearly, the point where one person's reasonable doubt ends and another's begins is not well-defined. What is obviously needed is a precisely stated, objective criterion that can tell us when to accept the null hypothesis and when to reject it. There are actually many criteria (or *decision rules*) that would meet these requirements. The following one, though, has come to be recognized as a standard in many areas of applied science.

> $P = .05$ **Decision Rule.** The null hypothesis, H, is rejected (that is, reasonable doubt is said to have been established) if, when H is assumed to be true, the probability of observing a sample mean as extreme or more extreme than what was actually found is less than .05.

Comment

If H is rejected by this decision rule, it is said to have been *rejected at the $P = .05$ level of significance*. Occasionally, 0.01 or 0.001 is substituted for 0.05. The choice of a "level of significance" will be discussed a little later.

Comment

The word "extreme" as it appears in the statement of the $P = .05$ Decision Rule needs some further explanation. If the hypotheses being tested were

H: $\mu = 6.8$ versus   A: $\mu < 6.8$

and if $\bar{x}$ equaled, say, 6.0, then another sample mean (say, $\bar{x}_1$) would be considered more extreme only if it was less than 6.0. But if the hypotheses were

$$H: \quad \mu = 6.8 \quad \text{versus} \quad A: \quad \mu > 6.8$$

and an $\bar{x}$ of 7.1 was observed, then any $\bar{x}_1$ greater than 7.1 would be termed more extreme. If the alternative was two-sided,

$$H: \quad \mu = 6.8 \quad \text{versus} \quad A: \quad \mu \neq 6.8$$

and the observed $\bar{x}$ was 6.4, then any $\bar{x}_1$ whose distance from 6.8 was greater than the distance of 6.4 from 6.8 — namely, 0.4 — would be considered more extreme. This would include any $\bar{x}_1$ *less than* 6.4 or *greater than* 7.2.

In general, the observed sample mean, together with the *form* of the alternative hypothesis, determines what range of $\bar{x}$ values is to be considered "more extreme."

Referring again to Example 4.2.2, note that the $P = .05$ Decision Rule does not tell us explicitly those particular values of the sample mean for which H is to be rejected, but it does indicate how they can be found. Recall the sampling distribution of $\bar{X}$ when H is true.

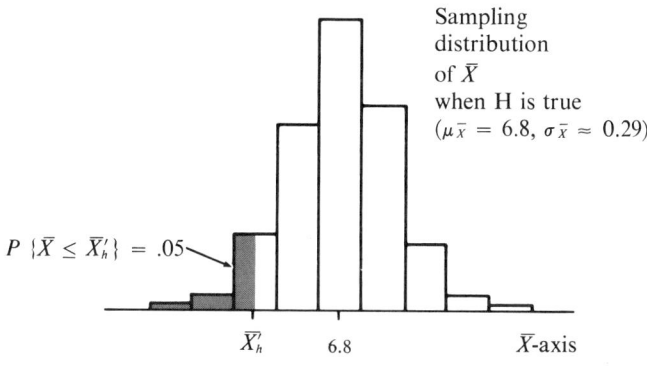

FIGURE 4.12

Somewhere along the $\bar{X}$-axis there is a point, call it $\bar{X}'_h$, having the property that the area under the histogram to its left is 0.05. Therefore, according to the $P = .05$ Decision Rule, H should be rejected if the observed sample mean is numerically equal to or less than $\bar{X}'_h$.

In general, $\bar{X}'_h$ is difficult to evaluate numerically, but a good "substitute" is the point $\bar{X}'$ that "cuts off" an area of 0.05 in the left-hand tail of the approximating normal curve.

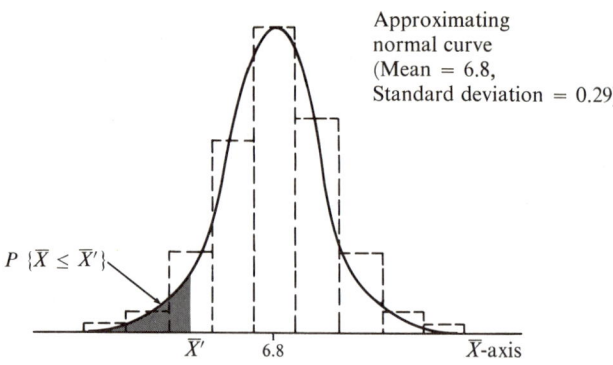

FIGURE 4.13

To find $\bar{X}'$, we use the table in Appendix I — but we use it backwards! Whatever is the value of $\bar{X}'$, it must satisfy the equation

$$P\{\bar{X} \leq \bar{X}'\} = .05$$

Since the mean and standard deviation of the $\bar{X}$ distribution (when H is true) are 6.8 and $1.7/\sqrt{35} = 0.29$, respectively,

$$P\{\bar{X} \leq \bar{X}'\} = P\left\{\frac{\bar{X} - 6.8}{0.29} \leq \frac{\bar{X}' - 6.8}{0.29}\right\}$$

$$\approx P\left\{Z \leq \frac{\bar{X}' - 6.8}{0.29}\right\} = .05$$

Also, recall from previous discussions of the standard normal curve (and Appendix I) that

$$P\{Z \leq -1.64\} = .05$$

But clearly, the similarity of these last two expressions,

$$P\left\{Z \leq \frac{\bar{X}' - 6.8}{0.29}\right\} = .05$$

and

$$P\{Z \leq -1.64\} = .05$$

implies that

$$-1.64 = \frac{\bar{X}' - 6.8}{0.29}$$

Solving for $\bar{X}'$ gives

$$\bar{X}' = 6.8 - 1.64(0.29)$$
$$= 6.3$$

Comment

This is not the first time that Appendix I has been used in this way. Question 3.9.4 and Review Exercises 3.4, 3.5, and 3.12 all required a similar sequence of steps.

The decision rule is now complete. If the average score of the maladjusted students is less than or equal to 6.3, we reject H: $\mu = 6.8$ and accept A: $\mu < 6.8$. But if $\bar{x} > 6.3$, H is accepted. For the data given, $\bar{x}$ was 6.0; so we reject H and conclude that deaf students who are *not* well-adjusted tend to perform, on the average, less capably in vocational training classes than students who *are* well-adjusted.

Comment

Usually, no distinction will be made between $\bar{X}'_h$ and $\bar{X}'$. So long as n is reasonably large and the distribution of X is more or less bell-shaped, the values of $\bar{X}'_h$ and $\bar{X}'$ will be numerically equal, for all practical purposes.

The example just presented was intended to be both an explanation of the principles of hypothesis testing and an exercise in their application. As such, it was longer and more involved than a typical hypothesis test needs to be. In practice, a large-sample, one-sided test at, say, the $P = .05$ level of significance would be done more concisely, step-by-step:

(1) From the experimental situation, determine H and A. If μ_o denotes the "status quo" or "untreated" value for the location parameter, then there are two possible one-sided hypothesis tests:

$$\text{H:} \quad \mu = \mu_o \quad \text{versus} \quad \text{A:} \quad \mu < \mu_o$$

or

$$\text{H:} \quad \mu = \mu_o \quad \text{versus} \quad \text{A:} \quad \mu > \mu_o$$

(2) Compute $\bar{x}$ and s.

(3) Sketch a diagram of the sampling distribution of $\bar{X}$ when H is true. Remember that $\mu_{\bar{x}} = \mu_o$ and $\sigma_{\bar{x}} \simeq s/\sqrt{n}$.

(4) Indicate on the diagram the location of the critical value $\bar{X}'$. If the alternative hypothesis is A: $\mu < \mu_o$, then H will be rejected if the sample mean $\bar{x}$ is much *less* than μ_o. In particular, H is rejected if $\bar{x} \leq \bar{X}'$, where $\bar{X}' = \mu_o - 1.64(s/\sqrt{n})$.

If the alternative hypothesis is A: $\mu > \mu_o$, then H will be rejected if the sample mean is much greater than μ_o. Here the critical value is in the right-hand tail and H is rejected if $\bar{x} \geq \bar{X}'$, where $\bar{X}' = \mu_o + 1.64(s/\sqrt{n})$.

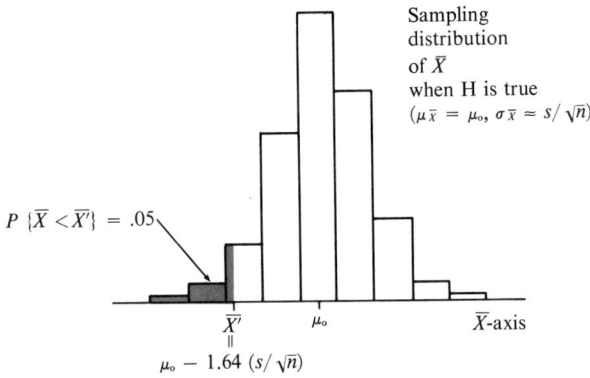

FIGURE 4.14

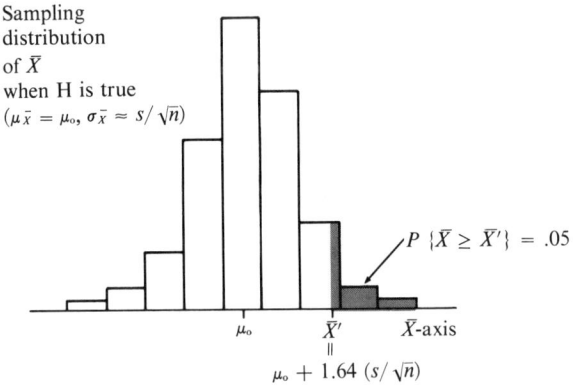

FIGURE 4.15

Comment

The expressions for these "critical" values ($\bar{X}'$) are easily derived. Consider the case where H: $\mu = \mu_o$ is being tested against A: $\mu > \mu_o$. By the nature of

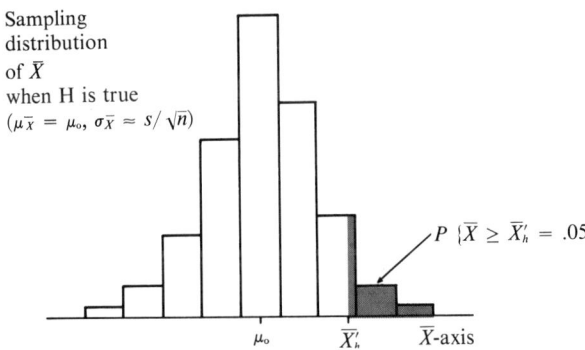

FIGURE 4.16

the $P = .05$ Decision Rule, it follows that the point $\bar{X}'$, which approximates $\bar{X}'_h$, is a number exceeded by chance only 5% of the time. Furthermore, the tail area under the $\bar{X}$ histogram to the right of $\bar{X}'_h$ can be approximated by the corresponding tail area to the right of $\bar{X}'$ under the normal curve with mean μ_o and standard deviation $s/\sqrt{n}$.

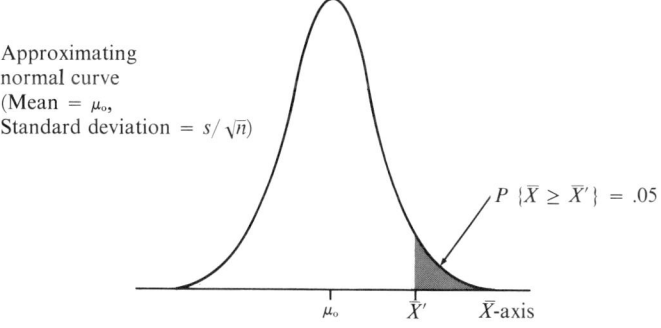

FIGURE 4.17

To determine $\bar{X}'$, we reduce the problem to one involving the standard normal curve. From Appendix I it can be verified that the area to the right of $Z = 1.64$ is 0.05. In terms of standard deviations, the distance from μ_o to $\bar{X}'$ must be the same as the distance from 0 to 1.64. And since the standard deviation of the standard normal curve is 1, it follows that $\bar{X}'$ must be 1.64 standard deviations (of $\bar{X}$) to the right of μ_o. However, the standard deviation of the $\bar{X}$ distribution is $s/\sqrt{n}$, so

$$\bar{X}' = \mu_o + 1.64\left(\frac{s}{\sqrt{n}}\right)$$

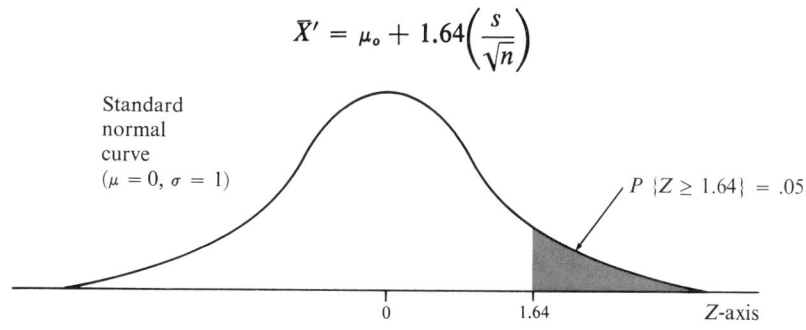

FIGURE 4.18

Comment

Note that from Appendix I the area under the standard normal curve to the right of 2.33 is approximately 0.01, as shown in Figure 4.19. Therefore, when testing H: $\mu = \mu_o$ against A: $\mu > \mu_o$ at the $P = .01$ level of significance, the critical value $\bar{X}'$ has the form

$$\bar{X}' = \mu_o + 2.33\left(\frac{s}{\sqrt{n}}\right)$$

140   Model Two — The One-Sample Problem   [4.2]

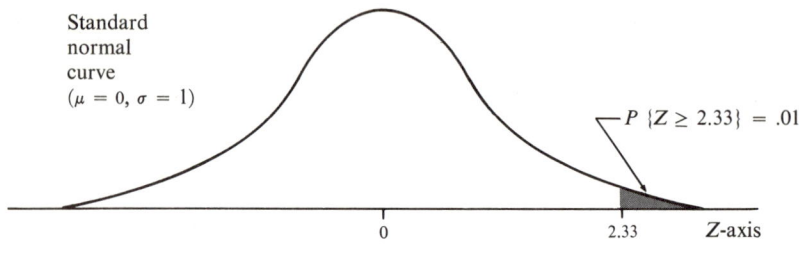

FIGURE 4.19

Question 4.2.2. What would $\bar{X}'$ equal if H: $\mu = \mu_0$ was being tested against A: $\mu > \mu_0$ at the $P = .10$ level of significance? At the $P = .025$ level of significance?

Question 4.2.3. If the null hypothesis in a given problem is rejected in favor of a one-sided alternative at the $P = .05$ level of significance, will it necessarily be rejected at the $P = .01$ level of significance?

Question 4.2.4. If H is rejected at $P = .01$, will it necessarily be rejected at $P = .05$? (Assume the alternative is one-sided.)

EXAMPLE 4.2.3. Synovial Fluid and pH

Synovial fluid is the clear, viscid secretion that lubricates joints and tendons. For some conditions, its hydrogen ion concentration (pH) has diagnostic significance. In healthy adults, the average pH for synovial fluid is 7.39. Listed below are synovial pH's measured for fluids drawn from the knees of 44 patients with various arthritic conditions (Treuhaft and McCarty, 1971).

7.02	7.26	7.31	7.14	7.45	7.32	7.21	7.36	7.36
7.35	7.25	7.24	7.20	7.39	7.40	7.33	7.09	6.60
7.32	7.35	7.34	7.41	7.28	6.99	7.28	7.32	7.29
7.33	7.38	7.32	7.77	7.34	7.10	7.35	6.95	7.31
7.15	7.20	7.34	7.12	7.22	7.30	7.24	7.35	

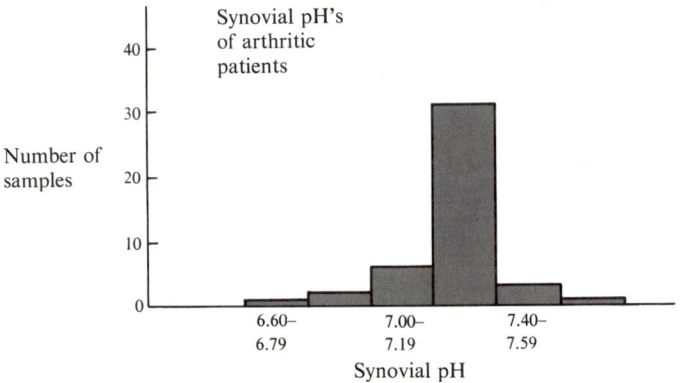

FIGURE 4.20

Can we conclude from these data that persons with similar conditions will have, on the average, a synovial pH lower than the 7.39 "norm"?

Let μ denote the true average synovial pH of persons with arthritis.

(1) The two hypotheses in question are

$$H: \quad \mu = 7.39 \quad \text{(No change in pH)}$$

versus

$$A: \quad \mu < 7.39 \quad \text{(Arthritis is accompanied by a lowered pH)}$$

(2) For these 44 observations,

$$\sum_{i=1}^{44} x_i = 319.63 \quad \text{and} \quad \sum_{i=1}^{44} x_i^2 = 2323.1419$$

so that

$$\bar{x} = \frac{319.63}{44} = 7.26$$

and

$$s = \sqrt{\frac{44(2323.1419) - (319.63)^2}{44(43)}}$$
$$= \sqrt{0.0290} = 0.17$$

(3) The sampling distribution of $\bar{X}$, if H is true, has

$$\mu_{\bar{X}} = 7.39 \quad \text{and} \quad \sigma_{\bar{X}} \approx \frac{0.17}{\sqrt{44}} = 0.026$$

(4) Also, for $P_\bullet = .05$,

$$\bar{X}' = \mu_o - 1.64\left(\frac{s}{\sqrt{n}}\right)$$
$$= 7.39 - 1.64\left(\frac{0.17}{\sqrt{44}}\right)$$
$$= 7.35$$

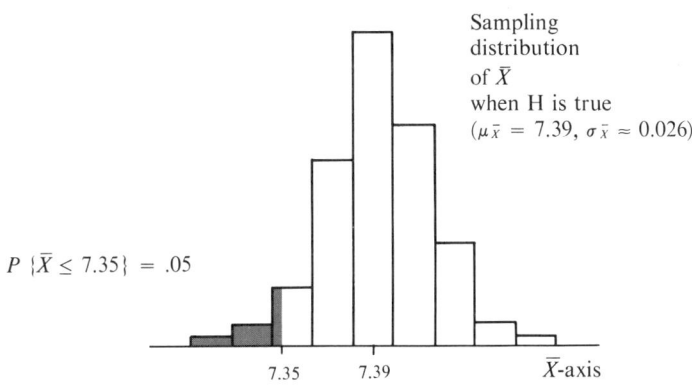

FIGURE 4.21

Therefore, H should be rejected at the $P = .05$ level of significance if the sample mean is less than or equal to 7.35. But $\bar{x}$ was 7.26, so H is rejected.

Question 4.2.5. Using these same data, test H: $\mu = 7.39$ against A: $\mu < 7.39$ at the $P = .01$ level of significance.

Two-sided hypothesis tests are carried out similarly except that "extreme" sample means on *either* side of μ_o will cause H to be rejected. The immediate consequence is that each two-sided hypothesis test has *two* critical values, one in each tail of the $\bar{X}$ distribution; and the combined tail areas cut off by these critical values must total the specified level of significance.

For example, suppose

$$\text{H:} \quad \mu = 100 \quad \text{versus} \quad \text{A:} \quad \mu \neq 100$$

is to be tested at the $P = .05$ level of significance. And suppose a sample of size 64 is drawn for which $\bar{x} = 108.3$ and $s = 40.2$. Let $\bar{X}'_1$ and $\bar{X}'_2$ denote the left-tail and right-tail critical values, respectively. Then

$$P\{\bar{X} \leq \bar{X}'_1\} + P\{\bar{X} > \bar{X}'_2\} = .05$$

when H is true. By convention, these two probabilities are set equal:

$$P\{\bar{X} \leq \bar{X}'_1\} = .025 \quad \text{and} \quad P\{\bar{X} \geq \bar{X}'_2\} = .025$$

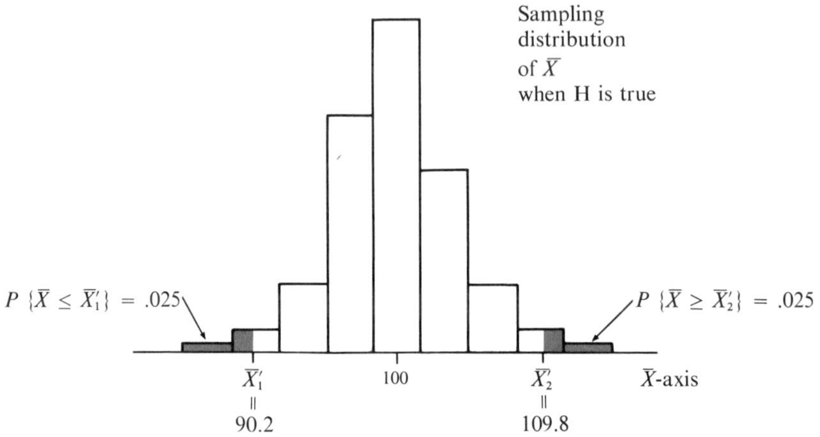

FIGURE 4.22

For the standard normal curve,

$$P\{Z \leq -1.96\} = .025 = P\{Z \geq 1.96\}$$

meaning that X'_1 and X'_2 are 1.96 standard deviations away from the value of μ stated in the null hypothesis. Therefore,

$$X'_1 = \mu_o - 1.96\left(\frac{s}{\sqrt{n}}\right)$$
$$= 100 - 1.96\left(\frac{40.2}{\sqrt{64}}\right)$$
$$= 90.2$$

and

$$X'_2 = \mu_o + 1.96\left(\frac{s}{\sqrt{n}}\right)$$
$$= 100 + 1.96\left(\frac{40.2}{\sqrt{64}}\right)$$
$$= 109.8$$

In this case, then, the $P = .05$ Decision Rule calls for H to be rejected if $\bar{x}$ is either *less than or equal to 90.2* or *greater than or equal to 109.8*. Since $\bar{x}$ was 108.3, H is accepted.

Comment

For two-sided (large-sample) hypothesis tests at the $P = .01$ level of significance,

$$X'_1 = \mu_o - 2.58\left(\frac{s}{\sqrt{n}}\right) \quad \text{and} \quad X'_2 = \mu_o + 2.58\left(\frac{s}{\sqrt{n}}\right)$$

since $P\{Z \leq -2.58\} + P\{Z \geq 2.58\} = .01$

Comment

The step-by-step procedure outlined earlier for doing one-sided hypothesis tests should also be followed in the case of two-sided tests. The major difference is the presence of two critical values rather than one. Listed below are the multiples of $s/\sqrt{n}$ used for computing critical values in large-sample, one- and two-sided tests at the $P = .05$ and $P = .01$ levels of significance.

Multiples of $s/\sqrt{n}$

	One-sided test	Two-sided test
$P = .05$	1.64	± 1.96
$P = .01$	2.33	± 2.58

The stated objective of this section was to develop a hypothesis test for μ when n, the sample size, was greater than 30. As we have just seen, the solution to such problems rests on the fact that a standard normal curve is a good approximation to the distribution of $(\bar{X} - \mu_o)/(s/\sqrt{n})$. But when n is less than or equal to 30, the distribution of $(\bar{X} - \mu_o)/(s/\sqrt{n})$ is better described by another curve, introduced in the next section. However, there is one exception to this general pattern. Sometimes, although very infrequently, the numerical value of σ is known for a given situation. When this is the case, the distribution $(\bar{X} - \mu_o)/(\sigma/\sqrt{n})$, regardless of the size of n, is approximated very well by a standard normal curve (provided the X distribution is more or less bell-shaped), and the methods of this section are quite appropriate.

EXAMPLE 4.2.4. Platelet Counts in the Elderly

Platelet counts for 24 elderly women were the subject of Example 3.3.2. The question was raised as to whether any differences could be discerned between *these* counts and what might be expected from the "normal" population. Let's suppose that experience has shown that the true mean and standard deviation of the distribution of platelet counts in the normal population are $250,000/mm^3$ and $75,000/mm^3$, respectively. Is the average platelet count for elderly women (μ) any different? (Let $P = .01$ be the level of significance).

(1) The hypotheses indicated are

$$H: \quad \mu = 250,000 \quad \text{versus} \quad A: \quad \mu \neq 250,000$$

(2) Since σ is known to be 75,000, there is no need to compute s. But

$$\bar{x} = \frac{1}{24}\sum_{i=1}^{24} x_i = \frac{4,645,000}{24}$$
$$= 193,000/mm^3$$

(3) The sampling distribution of $\bar{X}$, when H is true, will be approximated by a normal curve with $\mu_{\bar{x}} = 250,000$ and $\sigma_{\bar{x}} = \sigma/\sqrt{n} = 75,000/\sqrt{24} = 15,300$.

(4) Since

$$P\{Z \leq -2.58\} + \{Z \geq 2.58\} = .01$$

the two critical values are given by

$$X_1' = \mu_o - 2.58\left(\frac{\sigma}{\sqrt{n}}\right)$$
$$= 250,000 - 2.58(15,300)$$
$$= 210,500/mm^3$$

and

$$X_2' = \mu_o + 2.58\left(\frac{\sigma}{\sqrt{n}}\right)$$
$$= 250,000 + 2.58(15,300)$$
$$= 289,500/mm^3$$

Since the observed $\bar{x}$ ($= 193,500$) was less than X_1', we reject the null hypothesis, at the $P = .01$ level of significance.

[4.2] Large Sample Hypothesis Tests For μ 145

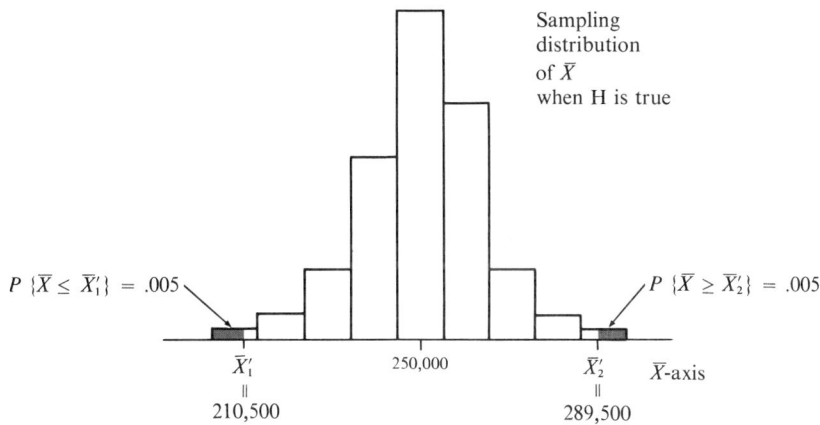

FIGURE 4.23

Question 4.2.6. Test H: $\mu = 250{,}000$ versus A: $\mu \neq 250{,}000$ at the $P = .001$ level of significance.

Question 4.2.7. The level of significance P that is used in any hypothesis testing problem is more or less arbitrary, although the most common choice, by far, is .05 — with .10, .01, and .001 being about the only other levels ever used. In what sort of situation might an experimenter choose P to be relatively large — say, .10?

Comment

There are actually several different, but equivalent, ways to do the same hypothesis test. The approach taken in this chapter and throughout this text, is to phrase the decision rule in terms of the values of the statistic (in this case, $\bar{x}$), that lead to the rejection of the null hypothesis. For example, in testing H: $\mu = \mu_o$ versus A: $\mu < \mu_o$ at the $P = .05$ level of significance, we would reject H is $\bar{x}$ is less than or equal to $\bar{X}' = \mu_o - 1.64(\sigma/\sqrt{n})$.

But the decision rule can also be expressed in terms of standardized Z values. Recall that for a given $\bar{x}$, the corresponding "Z-score" is

$$z = \frac{\bar{x} - \mu_o}{\frac{\sigma}{\sqrt{n}}}$$

Clearly, the same set of $\bar{x}$'s for which

$$\bar{x} \leq \mu_o - 1.64\left(\frac{\sigma}{\sqrt{n}}\right) = \bar{X}'$$

will also satisfy the inequality

$$\frac{\bar{x} - \mu_o}{\frac{\sigma}{\sqrt{n}}} \leq -1.64 = Z'$$

Therefore, the $P = .05$ Decision Rule for this particular one-sided alternative can also be written:

$$\text{Reject H if} \quad \frac{\bar{X} - \mu_0}{\frac{\sigma}{\sqrt{n}}} \leq -1.64$$

4.3
SMALL SAMPLE HYPOTHESIS TESTS FOR μ

If random samples of size n are drawn from a distribution whose mean is μ and whose standard deviation is σ, the Central Limit Theorem states that the distribution of $(\bar{X} - \mu)/(\sigma/\sqrt{n})$ will be closely approximated by a standard normal curve. The same is *not* always true of $(\bar{X} - \mu)/(s/\sqrt{n})$. *Its* sampling distribution is better described by another mathematical model, the *Student t curve*.

Comment

Actually, there is a *family* of Student t curves, one for every sample size. But as n increases, they all become more and more similar to the standard normal. In fact, for sample sizes over 30, the two mathematical models are so much alike that

$$\frac{\bar{X} - \mu}{\frac{s}{\sqrt{n}}}$$

is treated just as though it were a "Z-variable".

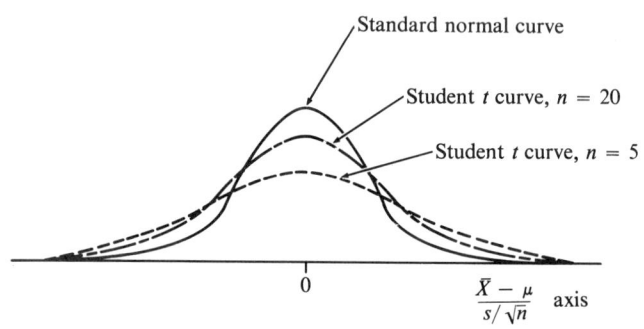

FIGURE 4.24

When n is less than or equal to 30, the particular t distribution that best describes the behavior of $(\bar{X} - \mu)/(s/\sqrt{n})$ is said to have $n - 1$ *degrees of freedom*. Just as μ and σ are parameters for the normal curve, "degrees of freedom" (abbreviated *df*) is a parameter of the Student t curve.

Finding areas under Student t curves is similar, in certain respects, to finding areas under standard normal curves. For example, all Student t curves are symmetric around 0. That means that if, say, 15% of the area under a particular curve lies *to the right* of some number t, then 15% of the area also lies *to the left* of $-t$.

Numerical values of points such as t that cut off tail areas of a given size are listed in Appendix II. Although the t-values being sought here are analogous to the Z-values of the previous section, the table in Appendix II is set up differently than the one in Appendix I. Each row in Appendix II corresponds to a Student t curve with a particular number of degrees of freedom, ranging from 1 to 29 (entries in the "30+" row are taken from the standard normal curve). For example, the numbers in the "16 df" row are 0.54, 0.86, ..., 2.92. These are the values on the horizontal axis that cut off, *to their left*, the areas shown at the top of each column: that is, the area under the curve to the left of $t = 0.54$ is 0.70; to the left of $t = 0.86$, 0.80; and so on.

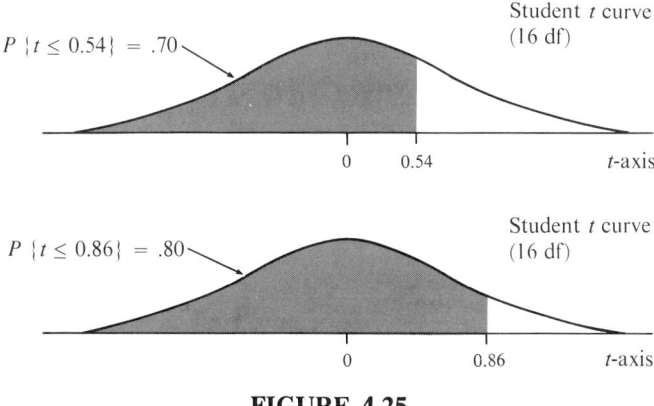

FIGURE 4.25

Of course, for hypothesis-testing applications, the most important of these numbers will be the ones in the extreme tail areas. For example, the number 1.75 cuts off to its left 95% of the area under a Student t curve having 16 degrees of freedom. This means that the area *to the right* of 1.75 (and *to the left* of -1.75) is .05. (Recall that the corresponding values for the standard normal curve were 1.64 and -1.64).

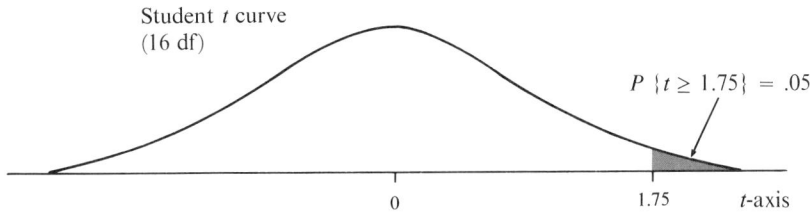

FIGURE 4.26

Comment

This example brings out the main difference between Student t curves and standard normal curves: the former are more "flattened" and have proportionately more area in their tails. For example, the area under a standard normal curve to the right of 1.64 is 0.05; but from Appendix II, the area to the right of 1.64 under a Student t curve with 16 degrees of freedom is between 0.05 and 0.10. The reason for this increased likelihood of extreme deviations is related to the fact that σ is being estimated by s. When σ is unknown and n is small, s will vary considerably from sample to sample. This results in the behavior of $(\bar{X} - \mu)/(s/\sqrt{n})$ being more variable than the behavior of $(\bar{X} - \mu)/(\sigma/\sqrt{n})$. Student t curves "account" for this additional variability by assigning greater probability to values of $(\bar{X} - \mu)/(s/\sqrt{n})$ much smaller or much larger than 0.

Comment

Note that the symbol being used for t curves is not consistent with our previous convention that random variables be designated by capital letters and particular values of random variables by small letters. In Figure 4.26, for example, the probability statement would have read $P\{T \geq 1.75\}$ instead of $P\{t \geq 1.75\}$ and the horizontal axis would have been labeled the T-axis rather than the t-axis. However, the use of a small t in this situation is so widespread that any attempts to do otherwise would only cause confusion. Hopefully, it will be clear from the context which meaning is intended.

It should be clear how the $\bar{X}'$ values are calculated when a Student t curve is used to approximate the distribution of $(\bar{X} - \mu)/(s/\sqrt{n})$. Suppose that in a one-sided test of

$$H: \quad \mu = 50 \quad \text{versus} \quad A: \quad \mu > 50$$

the sample size is 17 ($= 16\, df$), and the sample mean and sample standard deviation are 58.7 and 21.5, respectively. If .05 is chosen as the level of significance,

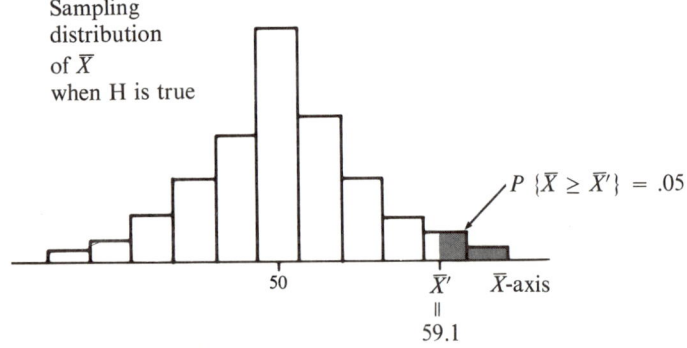

FIGURE 4.27

the critical value, $\bar{X}'$, will be 1.75, rather than 1.64, multiples of the standard deviation of $\bar{X}$ to the right of 50:

$$\bar{X}' = \mu_0 + 1.75\left(\frac{s}{\sqrt{n}}\right)$$

$$= 50 + 1.75\left(\frac{21.5}{\sqrt{17}}\right)$$

$$= 59.1$$

Since $\bar{x}$ was 58.7, we would *accept* H.

EXAMPLE 4.3.1. Air-Flow Rates

Recall the air-flow rates of the 19 workers involved in the manufacture of an enzyme detergent (Review Exercise 1.9).

Subject	FEV_1/VC	Subject	FEV_1/VC
RH	.61	WS	.78
RB	.70	RV	.84
MB	.63	EN	.83
DM	.76	WD	.82
WB	.67	FR	.74
RB	.72	PD	.85
BF	.64	EB	.73
JT	.82	PC	.85
PS	.88	RM	.87
RB	.82		

In the normal population it is known that the distribution of FEV_1/VC values has a mean of 0.80. But the *sample* mean for these 19 individuals is 0.77 (see step 2 below). That raises an obvious question: is the difference between 0.77 and 0.80 due simply to the sampling variability of X, or does it constitute substantial "proof" that the average air-flow rate for workers on this job will be reduced?

Let μ denote the true average air-flow rate in the population that is represented by these 19 individuals. Since σ is unknown and n is less than or equal to 30, the appropriate analysis for these data is a "t-test". As shown below, the steps involved are completely analogous to those used in Section 4.2. (Assume that $P = .01$ has been chosen to be the level of significance.)

(1) The hypotheses to be tested are

H: $\mu = 0.80$ versus A: $\mu < 0.80$

(2) Compute

$$\bar{x} = \frac{1}{19}\sum_{i=1}^{19} x_i = \frac{14.56}{19}$$

$$= 0.77$$

and

$$s = \sqrt{\frac{n(\sum x_i^2) - (\sum x_i)^2}{n(n-1)}}$$

$$= \sqrt{\frac{19(11.2904) - (14.56)^2}{19(18)}} = \sqrt{0.00738}$$

$$= 0.086$$

(3) Since $n = 19$, the appropriate multiple of $s/\sqrt{n}$ will come from a Student t curve with 18 df. From Appendix II,

$$P\{t \leq -2.55\} = .01$$

which makes

$$\bar{X}' = \mu_o - 2.55\left(\frac{s}{\sqrt{n}}\right)$$

$$= 0.80 - 2.55\left(\frac{.086}{\sqrt{19}}\right)$$

$$= 0.75$$

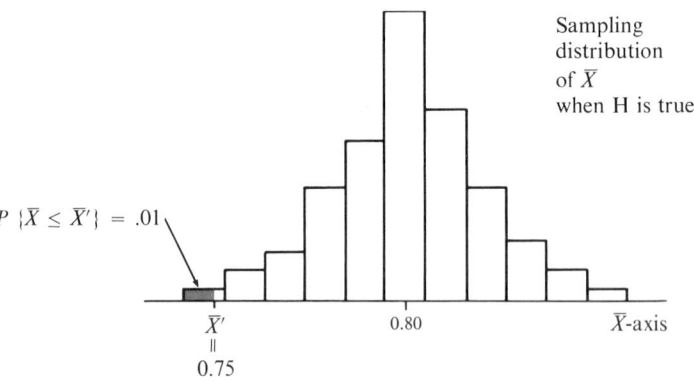

FIGURE 4.28

But the observed $\bar{x}$ was 0.77 so H is accepted, at the $P = .01$ level of significance.

Question 4.3.1. Why would a two-sided alternative not be used for these data?

Question 4.3.2. Suppose a similar study was done with 25 employees and it was found that $\bar{x} = 0.77$ and $s = 0.086$. Test H: $\mu = 0.80$ versus A: $\mu < 0.80$ at the $P = .05$ level of significance.

Question 4.3.3. Refer to the coordination study described in Example 3.7.2. Let μ denote the true average writing score that would be achieved by persons given this same amount of alcohol. Test H: $\mu = 0$ versus A: $\mu < 0$ at the $P = .05$ level of significance.

EXAMPLE 4.3.2. Noise-Induced Hearing Loss

One of the occupational hazards of being an airplane pilot is the hearing loss that results from being exposed to high noise levels. To better understand the magnitude of the problem, a team of researchers measured the cockpit noise levels of 18 aircraft (Kronoveter and Somerville, 1970). (The figures shown below are averages of the intensities recorded at frequencies of 500, 1000, and 2000 cycles per second.)

Plane	Cockpit noise level (Decibels)
1	74
2	77
3	80
4	82
5	82
6	85
7	80
8	75
9	75
10	72
11	90
12	87
13	73
14	83
15	86
16	83
17	83
18	80

One way to put these numbers in perspective is to compare them to some standard — for example, the lowest noise level that prohibits reliable voice communication. For pilots in a cockpit, approximately two feet apart, this "speech interference level" (SIL) is 76 decibels. Can we conclude from these data that the average cockpit noise in commercial aircraft exceeds the SIL?

Let μ be the true average cockpit noise of commercial aircraft (during cruising).

(1) The question just posed reduces to a test of

$$H: \quad \mu = 76 \quad \text{versus} \quad A: \quad \mu > 76$$

Let $P = .05$.

(2) The sum and the sum of the squares of the 18 observations are 1447 and 116,773, respectively, so

$$\bar{x} = \frac{1447}{18} = 80.4$$

and

$$s = \sqrt{\frac{18(116{,}773) - (1447)^2}{18(17)}} = \sqrt{26.49}$$
$$= 5.1$$

(3) Since $n = 18$, the multiple of $s/\sqrt{n}$ in the expression for $\bar{X}'$ will come from the Student t distribution with 17 degrees of freedom. More specifically,

$$P\{t \geq 1.74\} = .05$$

so

$$\bar{X}' = \mu_o + 1.74\left(\frac{s}{\sqrt{n}}\right)$$
$$= 76 + 1.74\left(\frac{5.1}{\sqrt{18}}\right)$$
$$= 78.1$$

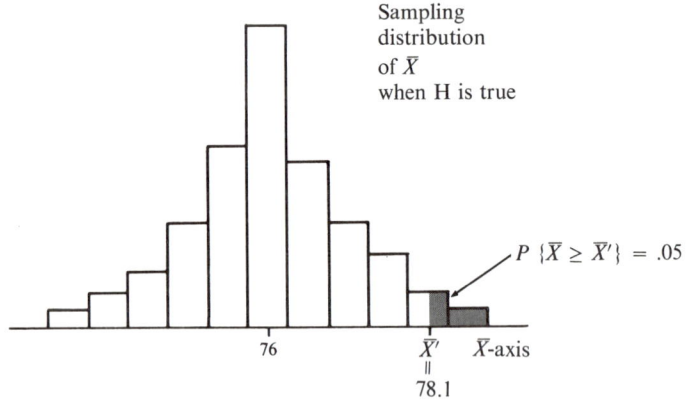

FIGURE 4.29

But the observed sample mean was 80.4, so H is rejected.

Comment

In published articles, space limitations prevent a statistical analysis from being presented in the detail that has been shown here. What is typically done is to give the observed sample mean, together with the computed t value. For example, the results of this particular study might appear as follows:

Cockpit noise level (Decibels)

80.4   ($t = 3.67$)

This means that $\bar{x}$ was 80.4 and

$$t = \frac{\bar{x} - \mu_o}{\frac{s}{\sqrt{n}}} = \frac{80.4 - 76}{\frac{5.1}{\sqrt{18}}} = 3.67$$

It is then left to the reader to "complete" the hypothesis test by deciding whether or not a t value of 3.67 is significant.

A better way to summarize an analysis, but one that is not used nearly as often as it should be, is to include information about (1) the variation in the data and (2) the sample size.

Cockpit noise level (Decibels)

$$80.4 \pm 1.20 \ (18) \qquad t = 3.67 \qquad P < .05$$

Statements of this sort mean that $\bar{x}$ was 80.4, the standard error of the mean $(s/\sqrt{n})$ was 1.20, the sample size was 18, the computed t statistic was 3.67, and the null hypothesis was rejected at the $P = .05$ level of significance.

Question 4.3.4. Suppose the 10 prothrombin times referred to in Example 2.6.4 were determined using a laboratory procedure that differed in certain respects from the standard procedure. And suppose that with the standard procedure it was known that, for normal blood, the average prothrombin time was 15 seconds. Can we conclude from these ten samples that the new procedure has a different average? Use a two-sided test and the .05 level of significance. (Refer to Sections 3.2 and 3.5 for the sample mean and the sample standard deviation.)

4.4 CONFIDENCE INTERVALS

Hypothesis tests for location make it possible to determine whether an observed sample mean, $\bar{x}$, is "compatible" with some *particular* value of μ (often the value associated with a standard). But for some experimental situations — for example, research done on new processes or under new conditions — there is *no* standard available. In cases like these, we construct a *confidence interval for* μ rather than do a hypothesis test.

Comment

Like hypothesis tests, the precise formulation of a confidence interval for μ depends on whether n is greater than 30 or less than or equal to 30. The development in this section focuses on the more typical situation — when $n \leq 30$. The modifications necessary for the case where $n > 30$ will be apparent.

To see how a confidence interval is formed, we need to appeal to the result that was used in the previous section — namely, if samples of size $n \ (\leq 30)$ are drawn from a bell-shaped distribution with unknown mean μ and unknown standard deviation σ, the behavior of $(\bar{X} - \mu)/(s/\sqrt{n})$ will be approximated by a Student t distribution with $n - 1$ degrees of freedom. This implies that two numbers, $-t$ and $+t$, can be found such that

$$P\left\{-t \leq \frac{\bar{X} - \mu}{\frac{s}{\sqrt{n}}} \leq t\right\} = .95$$

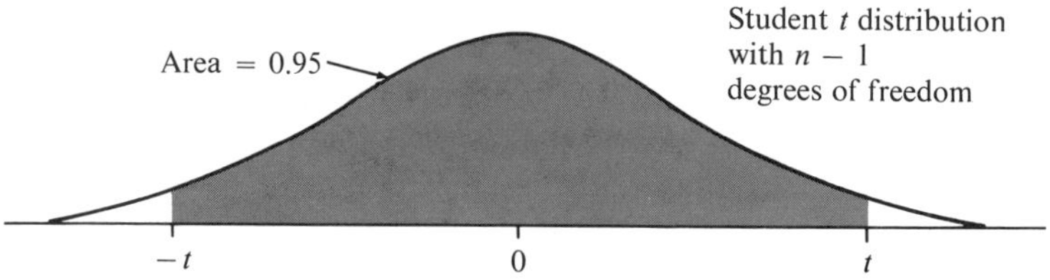

FIGURE 4.30

If n were 13, for example, the values satisfying this expression would be $-t = -2.18$ and $t = 2.18$ (see Appendix II).

Note that the inequalities inside the braces of the probability statement can be written in several different, but equivalent, ways:

$$-t \leq \frac{\bar{X} - \mu}{\frac{s}{\sqrt{n}}} \leq t$$

is the same as

$$-t\left(\frac{s}{\sqrt{n}}\right) \leq \bar{X} - \mu \leq t\left(\frac{s}{\sqrt{n}}\right)$$

or

$$-\bar{X} - t\left(\frac{s}{\sqrt{n}}\right) \leq -\mu \leq -\bar{X} + t\left(\frac{s}{\sqrt{n}}\right)$$

or

$$\bar{X} - t\left(\frac{s}{\sqrt{n}}\right) \leq \mu \leq \bar{X} + t\left(\frac{s}{\sqrt{n}}\right)$$

It must be true, then, that

$$P\left\{-t \leq \frac{\bar{X} - \mu}{\frac{s}{\sqrt{n}}} \leq t\right\} = .95 = P\left\{\bar{X} - t\left(\frac{s}{\sqrt{n}}\right) \leq \mu \leq \bar{X} + t\left(\frac{s}{\sqrt{n}}\right)\right\}$$

The right-hand expression can best be interpreted in a sampling context: if many samples of size n are drawn from the given probability distribution and if, for each one, $\bar{x}$ and s are computed, then approximately 95% of the intervals $\bar{x} - t(s/\sqrt{n})$ to $\bar{x} + t(s/\sqrt{n})$ would include the true value of the parameter μ. We call the numbers from $\bar{x} - t(s/\sqrt{n})$ to $\bar{x} + t(s/\sqrt{n})$ a 95% *confidence interval for μ*.

Comment

Figure 4.31 may clarify what is meant by a 95% confidence interval. Imagine taking many samples of size n and, for each, computing $\bar{x}$, s, and the corresponding 95% confidence interval. Note, first of all, that both the length and the location of these intervals would vary from sample to sample (since both $\bar{x}$

and s would vary from sample to sample). Also, note that somewhere along the horizontal axis is the *true* value of μ — say, μ_0. Being a parameter, μ_0 is a constant whose exact value always remains unknown. However, we *do* know that 95% of all the 95% confidence intervals that *could* be constructed would contain μ_0 as one of their values.

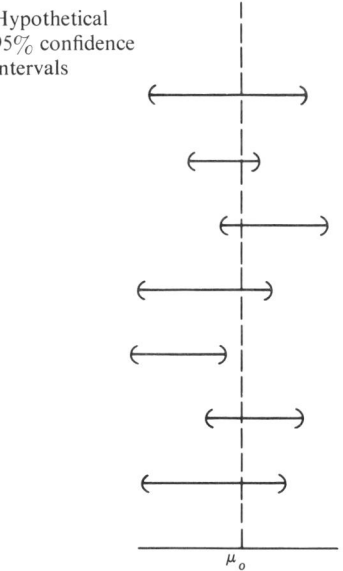

FIGURE 4.31

Comment

This is an instance where the distinction between a random variable and a particular realization of a random variable is of critical importance. Thinking of $\bar{X}$ (and s) as random variables, we can correctly say that, in the long run, intervals of the form $[\bar{X} - t(s/\sqrt{n}), \bar{X} + t(s/\sqrt{n})]$ will contain μ_0 95% of the time. But as soon as the data are collected and sample values for $\bar{x}$ and s are substituted, it no longer makes sense to say that the *particular* interval $[\bar{x} - t(s/\sqrt{n}), \bar{x} + t(s/\sqrt{n})]$ covers μ_0 95% of the time. Since μ_0 is a constant, any particular interval covers it either 100% of the time or 0% of the time.

Comment

In hypothesis testing, the most frequently chosen level of significance is .05 but certain other values of P — in particular, .10 and .01 — are also used. Similarly, in constructing confidence intervals, the "usual" *confidence coefficient* is 95%, but 90% and 99% are not uncommon (see Questions 4.4.1 and 4.4.3).

EXAMPLE 4.4.1. Spirometry

Methods for measuring various aspects of breathing are part of the science known as spirometry. One such aspect is the maximal breathing capacity

(MBC). This is defined to be the greatest volume of air a person can inhale and exhale in one minute. (Actually, the test is done for only a 15- to 20-second period and the results are extrapolated to one minute). The data below are maximal breathing capacities recorded for 22 healthy subjects (Bartels, 1963).

Subject	MBC (liters/min)	Subject	MBC (liters/min)
1	131	12	194
2	79	13	102
3	20	14	53
4	168	15	200
5	183	16	156
6	128	17	104
7	28	18	161
8	89	19	59
9	93	20	61
10	129	21	135
11	24	22	178

Here

$$\sum_{i=1}^{22} x_i = 2475 \quad \text{and} \quad \sum_{i=1}^{22} x_i^2 = 345503$$

so that

$$\bar{x} = \frac{2475}{22} = 112.5$$

and

$$s = \sqrt{\frac{22(345503) - (2475)^2}{22(21)}} = \sqrt{3193.60} = 56.5$$

From Appendix II, the numbers that cut off areas of 0.025 in either tail of the Student t curve with 21 ($= n - 1$) degrees of freedom are -2.08 and 2.08. Therefore, a 95% confidence interval for μ, the true average maximal breathing capacity, is the set of values

$$\left[\bar{x} - 2.08 \left(\frac{s}{\sqrt{n}} \right), \bar{x} + 2.08 \left(\frac{s}{\sqrt{n}} \right) \right]$$

or

$$\left[112.5 - 2.08 \left(\frac{56.5}{\sqrt{22}} \right), 112.5 + 2.08 \left(\frac{56.5}{\sqrt{22}} \right) \right]$$

which reduces to the interval from 87.5 to 137.5.

[4.4] Confidence Intervals

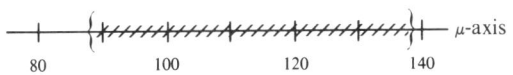

95% confidence interval

FIGURE 4.32

Comment

Confidence intervals are often misinterpreted. Here we would say that "the 95% confidence interval is the set of values from 87.5 to 137.5; in the long run, 95% of the intervals constructed in this fashion would include the true average MBC." For the reasons cited above, it would be incorrect to say that the interval 87.5 to 137.5 contains the true average MBC 95% of the time.

Question 4.4.1. Explain what a 99% confidence interval would be. For a given set of data, would a 99% confidence interval be longer or shorter than a 95% confidence interval?

EXAMPLE 4.4.2. Estimating Radiation Exposure

With the probable proliferation in the near future of nuclear reactors as a major source of power, the cumulative effects of low-level background radiation are being reexamined as a potential public health problem. Are the current levels safe? If so, how much higher can they go before becoming unsafe? As a first step towards answering these questions, studies have been undertaken to determine the levels of exposure typical of different parts of the country. The following data show the Ra^{226} concentrations found in the bones of long-time residents of Chicago (Holtzman, 1965). (Ra^{226} is a naturally-occurring isotope of radium.)

Person	Ra^{226} concentration (picocuries/g Ash)
1	.014
2	.005
3	.009
4	.025
5	.022
6	.028
7	.010
8	.021
9	.020
10	.008
11	.009
12	.007
13	.006
14	.022

Model Two — The One-Sample Problem [4.4]

There is so little known about low-level radiation that no real "standards" have emerged. This means that a confidence interval, rather than a hypothesis test, would be the most appropriate analysis for these data. Let μ denote the true average Ra[226] concentration that would be found for the population of all long-time Chicago residents. Since

$$\sum_{i=1}^{14} x_i = 0.206 \quad \text{and} \quad \sum_{i=1}^{14} x_i^2 = 0.00385$$

it follows that

$$\bar{x} = \frac{0.206}{14} = 0.015$$

and

$$s = \sqrt{\frac{14(.00385) - (.206)^2}{14(13)}} = \sqrt{.0000630} = 0.008$$

To construct a 95% confidence interval for μ, we need to use multiples from the Student t curve with 13 df. From Appendix II,

$$P\{t \leq -2.16\} + P\{t \geq 2.16\} = .05$$

implying that the 95% confidence interval should have the form

$$\left[\bar{x} - 2.16\left(\frac{s}{\sqrt{n}}\right), \bar{x} + 2.16\left(\frac{s}{\sqrt{n}}\right)\right]$$

or, in this case,

$$\left[0.015 - 2.16\left(\frac{0.008}{\sqrt{14}}\right), 0.015 + 2.16\left(\frac{0.008}{\sqrt{14}}\right)\right]$$

which reduces to

$$(0.010, 0.020)$$

Question 4.4.2. How might information of a similar nature collected from different parts of the country be used to assess the health effects of low-level radiation?

Question 4.4.3. Construct a 90% and a 99% confidence interval for these same data. Do these intervals support your answer to Question 4.4.1?

Comment

For sample sizes greater than 30 or for situations where σ is known, the t values in confidence interval expressions are replaced by Z values.

Question 4.4.4. Whether or not there is a standard value for μ, a "point" estimate can still be given for the location of a population distribution: namely, $\bar{x}$. What advantage is gained by estimating the unknown μ with, say, a 95% confidence interval rather than with a single point?

4.5
BINOMIAL DATA

Up to this point, the methods discussed in this chapter have been appropriate for continuous data — prothrombin times, air-flow rates, radiation levels, etc. But much of the data encountered in medical research is *not* continuous: patients live or die, a blood pressure is normal or abnormal, the public health facilities in a rural area are adequate or inadequate. Data like these are said to be *binomial* (that is, "nominal" with two classes), and their analysis requires procedures slightly different from those which would be used for continuous data.

Suppose a project is undertaken in a nursing home to investigate the effects of intensive psychological counseling in reducing senility. At the end of six weeks the progress of each patient is rated either satisfactory or unsatisfactory. If n patients are included in the study and a total of x respond favorably, then x/n is the sample proportion of "successes." (In more general terms, the patients would be referred to as a *sequence of n binomial trials*. Also, we will assume that these n trials (or patients) are "independent" — that is, the probability that the counseling will be successful for Patient i is not affected by whether or not it was successful for Patient j.)

Like $\bar{x}$, the proportion of successes will vary from sample to sample. If a second set of n patients were "treated," y of *them* would respond and, in general, y would be slightly different than x. The parameter that x/n estimates (as $\bar{x}$ estimates μ) is the proportion of favorable responses that would be observed if *all* nursing home patients were similarly counseled. We use the letter p to denote this *true* proportion of successes.

To make inferences about p on the basis of x/n, it is necessary to know the properties of the sampling distribution of X/n (just as it was necessary to know the properties of the sampling distribution of $\bar{X}$ in order to make generalizations about μ). The next result, which was historically the first formulation of the Central Limit Theorem, provides a very useful approximation to that distribution.

> *Binomial Approximation.* Let X be the number of "successes" in a sequence of n independent binomial trials, where the true probability of success is p. The sampling distribution of X/n is approximated by a normal curve with mean equal to p and standard deviation equal to
>
> $$\sqrt{\frac{p(1-p)}{n}}$$
>
> Or, equivalently, the variable
>
> $$\frac{\frac{X}{n} - p}{\sqrt{\frac{p(1-p)}{n}}}$$
>
> is approximated by the standard normal.

Comment

If the numerical value of p is not specified, the standard deviation of the X/n distribution can be estimated by

$$\sqrt{\frac{\frac{X}{n}\left(1 - \frac{X}{n}\right)}{n}}$$

in which case, the behavior of

$$\frac{\frac{X}{n} - p}{\sqrt{\frac{\frac{X}{n}\left(1 - \frac{X}{n}\right)}{n}}}$$

can also be described by a Z distribution.

Comment

The normal approximation to the binomial is only adequate when n is fairly large (greater than 50) and p is not too different from 0.5 — say, between 0.1 and 0.9. If either or both of these conditions is not met, it would be better to analyze the data in some other way.

The next two examples show how the Binomial Approximation can be used to test hypotheses about the parameter p.

EXAMPLE 4.5.1. DPT Immunization

In 1968, an immunization survey was carried out in a Model Cities area of Atlanta, Georgia (Center for Disease Control, 1968). Out of the sample of 537 persons under the age of 15, a total of 460 (or 85.7%) had had the usual sequence of diphtheria-pertussis-tetanus (DPT) vaccinations.

Suppose that public health officials had decided that any inner city community having fewer than 90% of their under-15 population vaccinated with the DPT series should be the target of an intensive immunization campaign. Should this particular Model Cities area be included in that category? Or can the difference between 0.857 and 0.90 be attributed to sampling variability?

Let p denote the true proportion of the under-15 population protected by the DPT series. In the language of hypothesis testing, the choices regarding p reduce to H: $p = 0.90$ or the one-sided alternative H: $p < 0.90$. (A two-sided alternative would not be used here because it does not matter if the community is "overimmunized," that is, if $p > 0.90$).

Following the same rationale used in hypothesis tests for μ, we will choose between H and A on the strength of the "compatibility" of the observed proportion $[(x/n) = 0.857]$ with the sampling distribution of X/n under the assumption that H is true. More specifically, if H is true, the binomial version of the Central Limit Theorem states that the sampling distribution of $X/537$ is approximated by a normal curve with mean 0.9 and standard deviation $\sqrt{[(0.9)(0.1)]/537} = 0.013$.

Suppose the hypotheses are to be tested at the $P = .05$ level of significance. It follows from the nature of the alternative hypothesis that the associated critical value, denoted $(X/n)'$, should be 1.64 standard deviations (of X/n) to the left of 0.90:

$$\left(\frac{X}{n}\right)' = p_0 - 1.64\sqrt{\frac{p_0(1-p_0)}{n}}$$

$$= 0.90 - 1.64\sqrt{\frac{0.9(0.1)}{537}}$$

$$= 0.88$$

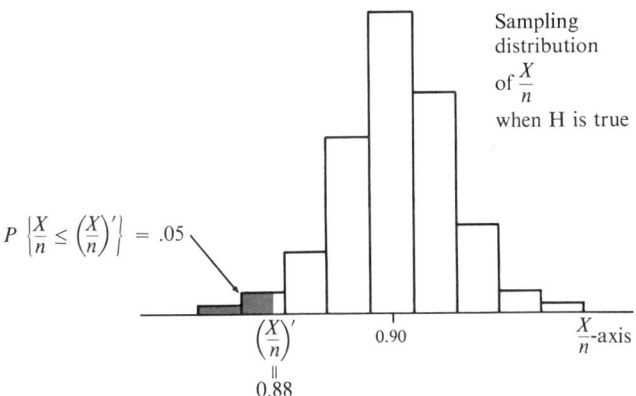

FIGURE 4.33

Since the sample proportion, x/n ($= 0.857$), was *less* than $(X/n)'$, our conclusion is to reject H. This particular area does *not* appear to be adequately immunized.

Question 4.5.1. As the sample size increases, the chances that a sample proportion will be within a fixed distance of the true proportion increase. Why?

Later chapters will bear out the statement that many different kinds of hypothesis tests can be handled very conveniently in the step-by-step fashion introduced in Section 4.2. This is certainly true for tests involving the binomial parameter.

EXAMPLE 4.5.2. ESP — Fact or Fiction?

Attempts to demonstrate statistically the existence of extrasensory perception (ESP) have been going on for many years. One of the still-classic results is an experiment done at Duke University in 1938 (Hansel, 1966). This particular study involved a total of 32 subjects and tested their ability to identify symbols on cards. There were five different symbols, each equally likely to appear, so the probability of simply *guessing* the right answer was 1/5. Altogether, the 32 subjects were shown 60,000 cards and scored a total of 12,489 correct answers.

Note that if random chance were the only factor involved, the expected number of correct answers would be 12,000 ($= 1/5 \times 60,000$). Does it follow, then, that these additional 489 correct answers "prove" the existence of ESP?

(1) Let the parameter p denote a subject's *true* probability of getting the right answer (if ESP has no effect, $p = 1/5$). To allow for the possibility that nonrandom influences might inhibit, as well as enhance, a subject's ability, a two-sided alternative will be used.

$$\text{H:} \quad p = \frac{1}{5} = 0.20 (= p_o) \quad \text{versus} \quad \text{A:} \quad p \neq \frac{1}{5}$$

Assume that $P = .01$ is chosen to be the level of significance.

(2) Compute the sample proportion.

$$\frac{x}{n} = \frac{\text{Number of "successful" trials}}{\text{Total number of trials}}$$
$$= \frac{12,489}{60,000}$$
$$= 0.208$$

(3) The sampling distribution of X/n, when H is true, has a mean equal to 0.200 and a standard deviation equal to

$$\sqrt{\frac{0.20(0.80)}{60,000}} = 0.0016$$

(4) Since the alternative hypothesis is two-sided, we need to find *two* critical values, each a distance of 2.58 standard deviations of X/n away from p_o (why?). Therefore,

$$\left(\frac{X}{n}\right)'_1 = p_o - 2.58\sqrt{\frac{p_o(1-p_o)}{n}}$$
$$= 0.200 - 2.58(0.0016)$$
$$= 0.196$$

and

$$\left(\frac{X}{n}\right)'_2 = p_o + 2.58\sqrt{\frac{p_o(1-p_o)}{n}}$$
$$= 0.200 + 2.58(0.0016)$$
$$= 0.204$$

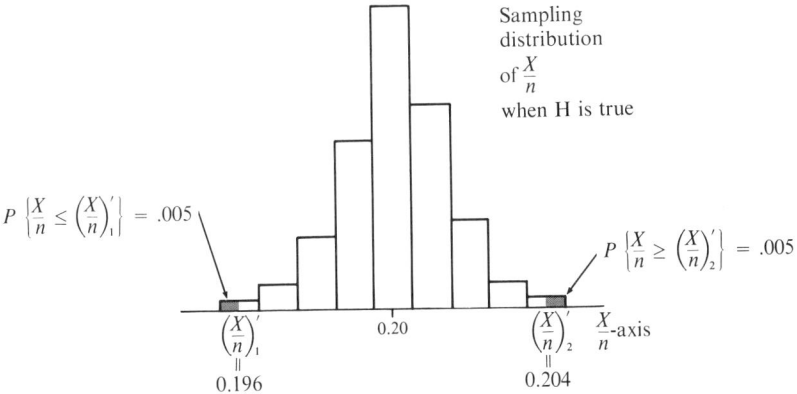

FIGURE 4.34

The observed proportion, 0.208, falls far to the right of $(X/n)'_2$ so we reject H, and conclude that something other than chance is necessary to account for so many correct answers.

Question 4.5.2. What is the *exact* probability that X/n will exceed the observed sample proportion, 0.208, if, in fact, H: $p = 1/5$ is true?

Example 4.5.3 shows how confidence intervals can be constructed for the binomial parameter p.

EXAMPLE 4.5.3. Electric Shock Therapy

Electric shock therapy (EST) is a somatic, rather than a psychotherapeutic, method of treating mental disorders. Although its mechanism is still unknown, EST has proven to be quite effective for certain conditions. For example, data accumulated on 788 patients with paranoia showed that 76.3% were considered "improved" following electric shock therapy (Hutt and Gibby, 1957).

The best way to make a statement about the *true* effectiveness (p) of EST in treating paranoia would be to construct a confidence interval. In particular, a 95% confidence interval for p would be

$$\left[\frac{x}{n} - 1.96\sqrt{\frac{\frac{x}{n}\left(1-\frac{x}{n}\right)}{n}},\ \frac{x}{n} + 1.96\sqrt{\frac{\frac{x}{n}\left(1-\frac{x}{n}\right)}{n}}\right]$$

or

$$\left[0.763 - 1.96\sqrt{\frac{0.763(0.237)}{788}},\ 0.763 + 1.96\sqrt{\frac{0.763(0.237)}{788}}\right]$$

which reduces to

$$(0.733,\ 0.793)$$

That is, a 95% confidence interval for the true proportion of people with paranoia whose conditions would be improved by electric shock therapy is the interval (0.733, 0.793). Whether or not this particular set of numbers actually includes p can never be known but, as usual, we have the reassurance that 95% of all the intervals constructed in this way *will* contain p.

Question 4.5.3. Using the data of Example 2.5.2, construct a 99% confidence interval for the true proportion of student nurses who have used marihuana at least once. What assumptions regarding the sample and the population must be made in interpreting this interval?

4.6
TYPE I AND II ERRORS

The material in this section should be considered optional. Knowing how to compute and interpret the probability of a Type II error is *not* a prerequisite for doing any of the problems later in the book. However, the ideas presented here will put the problem of hypothesis testing in a more meaningful perspective.

To begin, we should recall the definitions of Type I and Type II errors. A Type I error is committed whenever the data and the decision rule lead us to reject the null hypothesis, H, even though it is really true. A Type II error is committed when the decision is to accept H when, in fact, the alternative is true.

For any test involving μ, the likelihood of committing either type of error is determined by the probability of $\bar{X}$ falling into a certain interval. Take, for instance, the problem discussed in Example 4.2.2. The hypotheses were

$$\text{H:} \quad \mu = 6.8 \quad \text{versus} \quad \text{A:} \quad \mu < 6.8$$

It was decided, using the $P = .05$ Decision Rule, that H should be rejected if $\bar{x} \leq 6.3$.

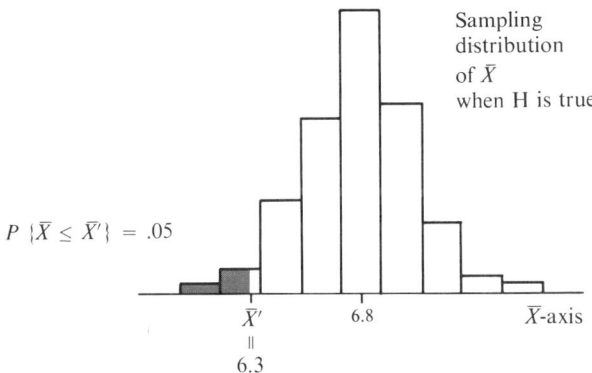

FIGURE 4.35

Now, the fact that $\bar{X}$ will, by chance, be less than 6.3, 5% of the time (when H is true) means that the probability of committing a Type I error is 5%. Of course, this comes as no surprise since the critical value, $\bar{X}' = 6.3$, was chosen specifically to meet the condition that $P\{\bar{X} \leq \bar{X}'\} = .05$. It follows, then, that for *any* hypothesis test, the probability of committing a Type I error is equal to the specified level of significance.

Computing the probability of a Type II error is not quite so straightforward. Notice that if H is assumed to be true, the exact value of μ is known (in this case, 6.8). But if A is assumed to be true, nothing definite is known about μ except that it is *less* than 6.8. The consequence of this "composite" nature of A is that for every different value of μ less than 6.8, there is a different probability of committing a Type II error.

Suppose, for example, that μ was actually equal to 6.5. Then, by definition, the probability of committing a Type II error is equal to the shaded area to the right of $\bar{X}' = 6.3$ under the sampling distribution of $\bar{X}$ when $\mu = 6.5$.

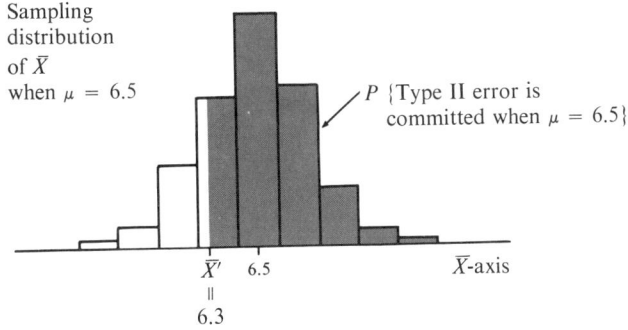

FIGURE 4.36

In probability notation,

P {a Type II error is committed when $\mu = 6.5$}
$\quad = P$ {H: $\quad \mu = 6.8$ is accepted when $\mu = 6.5$}
$\quad = P$ {$\bar{X} > 6.3$ when $\mu = 6.5$}

This last statement can be evaluated numerically by relating the area in question to an equivalent area under a standard normal curve (see Section 4.2). That is, since $s = 1.7$ and $n = 35$ (see p. 132),

$$P\{\bar{X} > 6.3 \text{ when } \mu = 6.5\} = P\left\{\frac{\bar{X} - 6.5}{\frac{1.7}{\sqrt{35}}} > \frac{6.3 - 6.5}{\frac{1.7}{\sqrt{35}}}\right\}$$
$$\approx P\{Z > -0.70\}$$
$$= 1 - P\{Z \leq -0.70\} = 1 - 0.2420$$
$$= 0.7580 \approx 0.76$$

This means that *if μ were 6.5*, the $P = .05$ Decision Rule would lead us to accept H: $\quad \mu = 6.8$ 76% of the time (and commit a Type II error 76% of the time).

But suppose μ was actually 6.0. Then

P {a Type II error is committed when $\mu = 6.0$}
$$= P\{\bar{X} > 6.3 \text{ when } \mu = 6.0\}$$
$$= P\left\{\frac{\bar{X} - 6.0}{\frac{1.7}{\sqrt{35}}} > \frac{6.3 - 6.0}{\frac{1.7}{\sqrt{35}}}\right\}$$
$$\approx P\{Z > 1.04\}$$
$$= 1 - P\{Z \leq 1.04\} = 1 - 0.8508$$
$$= 0.1492 \approx 0.15$$

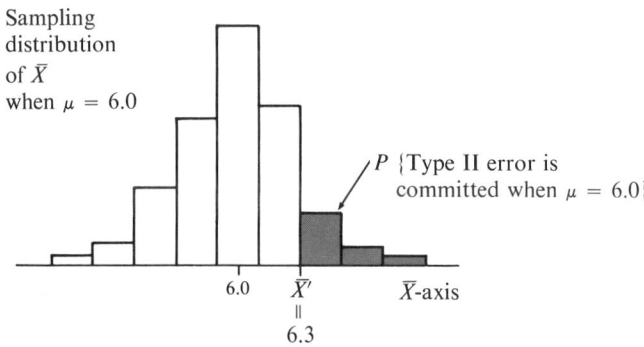

FIGURE 4.37

That is, if μ were actually 6.0 we would fail to recognize that H was false (i.e., commit a Type II error) only 15% of the time. Note that as the true value of μ gets further away from the "H" value of μ, the probability of committing a

Type II error diminishes. This makes sense since the further away the true μ gets from μ_o, the more likely it is that the observed sample mean will be incompatible with the particular sampling distribution of $\bar{X}$ associated with H. [In this case, incompatible means that $\bar{x} \leq 6.3 \, (= \bar{X}')$].

Suppose that calculations like these were done for a *set* of μ values, each less than 6.8. The results could then be graphed by plotting (on the vertical axis) the probability of committing a Type II error against (on the horizontal axis) the presumed value for μ. Graphs of this sort are called *operating characteristic curves*. They reflect the ability of the test procedure to detect the alternative hypothesis.

Comment

Keep in mind that μ is *not* a variable; it has only one value. However, that value is never known. The purpose of an operating characteristic curve is to indicate how sensitive the hypothesis test would be (in terms of committing Type II errors) *if* the true value of μ were 6.5, or 6.0, or any other value.

The operating characteristic curve for the test used on the data of Example 4.2.2 is shown in Figure 4.38. The two X's on the curve are the points calculated in the preceding discussion.

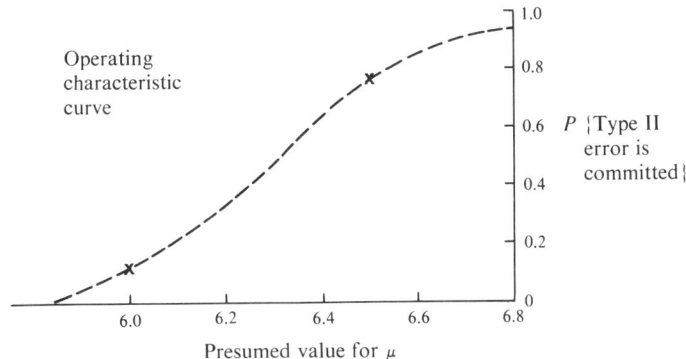

FIGURE 4.38

Comment

Two points on the operating characteristic curve can be derived without any calculation. When $\mu = \mu_o$, the probability of committing a Type II error is simply 1 minus the level of significance (in this case, $1 - 0.05 = 0.95$). Also, when $\mu = \bar{X}'$, the probability of committing a Type II error is 0.50, by virtue of the symmetry of the sampling distribution of $\bar{X}$. These two points, together with two or three calculated points, are usually adequate for approximating the shape of the curve.

Superimposing the normal curves that approximate the sampling distributions of $\bar{X}$ when H is true ($\mu = 6.8$) and when some particular alternative is true (say, $\mu = 6.0$) brings out an important relationship between Type I and Type II errors. *Decreasing* the probability of committing one kind of error *increases* the probability of committing the other. For this situation,

$$P\{\text{Type I error}\} = P\{\bar{X} \leq 6.3 \text{ when } \mu = 6.8\}$$
$$= .05$$

and

$$P\{\text{Type II error}\} = P\{\bar{X} > 6.3 \text{ when } \mu = 6.0\}$$
$$= .15$$

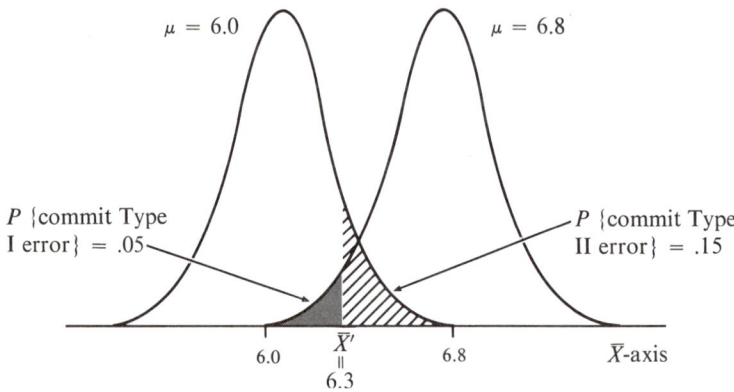

FIGURE 4.39

Clearly, the chances of making a Type I error could be lessened by moving $\bar{X}'$ *to the left*. In particular, if $\bar{X}'$ were located 2.33, instead of 1.64, standard deviations of $\bar{X}$ to the left of 6.8, the probability of committing a Type I error (and the level of significance) would be .01. That would make

$$\bar{X}' = 6.8 - 2.33\left(\frac{1.7}{\sqrt{35}}\right)$$
$$= 6.1$$

but *now* the probability of committing a Type II error (for $\mu = 6.0$) would be

$$P\{\bar{X} > 6.1 \text{ when } \mu = 6.0\} = P\left\{\frac{\bar{X} - 6.0}{\frac{1.7}{\sqrt{35}}} > \frac{6.1 - 6.0}{\frac{1.7}{\sqrt{35}}}\right\}$$
$$\approx P\{Z > 0.35\}$$
$$= 1 - P\{Z \leq 0.35\} = 1 - 0.6368$$
$$= 0.3632 \approx 0.36$$

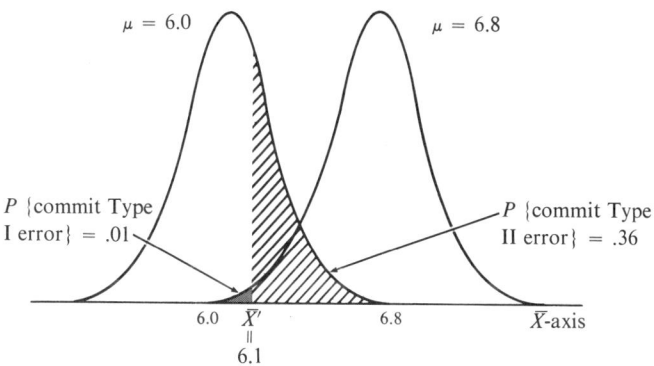

FIGURE 4.40

Thus, in *reducing* the probability of committing a Type I error from .05 to .01 we have, at the same time, *increased* the probability of committing a Type II error from .15 to .36 (for the particular alternative that $\mu = 6.0$).

Comment

Theoretically, decision rules should be constructed so that the probabilities of making either type of error reflect the *consequences* of those errors. For example, in the polygraph data of Example 3.7.1, it is certainly worse to convict an innocent defendant (commit a Type I error), than it is to acquit a guilty defendant (commit a Type II error). In most cases, though, the consequences — whether economic, medical, or moral — of making Type I or Type II errors are extremely difficult, if not impossible, to determine.

Question 4.6.1. Find the probability of committing a Type II error when $\mu = 300{,}000$ for the hypothesis test described in Example 4.2.4.

Question 4.6.2. There is one way to simultaneously decrease the probabilities of committing both Type I and Type II errors: by increasing the sample size. Explain why that should be true.

Comment

Question 4.6.2 suggests how operating characteristic curves can contribute to the planning stage of an experiment. Suppose we intend to do a hypothesis test of H: $\mu = \mu_o$ against A: $\mu < \mu_o$, using a sample of size n. If, after computing the corresponding operating characteristic curve, it seems clear that the test, as proposed, would result in too great a chance of committing a Type II error, we have the option of redesigning the experiment to include a *larger* sample size — thereby reducing the probability of committing a Type II error. On the other hand, it may be apparent that the original experiment would be *too* precise for its intended purpose and that a smaller sample size would be quite adequate.

Question 4.6.3. Construct an operating characteristic curve for the study described in Example 4.2.3. Suppose the experimenter wanted to commit a Type II error less than 10% of the time when, in fact, the true mean was 7.33. Is the sample size ($n = 44$) large enough?

4.7
SUMMARY

In reviewing Chapter 4 it would be good to keep in mind the sequence of steps in which the analysis of a Model Two problem usually proceeds. Step 1, after the data have been collected (and if the sample size is fairly large), is to draw a histogram, to provide some idea of the overall pattern in the data and, at the same time, to suggest how the data might best be analyzed mathematically. If the sample distribution is more or less bell-shaped, $\bar{x}$ and s should be calculated as measures of location and dispersion. (If the sample is small — say, less than 15 — a histogram will not be of much value. Usually in these cases we simply calculate $\bar{x}$ and s and do not do anything graphical.)

The final step of most Model Two problems involves inference. Having described the sample graphically and numerically, it seems only natural to want to "generalize" to some larger population. Most commonly, inference in the one-sample problem concerns $\bar{x}$ and what it implies about μ. This can be accomplished with either of two formats — *hypothesis tests* or *confidence intervals*. The two are actually very similar, mathematically, but they tend to arise in somewhat different contexts, experimentally. If the data relate to a process or situation where a recognized value for μ has already been established, then the more appropriate analysis would be a hypothesis test. But if nothing specific is known about the variable being measured, the confidence interval approach makes more sense.

The step-by-step details of doing a hypothesis test are fairly straightforward. First, the null and alternative hypotheses are formulated and a level of significance is chosen. (These, for the most part, are nonstatistical decisions and arise out of the physical context of the problem.) Then the sampling distribution of the statistic being used (say, $\bar{X}$) is conceptualized under the assumption that the null hypothesis is true. The appropriate critical value (or values, if the alternative hypothesis is two-sided) are found. The test statistic is then compared to the critical value, and a conclusion is reached.

To construct a confidence interval, we first choose a *confidence coefficient* (say, 95% or 99%) and then determine the upper and lower bounds according to the format set out in Section 4.4. The multiples of the standard error come from either the student t distribution with $(n - 1)$ degrees of freedom or the standard normal distribution, depending on what is known about n and σ. In particular, if n is less than or equal to 30 and if σ is unknown, the t distribution is used. In all other situations, the multiples come from the standard normal.

In some instances, the variable of interest is the *proportion* of times a certain event occurs — such as the proportion of patients for which a certain treatment is effective, or the proportion of admissions to an emergency room that are not really emergencies. These are examples of *binomial* variables. Their analysis parallels the analysis for continuous data, but the details, as indicated in Section 4.5, are slightly different. Once again, though, the Central Limit Theorem plays a key role.

The final section in this chapter takes a closer look at the *theory* of hypothesis testing. Type I and Type II errors are examined, and the construction of *operating characteristic curves* is explained.

Definitions

Binomial data. Data involving the number of "successes" recorded in n independent "trials," where each trial can have only one of two possible outcomes.

Central Limit Theorem. A result that states that the sampling distribution of $\bar{X}$ can be approximated by a normal curve; probably the single most important result in all of statistics.

Confidence interval. An interval having a high a priori probability (typically, 0.95 or 0.99) of containing an unknown parameter (often μ or p).

Critical value $(\bar{X}', (X/n)',$ etc.). In hypothesis testing, that particular number, which, if equalled or "exceeded" by $\bar{x}$ (or x/n), leads to the rejection of H; for two-sided alternatives, there are two such numbers.

Decision rule. In hypothesis testing, a statement indicating which values of $\bar{x}$ (or x/n) will result in H being rejected.

Degrees of freedom (df). A parameter associated with the family of Student t curves; given a sample of size n, the particular Student t curve that best approximates the distribution of $(\bar{X} - \mu)/(s/\sqrt{n})$ has $(n - 1)$ degrees of freedom.

Level of significance. The probability of committing a Type I error; generally set routinely by the experimenter at either .05 or .01.

Operating characteristic curve. For a given decision rule, a graph showing the probability of committing a Type II error for the various values of μ (or p) belonging to the alternative hypothesis.

Standard error of the mean $(\sigma_{\bar{X}})$. A term referring to the standard deviation of the sampling distribution of $\bar{X}$; in particular, $\sigma_{\bar{X}} = \sigma/\sqrt{n}$.

Student t curve. The mathematical model describing the behavior of $(\bar{X} - \mu)/(s/\sqrt{n})$; especially important when $n \leq 30$ (when $n > 30$, the distribution of $(\bar{X} - \mu)/(s/\sqrt{n})$ is approximated by the standard normal). Areas under Student t curves are tabulated in Appendix II. Hypothesis tests using this model are referred to as t tests.

Review Exercises

4.1 Food poisoning outbreaks are quite often the result of contaminated salads. In 1967, the New York City Department of Health established the following standards for bacterial counts in salads:

    Total plate count: less than 100,000 organisms/gram
    Enterococci: less than 1000 organisms/gram
    Coliforms: less than 100 organisms/gram
    Staphylococci (coagulase positive): 0 organisms/gram

That same year the department routinely examined 220 tuna salads marketed by various retail and wholesale outlets. A total of 179 were found to be unsatisfactory according to at least one of these criteria (Sharidi, et al., 1970). Construct a 95% confidence interval for the true proportion of contaminated tuna salads in New York City.

4.2 Years of testing have shown that College Entrance Examination Board scores are normally distributed with a mean of 500 and a standard deviation of 100. Suppose the average CEEB score of 64 randomly selected students is computed. What specific properties would the corresponding sampling distribution of $\bar{X}$ have? Find the probability that the average of these 64 scores will exceed 510. What is the probability that a *single* score will exceed 510?

4.3 Construct a 99% confidence interval for the true average radiation exposure characteristic of display areas where color televisions are sold. Use the data of Example 1.6.1 (and Review Exercise 3.6).

4.4 There is a theory that people tend to "postpone" their deaths until after some special event has occurred — say, a birthday. For example, the birth and death months of 348 persons listed in *Four Hundred Notable Americans* were examined, and it was found that only 16 (or $16/348 \times 100 = 4.6\%$) had died during the month immediately preceding their birth month (Tanur, 1972). If, in fact, their deaths had occurred at random, each month should have been represented 1/12 (or 8.3%) of the time. Let p denote the true probability of a person dying during the month preceding his birth month. Test, at the $P = .05$ level of significance, the null hypothesis H: $p = 1/12$ against the alternative A: $p < 1/12$.

4.5 Convert the mosquito data of Example 1.6.2 to minutes, and construct a 90% confidence interval for the true average bite duration.

4.6 The blood sugar levels of seven rabbits were measured one and one-half hours after each had been injected with 0.8 units of insulin (Rumke and deJonge, 1964).

Rabbit	Blood sugar level (mg/100 ml)
1	45
2	34
3	32
4	48
5	39
6	45
7	41

Suppose that similar studies had shown that after three hours the average blood sugar level is 50 mg per 100 ml. Can it be concluded at the $P = .05$ level of significance that the true average blood sugar level after one and one-half hours is different than the average level after three hours?

4.7 Construct an operating characteristic curve for testing whether or not synovial pH is lowered in arthritic conditions. The hypotheses are

$$H: \quad \mu = 7.39 \quad \text{versus} \quad A: \quad \mu < 7.39$$

Let $P = .05$ be the level of significance. Use the same sample size and the same estimate of the standard deviation that were given in Example 4.2.3.

4.8 What would an operating characteristic curve look like if the alternative hypothesis was two-sided?

4.9 To hunt flying insects, bats emit high frequency sounds and then listen for their echoes. Until an insect is "located," these signals are emitted at intervals of from 50 to 100 milliseconds. But when an insect *is* detected, the signal-to-signal interval suddenly decreases, so the bat can better pinpoint its prey's position. Using an elaborate photographic procedure, scientists have been able to measure this "detection" distance — that is, the bat-to-insect separation when the bat's signals first become noticeably more rapid (Griffin, Webster, and Michael, 1960). The results for 11 "catches" are listed below. Construct a 95% confidence interval for the true average bat detection distance.

Catch #	Detection distance (cm)
1	62
2	52
3	68
4	23
5	34
6	45
7	27
8	42
9	83
10	56
11	40

5

MODEL THREE
The Two-Sample Problem

*Man's most valuable trait is a
judicious sense of what not to believe.*
                                    Euripides

5.1
INTRODUCTION

Is Bufferin *really* better than "just plain aspirin"? Are marihuana smokers more likely to develop neuroses than nonsmokers? Do women tend to be more emotional than men? All of these are questions that, theoretically, can be answered with the methods of Model Three. Conceptually, there is little that is new in this chapter; to build a theory suitable for two-sample problems we need only adapt the principles already developed in chapter 4.

In every two-sample problem there will be two treatments (T_X and T_Y), each associated with a theoretical response distribution (P_X and P_Y). The usual objective will be to test whether or not T_X and T_Y are equally effective. For example, T_X and T_Y might be two levels of crowding in an experiment investigating the effects of environment on behavior. The target population might be "all adults," with P_X and P_Y being the hypothetical distributions of some observable measure of aggression.

As a way of comparing T_X and T_Y, we will look for differences between P_X and P_Y — in particular, whether or not the mean (μ_X) or P_X has "shifted" rela-

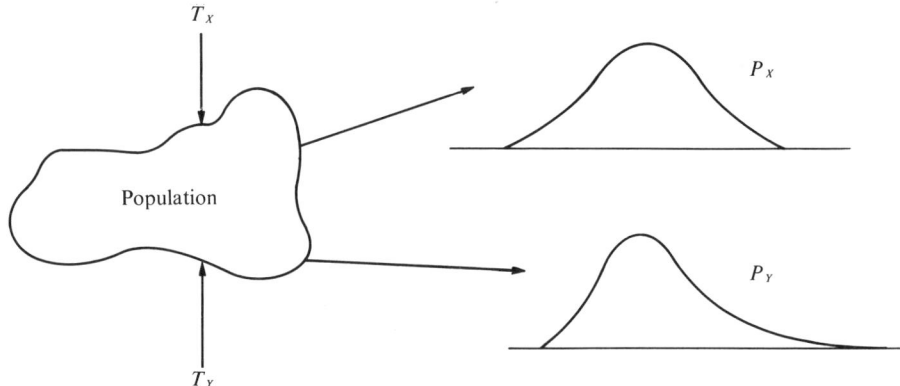

FIGURE 5.1

tive to the mean (μ_Y) of P_Y. Consequently, a typical hypothesis test for a two-sample problem would be

$$H: \quad \mu_X = \mu_Y \quad \text{versus} \quad A: \quad \mu_X \neq \mu_Y$$

As in the case of Model Two, A can be either two-sided (as above) or one-sided (A: $\mu_X < \mu_Y$ or A: $\mu_X > \mu_Y$), the choice depending on the nature of the problem.

Comment

P_X and P_Y can differ, of course, in ways other than location. But in many situations, location *is* the characteristic of the response distribution most affected by treatment differences. (A notable exception to this is discussed in Section 5.3.)

The data in problems of this sort will consist of a first sample $(x_1, x_2, \ldots, x_{n_X})$ of size n_X representing P_X and a second sample $(y_1, y_2, \ldots, y_{n_Y})$ of size n_Y representing P_Y. The sample sizes n_X and n_Y need not be equal.

Comment

Note that in both one-sample and two-sample problems, the existence of *two* population distributions is assumed (recall the discussion of Section 3.7). In Model Three, though, *both* distributions are sampled; whereas in Model Two only *one* is, with properties of the second distribution being estimated in other ways (similar studies, conjecture, past experience, etc.).

Because of certain superficial similarities, Model Three is sometimes confused with Models Four and Five. For that reason it is good to keep in mind those particular features of the sample-population structure that characterize Model Three. First of all, both sets of observations, the x's and the y's, must be "similar" so that differences such as $x_i - y_i$ have physical meaning. (If the x's were blood pressures and the y's were temperatures, $x_i - y_i$ would be meaningless, and the data could not belong to Model Three.) Secondly, in a Model Three problem, the individuals forming the first sample must be similar, but unrelated, to those making up the second sample. (If the effects of two vitamin supplements are to be compared, and we decide to test one on males between the ages of 40 and 65, then we should test the other on a sample of males in the same age bracket. However, none of the subjects can be included in both groups.)

In Sections 5.2 and 5.3, hypothesis tests are developed for the two-sample problem. We introduce the *two-sample t-test* for comparing μ_X and μ_Y and the *F-test* for comparing σ_X and σ_Y. Confidence intervals for the difference between population means $(\mu_X - \mu_Y)$ are constructed in Section 5.4.

5.2
THE TWO-SAMPLE *t*-TEST FOR MEANS (EQUAL STANDARD DEVIATIONS)

Section 5.1 has said that hypothesis testing in Model Three generally involves one of the following three situations:

(1) H: $\mu_X = \mu_Y$ versus A: $\mu_X \neq \mu_Y$
(2) H: $\mu_X = \mu_Y$ versus A: $\mu_X < \mu_Y$
(3) H: $\mu_X = \mu_Y$ versus A: $\mu_X > \mu_Y$

where μ_X and μ_Y are the unknown means of the two population distributions being studied. In each case, the appropriate test procedure is a modification of the *t*-test developed in Chapter 4.

Suppose that two random samples are drawn: $(x_1, x_2, \ldots, x_{n_X})$ and $(y_1, y_2, \ldots, y_{n_Y})$, representing P_X and P_Y, respectively. Let $\bar{x}$ and $\bar{y}$ denote the two sample means:

$$\bar{x} = \frac{1}{n_X} \sum_{i=1}^{n_X} x_i \quad \text{and} \quad \bar{y} = \frac{1}{n_Y} \sum_{i=1}^{n_Y} y_i$$

To test the equality of the two *population* means — H: $\mu_X = \mu_Y$ (or, equivalently, H: $\mu_X - \mu_Y = 0$) — it would seem reasonable to look at the difference between the two *sample* means, $\bar{x} - \bar{y}$. If the alternative hypothesis were two-sided, values of $\bar{x} - \bar{y}$ either *much smaller* or *much larger* than zero would tend to discredit H and lead to the acceptance of A: $\mu_X \neq \mu_Y$. If the alternative were A: $\mu_X < \mu_Y$ (or, A: $\mu_X - \mu_Y < 0$), then H would be rejected only if $\bar{x} - \bar{y}$ were *much smaller* than 0; similarly, if the alternative were A: $\mu_X > \mu_Y$, H would be rejected only if $\bar{x} - \bar{y}$ were *much larger* than 0.

Consider the two-sided test,

H: $\mu_X = \mu_Y$ versus A: $\mu_X \neq \mu_Y$

In order to know when to reject the null hypothesis it is necessary to make the definitions of "much smaller" and "much larger" more precise. In analogy with Model Two, this means finding two critical values, $(\bar{X} - \bar{Y})'_1$ and $(\bar{X} - \bar{Y})'_2$,

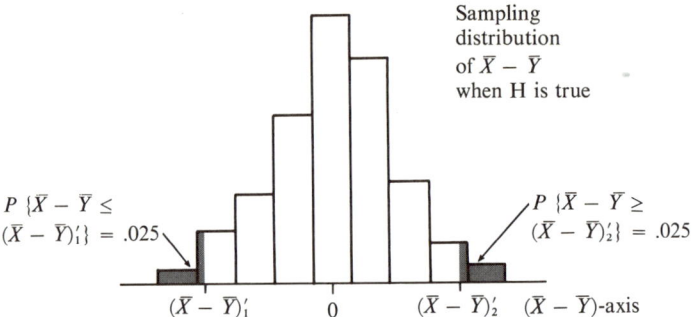

FIGURE 5.2

having the property that $\bar{X} - \bar{Y}$ will be less than or equal to $(\bar{X} - \bar{Y})'_1$ or greater than or equal to $(\bar{X} - \bar{Y})'_2$ by *chance* only, say, 5% of the time when H is true. Once again, finding the numerical values of the critical points is not difficult once the properties of the appropriate sampling distribution are known — in this case, the sampling distribution of $\bar{X} - \bar{Y}$. Theorem 5.2.1 gives those properties.

Theorem 5.2.1. Suppose two random samples, $(x_1, x_2, \ldots, x_{n_X})$ and $(y_1, y_2, \ldots, y_{n_Y})$, are drawn from two bell-shaped distributions having means μ_X and μ_Y and the same standard deviation, σ ($= \sigma_X = \sigma_Y$). If H: $\mu_X = \mu_Y$ is true, the sampling distribution of $\bar{X} - \bar{Y}$ has
(1) Mean equal to 0 and
(2) Standard deviation approximately equal to

$$s_p \sqrt{\frac{1}{n_X} + \frac{1}{n_Y}}$$

where

$$s_p = \sqrt{\frac{(n_X - 1)s_X^2 + (n_Y - 1)s_Y^2}{n_X + n_Y - 2}}$$

$$s_X^2 = \frac{n_X \sum_{i=1}^{n_X} x_i^2 - \left(\sum_{i=1}^{n_X} x_i\right)^2}{n_X(n_X - 1)}$$

$$s_Y^2 = \frac{n_Y \sum_{i=1}^{n_Y} y_i^2 - \left(\sum_{i=1}^{n_Y} y_i\right)^2}{n_Y(n_Y - 1)}$$

Also, the distribution of

$$\frac{\bar{X} - \bar{Y}}{s_p \sqrt{\frac{1}{n_X} + \frac{1}{n_Y}}}$$

is approximated by a Student t-curve with $n_X + n_Y - 2$ degrees of freedom.

Comment

The quantity s_p appearing in the denominator of the "t-statistic" is called the *pooled standard deviation*. It estimates σ.

Comment

The assumption in Theorem 5.2.1 that the x's and y's have both come from bell-shaped distributions does not, in practice, severely limit the applicability of the two-sample t-test. As we have already seen in Chapters 2 and 3, the distributions of many laboratory measurements do, in fact, have this particular shape. More importantly, though, the behavior of the t-statistic is not strongly affected by violations of this assumption unless the sample sizes are very small and the distributions in question deviate markedly from a bell-shape.

(In statistical terminology, a procedure whose validity is not strongly contingent on certain assumptions relating to the nature of the population(s) being sampled is said to be "robust." The t-test is robust with respect to the population distribution having something other than a bell shape.)

The next two examples show how Theorem 5.2.1 is applied. Notice the similarities between the reasoning used here and that used in Chapter 4.

EXAMPLE 5.2.1. Hospital Carpeting

The use of carpeting in hospitals has obvious esthetic merits, but is a vacuumed rug as sanitary as a washed floor? Recently a number of studies, like the one described below, have tried to answer that question by comparing bacterial counts in carpeted and uncarpeted rooms.

Airborne bacteria can be counted by passing air at a known rate over a growth medium, incubating that medium, and then counting the number of bacterial colonies that form. In this study, done in a Montana hospital, room air was forced over two Petri dishes at the rate of 1 cubic foot per minute (Walter and Stobie, 1963). One Petri dish contained blood agar; the other, a medium favorable to the growth of *Staphylococcus aureus*. This was done in 16 patient rooms, 8 carpeted and 8 uncarpeted. The results, expressed in terms of "bacteria per cubic foot of air," are listed in the accompanying table.

Carpeted rooms	Bacteria/ft³	Uncarpeted rooms	Bacteria/ft³
#212	$x_1 = 11.8$	#210	$y_1 = 12.1$
#216	$x_2 = 8.2$	#214	$y_2 = 8.3$
#220	$x_3 = 7.1$	#215	$y_3 = 3.8$
#223	$x_4 = 13.0$	#217	$y_4 = 7.2$
#225	$x_5 = 10.8$	#221	$y_5 = 12.0$
#226	$x_6 = 10.1$	#222	$y_6 = 11.1$
#227	$x_7 = 14.6$	#224	$y_7 = 10.1$
#228	$x_8 = 14.0$	#229	$y_8 = 13.7$

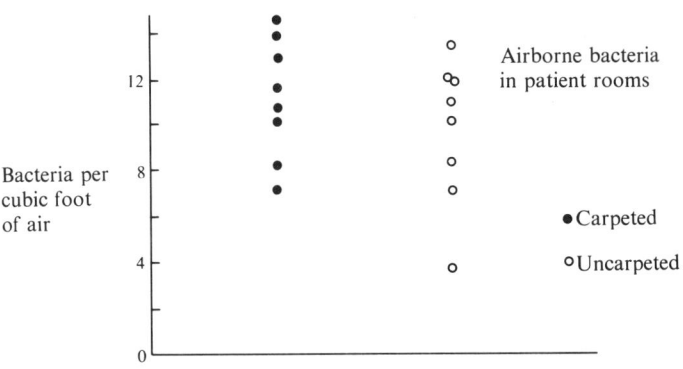

FIGURE 5.3

Suppose P_X and P_Y denote the population distributions of bacterial counts for carpeted rooms and uncarpeted rooms, respectively. Let μ_X and μ_Y denote the (unknown) means of P_X and P_Y.

(1) The problem is to choose between

$$H: \quad \mu_X = \mu_Y \quad \text{(Carpeting has no effect)}$$

versus

$$A: \quad \mu_X \neq \mu_Y \quad \text{(Carpeting } does \text{ have an effect)}$$

(Is it reasonable to use a two-sided alternative here?) Let $P = .05$ be the level of significance.

(2) The computations required for a two-sample problem are rather lengthy. First, the sums and the sums of the squares of the observations in each of the samples are found:

$$\sum_{i=1}^{8} x_i = 89.6 \qquad \sum_{i=1}^{8} x_i^2 = 1053.70$$

$$\sum_{i=1}^{8} y_i = 78.3 \qquad \sum_{i=1}^{8} y_i^2 = 838.49$$

Then the sample means and the pooled standard deviation can be computed:

$$\bar{x} = \frac{89.6}{8} = 11.2$$

$$\bar{y} = \frac{78.3}{8} = 9.8$$

$$s_X^2 = \frac{8(1053.70) - (89.6)^2}{8(7)} = 7.17$$

$$s_Y^2 = \frac{8(838.49) - (78.3)^2}{8(7)} = 10.30$$

The Two-Sample t-Test for Means (Equal Standard Deviations)

and

$$s_p = \sqrt{\frac{7(7.17) + 7(10.30)}{8 + 8 - 2}} = \sqrt{8.74}$$
$$= 3.0$$

(3) If H: $\mu_X = \mu_Y$ is true, the sampling distribution of
(4)

$$\frac{\bar{X} - \bar{Y}}{s_p\sqrt{\frac{1}{8} + \frac{1}{8}}}$$

is approximated by a Student t-curve with 14 (= 8 + 8 − 2) degrees of freedom. From Appendix II,

$$P\left\{-2.14 < \frac{\bar{X} - \bar{Y}}{s_p\sqrt{\frac{1}{8} + \frac{1}{8}}} < 2.14\right\} = .95$$

$$= P\left\{-2.14\, s_p\sqrt{\frac{1}{8} + \frac{1}{8}} < \bar{X} - \bar{Y} < 2.14\, s_p\sqrt{\frac{1}{8} + \frac{1}{8}}\right\} = .95$$

so that

$$(\bar{X} - \bar{Y})'_1 = -2.14(3.0)\sqrt{\frac{1}{8} + \frac{1}{8}} = -6.42\sqrt{.25}$$
$$= -3.21$$

and

$$(\bar{X} - \bar{Y})'_2 = 2.14(3.0)\sqrt{\frac{1}{8} + \frac{1}{8}}$$
$$= 3.21$$

Since the observed $\bar{x} - \bar{y} = 11.2 - 9.8 = 1.4$ lies *between* $(\bar{X} - \bar{Y})'_1$ and $(\bar{X} - \bar{Y})'_2$, H: $\mu_X = \mu_Y$ is accepted. There is no reason to believe (at the $P = .05$ level of significance) that the average bacterial counts in carpeted and uncarpeted rooms are different.

Question 5.2.1. Using these same data, test

H: $\mu_X = \mu_Y$ versus   A: $\mu_X \neq \mu_Y$

at the $P = .10$ level of significance.

Question 5.2.2. In steps (3) and (4), what was the reason for setting up the equation

$$P\left\{-2.14 < \frac{\bar{X} - \bar{Y}}{s_p\sqrt{\frac{1}{8} + \frac{1}{8}}} < 2.14\right\} = .95?$$

EXAMPLE 5.2.2. The Thematic Apperception Test (TAT)

One of the standard personality inventories used by psychologists is the Thematic Apperception Test. It consists of a series of pictures depicting a variety of everyday experiences. The subject is asked to examine the pictures carefully and to make up a story about each one. Interpreted properly, the content of these stories can provide valuable insights into the subject's mental well-being.

The following study was designed to see whether mothers of schizophrenic children would respond differently to the Thematic Apperception Test than mothers of normal children (Werner, Stabenau, and Pollin, 1970). A total of 40 mothers participated, 20 of whom had schizophrenic children. Each mother was shown the same set of 10 pictures. The 10 stories told by each of the mothers were then categorized according to the sort of parent–child relationship each one exhibited. The data shown here give the number of those stories showing a "positive" parent–child relationship, one where the mother was clearly capable of interacting with her child in a flexible, open-minded way.

Number of stories showing a "positive" parent–child relationship (out of 10)

Normal children		Schizophrenic children	
Mother	Score	Mother	Score
1	$x_1 = 8$	21	$y_1 = 2$
2	$x_2 = 4$	22	$y_2 = 1$
3	$x_3 = 6$	23	$y_3 = 1$
4	$x_4 = 3$	24	$y_4 = 3$
5	$x_5 = 1$	25	$y_5 = 2$
6	$x_6 = 4$	26	$y_6 = 7$
7	$x_7 = 4$	27	$y_7 = 2$
8	$x_8 = 6$	28	$y_8 = 1$
9	$x_9 = 4$	29	$y_9 = 3$
10	$x_{10} = 2$	30	$y_{10} = 1$
11	$x_{11} = 2$	31	$y_{11} = 0$
12	$x_{12} = 1$	32	$y_{12} = 2$
13	$x_{13} = 1$	33	$y_{13} = 4$
14	$x_{14} = 4$	34	$y_{14} = 2$
15	$x_{15} = 3$	35	$y_{15} = 3$
16	$x_{16} = 3$	36	$y_{16} = 3$
17	$x_{17} = 2$	37	$y_{17} = 0$
18	$x_{18} = 6$	38	$y_{18} = 1$
19	$x_{19} = 3$	39	$y_{19} = 2$
20	$x_{20} = 4$	40	$y_{20} = 2$

(1) Since it seems unlikely that the mother of a schizophrenic child will, in general, have a *better* relationship with her child than the mother of a normal child, the appropriate hypothesis test would be one-sided. If μ_X and μ_Y denote the true average numbers of "positive" stories told by

mothers of schizophrenic children, respectively, the hypotheses to be tested are

$$H: \mu_X = \mu_Y \quad \text{versus} \quad A: \mu_X > \mu_Y$$

Let $P = .05$.

(2) After computing

$$\sum_{i=1}^{20} x_i = 71 \quad \sum_{i=1}^{20} x_i^2 = 319$$

$$\sum_{i=1}^{20} y_i = 42 \quad \sum_{i=1}^{20} y_i^2 = 134$$

it follows that

$$\bar{x} = \frac{71}{20} = 3.6$$

$$\bar{y} = \frac{42}{20} = 2.1$$

$$s_X^2 = \frac{20(319) - (71)^2}{20(19)} = 3.52$$

$$s_Y^2 = \frac{20(134) - (42)^2}{20(19)} = 2.41$$

and

$$s_p = \sqrt{\frac{19(3.52) + (19)(2.41)}{20 + 20 - 2}} = \sqrt{2.96}$$

$$= 1.7$$

(3) When H is true, the sampling distribution of
(4)

$$\frac{\bar{X} - \bar{Y}}{s_p\sqrt{\frac{1}{20} + \frac{1}{20}}}$$

is approximated by a Student t-curve with 38 ($= 20 + 20 - 2$) degrees of freedom. But in keeping with the convention established in the previous chapter, any Student t-curve having 30 or more degrees of freedom will be treated as though it were a standard normal. Therefore,

$$P\left\{\frac{\bar{X} - \bar{Y}}{s_p\sqrt{\frac{1}{20} + \frac{1}{20}}} \geq 1.64\right\} = .05$$

or, equivalently,

$$P\left\{\bar{X} - \bar{Y} \geq 1.64\, s_p\sqrt{\frac{1}{20} + \frac{1}{20}}\right\} = .05$$

in which case the critical value is

$$(\bar{X} - \bar{Y})' = 1.64(1.7)\sqrt{\frac{1}{20} + \frac{1}{20}} = 2.79\sqrt{0.10}$$
$$= 0.9$$

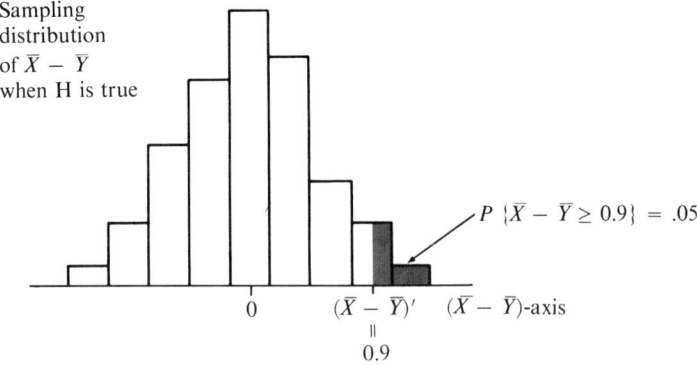

FIGURE 5.4

Therefore, since $\bar{x} - \bar{y} = 3.6 - 2.1 = 1.5$ exceeds $(\bar{X} - \bar{Y})'$, our conclusion would be to reject the null hypothesis.

Question 5.2.3. Since H: $\mu_X = \mu_Y$ was rejected in favor of A: $\mu_X > \mu_Y$ at the $P = .05$ level of significance, can it be concluded that mothers of schizophrenic children tend to be the "cause" of their parent–child relationships being less favorable?

5.3
THE TWO-SAMPLE t-TEST FOR MEANS (UNEQUAL STANDARD DEVIATIONS)

It was assumed in Section 5.2 (and in Theorem 5.2.1) that the standard deviations (σ_X and σ_Y) of the two populations being sampled (P_X and P_Y) were equal. Should that not be the case, the distribution of

$$\frac{\bar{X} - \bar{Y}}{S_p\sqrt{\frac{1}{n_X} + \frac{1}{n_Y}}}$$

will no longer be described by a Student t-curve with $n_X + n_Y - 2$ degrees of freedom and the methods of the last section will not be strictly valid. In the first part of this section, a procedure is developed for actually testing the assumption that σ_X equals σ_Y. Then, in the last part, a modified two-sample t-test is presented that can be used to test H: $\mu_X = \mu_Y$ in situations where H: $\sigma_X = \sigma_Y$ is rejected.

[5.3] The Two-Sample t-Test for Means (Unequal Standard Deviations)

Like μ_X and μ_Y, the values of σ_X and σ_Y are never known; but if the assumption of their equality is true, it seems reasonable to expect s_X to be fairly close to s_Y. For mathematical reasons, testing H: $\sigma_X = \sigma_Y$ is best accomplished by looking at the ratio of the squares of the sample standard deviations, s_X^2/s_Y^2. Of course, if the null hypothesis is true, s_X^2/s_Y^2 should be close to 1.

Since both s_X and s_Y will vary from sample to sample, it makes sense to talk about the *sampling distribution* of s_X^2/s_Y^2. More specifically, when $\sigma_X = \sigma_Y$ (and when P_X and P_Y are both bell-shaped) the sampling distribution of s_X^2/s_Y^2 can be approximated by a particular mathematical model known as the *F-distribution*.

Comment

The F-distribution is quite different than the normal and Student t-distributions. First, it is not symmetrical; second, being a ratio of squares, it cannot take on negative values.

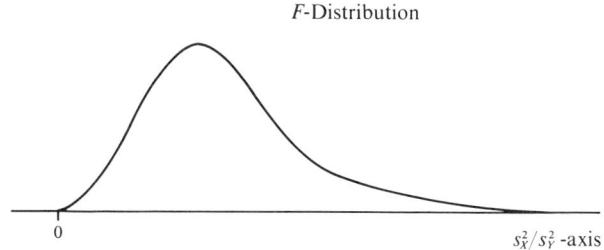

FIGURE 5.5

As was the case with the Student t-distribution, there is actually a *family* of F-distributions. But here the shape of each one is determined by *two* parameters N and D, where N equals $n_X - 1$ and D equals $n_Y - 1$. Both N and D are referred to as degrees of freedom; so if n_X was 10 and n_Y was 6, the sampling distribution of s_X^2/s_Y^2 would be approximated by the particular F-distribution having "9 and 5" degrees of freedom.

In deciding how the hypothesis that σ_X equals σ_Y should be tested, it follows, first of all, that the alternative should be two-sided. Secondly, it can be shown that the t-test of Section 5.2 is fairly robust to σ_X not being equal to σ_Y, which means that unless s_X is *much* different than s_Y, no modifications in that procedure need to be made. Therefore, no matter how the standard deviations are to be tested, the probability of committing a Type I error should be kept small.

Based on these considerations, we will verify (or not verify, as the case may be) the dispersion assumption of Theorem 5.2.1 by testing

$$\text{H:} \quad \sigma_X = \sigma_Y \quad \text{versus} \quad \text{A:} \quad \sigma_X \neq \sigma_Y$$

at the $P = .01$ level of significance. This requires that two critical values, $(s_X^2/s_Y^2)_1'$ and $(s_X^2/s_Y^2)_2'$, be found such that

$$P\left\{\left(\frac{s_X^2}{s_Y^2}\right) \leq \left(\frac{s_X^2}{s_Y^2}\right)_1'\right\} = .005 \quad \text{and} \quad P\left\{\left(\frac{s_X^2}{s_Y^2}\right) \geq \left(\frac{s_X^2}{s_Y^2}\right)_2'\right\} = .005$$

when H is true. The null hypothesis will be rejected if s_X^2/s_Y^2 is either *less than or equal to* $(s_X^2/s_Y^2)_1'$ or *greater than or equal to* $(s_X^2/s_Y^2)_2'$.

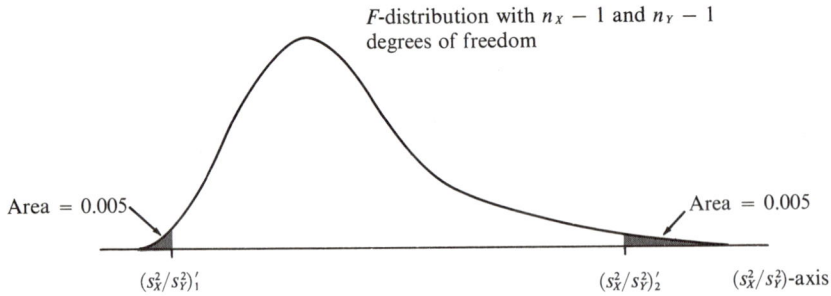

FIGURE 5.6

Values for $(s_X^2/s_Y^2)_1'$ and $(s_X^2/s_Y^2)_2'$ can be found directly from Appendix III. Suppose, for example, the $n_X = 9$ and $n_Y = 11$. Then $N = 8$ and $D = 10$, and from the body of the table $(s_X^2/s_Y^2)_1' = 0.139$ and $(s_X^2/s_Y^2)_2' = 6.12$. Similarly, if $n_X = 25$ and $n_Y = 16$, then $N = 24$, $D = 15$, $(s_X^2/s_Y^2)_1' = 0.308$, and $(s_X^2/s_Y^2)_2' = 3.79$.

Question 5.3.1. From the two numerical examples just given, and by looking at the values in Appendix III, it seems clear that as the sample sizes increase, the critical values in both the left-hand and right-hand tails converge to 1. Why should this be so?

EXAMPLE 5.3.1. Alpha Waves

Electroencephalograms are records showing fluctuations in electrical activity in the brain. In healthy individuals these fluctuations are quite rhythmic; but certain abnormalities, like epilepsy or brain tumors, can cause them to become very irregular. Actually, there are several different brain wave patterns produced simultaneously, with the dominant component usually being alpha waves. These have a characteristic frequency of anywhere from 8 to 13 cycles per second.

The objective of the following experiment was to see whether sensory deprivation over an extended period of time has any effect on a person's alpha-wave frequency (Gendreau et al., 1972). The subjects were 20 inmates of a maximum security prison in Kingston, Ontario. They were randomly split into two groups. The members of one group were put into solitary confinement; the inmates in the other group remained in their own cells. Seven days later, alpha-wave frequencies were measured for all 20 of the subjects.

[5.3] The Two-Sample t-Test for Means (Unequal Standard Deviations)

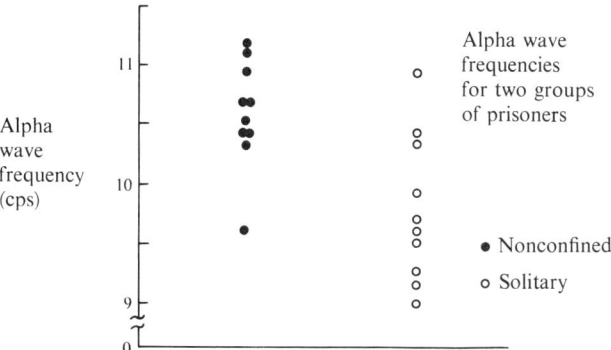

Alpha-wave frequencies (cps)

Nonconfined (x_i)	Solitary confinement (y_i)
10.7	9.6
10.7	10.4
10.4	9.7
10.9	10.3
10.5	9.2
10.3	9.3
9.6	9.9
11.1	9.5
11.2	9.0
10.4	10.9

FIGURE 5.7

From the graph, there is an apparent *decrease* in the alpha-wave frequency for persons in solitary confinement. It also seems that there might be an *increase* in the variability for that same group. The question is whether or not that increase is statistically significant.

(1) Let σ_X and σ_Y be the true standard deviations of alpha wave frequencies for nonconfined and solitary-confined groups, respectively. We want to test

$$H: \quad \sigma_X = \sigma_Y \quad \text{versus} \quad A: \quad \sigma_X \neq \sigma_Y$$

at the $P = .01$ level of significance.

(2) Since

$$\sum_{i=1}^{10} x_i = 105.8 \qquad \sum_{i=1}^{10} x_i^2 = 1121.26$$

$$\sum_{i=1}^{10} y_i = 97.8 \qquad \sum_{i=1}^{10} y_i^2 = 959.70$$

it follows that

$$s_X^2 = \frac{10(1121.26) - (105.8)^2}{10(9)} = 0.21$$

and

$$s_Y^2 = \frac{10(959.70) - (97.8)^2}{10(9)} = 0.36$$

(3) For these data, $n_X = 10$ and $n_Y = 10$, so N and D are 9 and 9, respectively.
(4) Therefore, the sampling distribution of s_X^2/s_Y^2, under the assumption that H: $\sigma_X = \sigma_Y$ is true, will be approximated by an F-curve with 9 and 9 degrees of freedom. Using Appendix III, note that the values cutting off areas of 0.005 in either tail of that distribution are 0.153 $[= (s_X^2/s_Y^2)_1']$ and 6.54 $[= (s_X^2/s_Y^2)_2']$. But

$$\frac{s_X^2}{s_Y^2} = \frac{0.21}{0.36} = 0.58$$

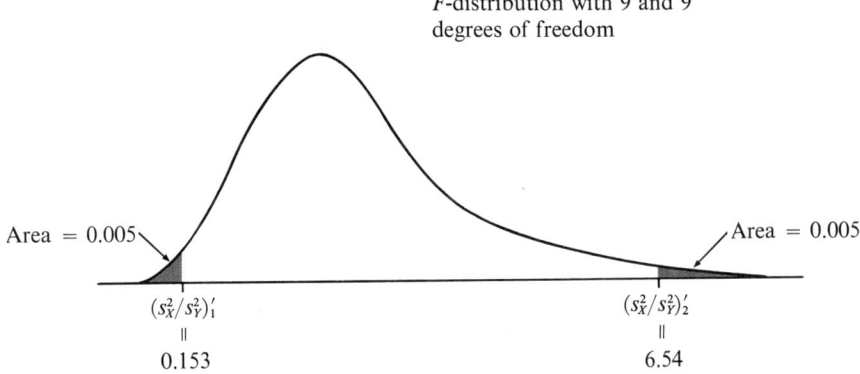

FIGURE 5.8

falls between $(s_X^2/s_Y^2)_1'$ and $(s_X^2/s_Y^2)_2'$ so H: $\sigma_X = \sigma_Y$ is accepted. The difference between the two sample standard deviations is not sufficiently large to warrant the conclusion that the population standard deviations are different. (Having reached this conclusion, it would now be appropriate to test the equality of μ_X and μ_Y with the two-sample t-test as described in Section 5.2.)

Question 5.3.2. Suppose that for two samples of sizes $n_X = 21$ and $n_Y = 15$, respectively, $s_X = 42.5$ and $s_Y = 19.6$. Test

H: $\sigma_X = \sigma_Y$ versus A: $\sigma_X \neq \sigma_Y$

at the $P = .01$ level of significance.

In the event that the standard deviations of the X and Y samples are so different that an F-test requires that H: $\sigma_X = \sigma_Y$ be rejected, a t-test for comparing μ_X and μ_Y can still be used — but only after certain modifications are made. These modifications are outlined in Theorem 5.3.1.

[5.3] The Two-Sample t-Test for Means (Unequal Standard Deviations)

> *Theorem 5.3.1.* Suppose two random samples, $(x_1, x_2, \ldots, x_{n_X})$ and $(y_1, y_2, \ldots, y_{n_Y})$, are drawn from two bell-shaped probability distributions having means μ_X and μ_Y and standard deviations σ_X and σ_Y. If H: $\sigma_X = \sigma_Y$ is rejected by an F-test, the sampling distribution of
>
> $$\frac{\bar{X} - \bar{Y}}{s_u} \quad \text{where} \quad s_u = \sqrt{\frac{s_X^2}{n_X} + \frac{s_Y^2}{n_Y}}$$
>
> can be approximated by a Student t-curve with f degrees of freedom, where f is the smallest integer larger than
>
> $$\frac{s_u^4}{\dfrac{\left(\dfrac{s_X^2}{n_X}\right)^2}{n_X - 1} + \dfrac{\left(\dfrac{s_Y^2}{n_Y}\right)^2}{n_Y - 1}}$$

The next example shows how Theorem 5.3.1 is applied.

EXAMPLE 5.3.2. Potential Differences as a Diagnostic Aid

Potential differences (PD) measured across certain parts of the intestinal tract have proven to be useful in diagnosing gastrointestinal disorders. With this as a precedent, an experiment was set up to see whether PD's could, in a similar way, distinguish diseases involving the esophagus (Vidins, Fox and Beck, 1971). Ten patients with clinically established esophagitis and 23 with no diseases of the esophagus were among those studied. The following table lists their esophageal PD's (in millivolts).

Potential differences (mV)							
Patients with esophagitis (x_i)		Controls (y_i)					
26	26	7	5	9	3	9	
15	39	4	7	16	3	6	
18	16	10	6	5	7	7	
32	10	2	6	1	6		
12	19	2	3	5	4		

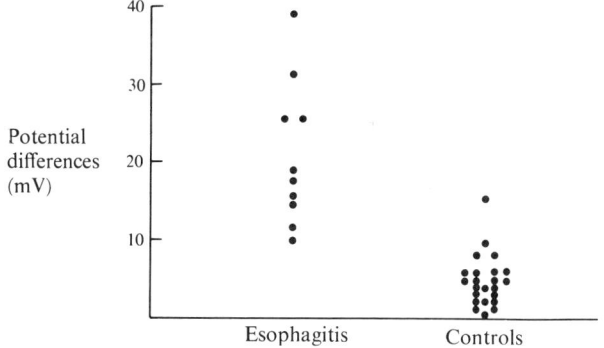

FIGURE 5.9

Model Three — The Two-Sample Problem [5.3]

Most likely, the ultimate concern here would be whether or not $\mu_X = \mu_Y$, but a quick look at the data indicates that s_X is considerably larger than s_Y — perhaps so much larger that H: $\sigma_X = \sigma_Y$ would have to be rejected, making the standard two-sample t-test invalid.

(1) First, then, we should do an F-test of

$$\text{H:} \quad \sigma_X = \sigma_Y \quad \text{versus} \quad \text{A:} \quad \sigma_X \neq \sigma_Y$$

(2) Since

$$\sum_{i=1}^{10} x_i = 213 \qquad \sum_{i=1}^{10} x_i^2 = 5307$$

$$\sum_{i=1}^{23} y_i = 129 \qquad \sum_{i=1}^{23} y_i^2 = 921$$

$$s_X^2 = \frac{10(5307) - (213)^2}{(10)9} = 85.6$$

and

$$s_Y^2 = \frac{23(921) - (129)^2}{(23)22} = 9.0$$

(3) If H: $\sigma_X = \sigma_Y$ is true, the sampling distribution of (s_X^2/s_Y^2) will be
(4) approximated by an F-curve with $N = 9$ and $D = 22$ degrees of freedom. That particular curve is not included in Appendix III, but a similar one has $N = 9$ and $D = 20$.

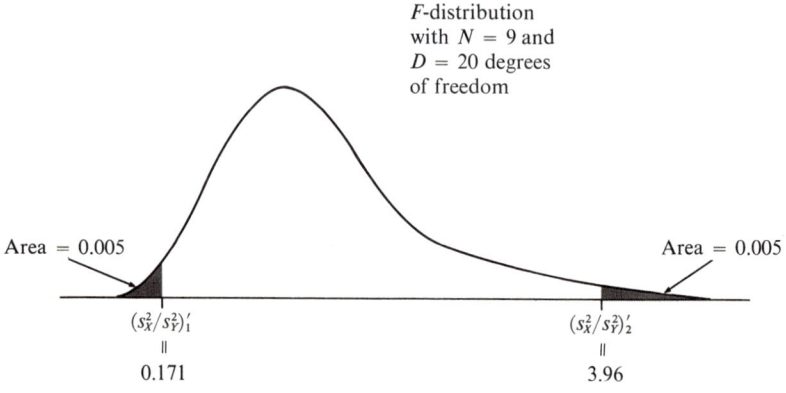

FIGURE 5.10

Since the observed ratio

$$\left(\frac{s_X^2}{s_Y^2}\right) = \frac{85.6}{9.0} = 9.4$$

exceeds the upper critical value, H: $\sigma_X = \sigma_Y$ should be rejected.

[5.3] The Two-Sample t-Test for Means (Unequal Standard Deviations)

At this point, with the assumption of Theorem 5.2.1 having been rejected, there is only one direction the analysis can take. It must appeal to Theorem 5.3.1.

(1) The hypotheses to be tested are

$$H: \quad \mu_X = \mu_Y \quad \text{versus} \quad A: \quad \mu_X \neq \mu_Y$$

Let $P = .05$.

(2) Note that

$$S_u = \sqrt{\frac{s_X^2}{n_X} + \frac{s_Y^2}{n_Y}} = \sqrt{\frac{85.6}{10} + \frac{9.0}{23}}$$
$$= \sqrt{8.56 + 0.39} = \sqrt{8.85} = 3.0$$

so that

$$f \approx \frac{s_u^4}{\dfrac{\left(\dfrac{s_X^2}{n_X}\right)^2}{n_X - 1} + \dfrac{\left(\dfrac{s_Y^2}{n_Y}\right)^2}{n_Y - 1}}$$

$$= \frac{(3.0)^4}{\dfrac{\left(\dfrac{85.6}{10}\right)^2}{10 - 1} + \dfrac{\left(\dfrac{9.0}{23}\right)^2}{23 - 1}} = \frac{81.0}{\dfrac{71.64}{9} + \dfrac{0.15}{22}}$$

$$= \frac{81.0}{7.96 + 0.01} = \frac{81.0}{7.97} = 10.2$$

$$\approx 11 \text{ (rounded up)}$$

(3) By Theorem 5.3.1, the sampling distribution of
(4)

$$\frac{\bar{X} - \bar{Y}}{S_u}$$

can be approximated by a Student t-curve with 11 degrees of freedom. From Appendix II,

$$P\left\{-2.20 < \frac{\bar{X} - \bar{Y}}{S_u} < 2.20\right\} = .95$$

so the two critical values for $\bar{x} - \bar{y}$ are

$$(\bar{X} - \bar{Y})_1' = -2.20 \, s_u = -2.20 \, (3.0) = -6.6$$

and

$$(\bar{X} - \bar{Y})_2' = 2.20 \, s_u = 6.6$$

194 Model Three — The Two-Sample Problem [5.4]

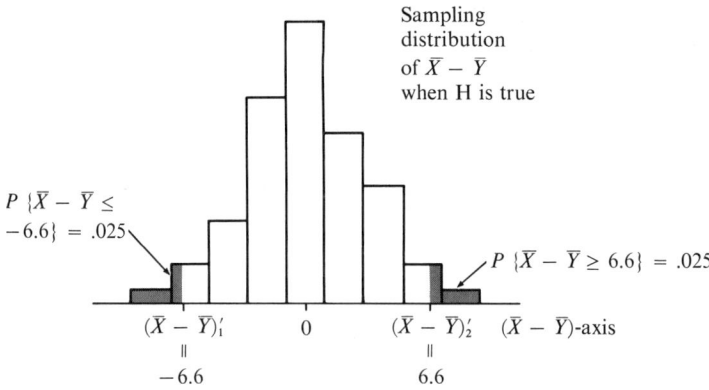

FIGURE 5.11

For these data, $\bar{x} = 213/10 = 21.3$ and $\bar{y} = 129/23 = 5.6$, making $\bar{x} - \bar{y} = 21.3 - 5.6 = 15.7$. Therefore, H: $\mu_X = \mu_Y$ should be rejected. There is a statistically significant increase in the characteristic esophageal potential difference of persons with esophagitis.

Comment

In a sense, the "price" that was paid as a result of σ_X not being equal to σ_Y was 20 degrees of freedom. Had the usual t-test been appropriate, the sampling distribution of

$$\frac{\bar{X} - \bar{Y}}{S_p\sqrt{\frac{1}{n_X} + \frac{1}{n_Y}}}$$

would have had 31 degrees of freedom.

Question 5.3.3. All other factors being equal, why is it better to do a t-test with 31, rather than 11, degrees of freedom?

5.4
CONFIDENCE INTERVALS FOR $\mu_X - \mu_Y$

Having discussed in the previous two sections how to test the equality of two means, H: $\mu_X = \mu_Y$, it remains a simple matter to construct a confidence interval for their difference, $\mu_X - \mu_Y$. If $\sigma_X = \sigma_Y$, and if both P_X and P_Y are essentially bell-shaped, it can be shown that the sampling distribution of

$$\frac{\bar{X} - \bar{Y} - (\mu_X - \mu_Y)}{S_p\sqrt{\frac{1}{n_X} + \frac{1}{n_Y}}}$$

is approximated by a Student t-curve with $n_X + n_Y - 2$ degrees of freedom.

Comment

The preceding statement is actually a more general result than that given in Theorem 5.2.1. In the particular case where $\mu_X = \mu_Y$,

$$\frac{\bar{X} - \bar{Y} - (\mu_X - \mu_Y)}{S_p\sqrt{\frac{1}{n_X} + \frac{1}{n_Y}}}$$

reduces to the more familiar

$$\frac{\bar{X} - \bar{Y}}{S_p\sqrt{\frac{1}{n_X} + \frac{1}{n_Y}}}$$

If $-t$ and $+t$ are numbers that cut off areas of, say 0.025 in either tail of the Student t-curve with $n_X + n_Y - 2$ degrees of freedom, then

$$P\left\{-t \leq \frac{\bar{X} - \bar{Y} - (\mu_X - \mu_Y)}{S_p\sqrt{\frac{1}{n_X} + \frac{1}{n_Y}}} \leq t\right\} = .95$$

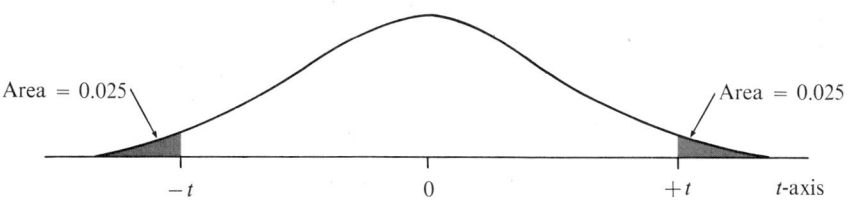

FIGURE 5.12

Multiplying every term by the denominator of the center expression gives

$$P\left\{-t \cdot S_p\sqrt{\frac{1}{n_X} + \frac{1}{n_Y}} \leq \bar{X} - \bar{Y} - (\mu_X - \mu_Y) \leq t \cdot S_p\sqrt{\frac{1}{n_X} + \frac{1}{n_Y}}\right\} = .95$$

Subtracting $\bar{X} - \bar{Y}$ from each expression and multiplying what is left by -1 gives

$$P\left\{\bar{X} - \bar{Y} - t \cdot S_p\sqrt{\frac{1}{n_X} + \frac{1}{n_Y}} \leq \mu_X - \mu_Y \leq \bar{X} - \bar{Y} + t \cdot S_p\sqrt{\frac{1}{n_X} + \frac{1}{n_Y}}\right\} = .95$$

The set of values from $\bar{x} - \bar{y} - t \cdot s_p\sqrt{(1/n_X) + (1/n_Y)}$ to $\bar{x} - \bar{y} + t \cdot s_p\sqrt{(1/n_X) + (1/n_Y)}$ is said to be a *95% confidence interval for* $\mu_X - \mu_Y$. In the long run, 95% of the intervals constructed in this fashion will include the true value of $\mu_X - \mu_Y$.

Question 5.4.1. If σ_X were *not* equal to σ_Y, according to an F-test, what quantity would be used in place of

$$\frac{\bar{X} - \bar{Y} - (\mu_X - \mu_Y)}{S_p\sqrt{\frac{1}{n_X} + \frac{1}{n_Y}}}$$

in the confidence interval derivation and what mathematical model would be used to describe its behavior?

Comment

If $n_X + n_Y - 2$ is 30 or more, or if σ_X and σ_Y are known, Z-values are substituted for t-values in the expressions for the upper and lower confidence limits.

EXAMPLE 5.4.1. Sexual Differences in Human Teeth

Occasionally in forensic medicine, or in the aftermath of a bad accident, identifying the sex of a victim can be very difficult. In some of these cases, dental structure can provide a useful criterion, since individual teeth will remain in good condition long after other tissues have deteriorated. Furthermore, studies have shown that female teeth and male teeth have different physical and chemical characteristics.

The extent to which X-rays can penetrate tooth enamel, for instance, is different for men and women. Listed below are "spectropenetration gradients" for eight female teeth and eight male teeth (Furuhata and Yamamoto, 1967). This particular variable is a measure of the rate of change in the amount of X-ray penetration through a 500-micron section of tooth enamel at a wavelength of 600 mμ as opposed to 400 mμ.

Enamel spectropenetration gradients	
Male	Female
4.9	4.8
5.4	5.3
5.0	3.7
5.5	4.1
5.4	5.6
6.6	4.0
6.3	3.6
4.3	5.0

Let μ_X and μ_Y be the population means of the spectropenetration gradients associated with male teeth and with female teeth, respectively. To find a 95% confidence interval for $\mu_X - \mu_Y$, note that

$$\sum_{i=1}^{8} x_i = 43.4 \qquad \sum_{i=1}^{8} x_i^2 = 239.32$$

from which
$$\bar{x} = \frac{43.4}{8} = 5.4$$
and
$$s_X^2 = \frac{8(239.32) - (43.4)^2}{8(7)} = 0.55$$
Similarly,
$$\sum_{i=1}^{8} y_i = 36.1 \qquad \sum_{i=1}^{8} y_i^2 = 166.95$$
so that
$$\bar{y} = \frac{36.1}{8} = 4.5$$
and
$$s_Y^2 = \frac{8(166.95) - (36.1)^2}{8(7)} = 0.58$$

Therefore, the pooled standard deviation is equal to
$$s_p = \sqrt{\frac{(n_X - 1)s_X^2 + (n_Y - 1)s_Y^2}{n_X + n_Y - 2}} = \sqrt{\frac{7(0.55) + 7(0.58)}{8 + 8 - 2}}$$
$$= \sqrt{0.565} = 0.75$$

The quantity
$$\frac{\bar{X} - \bar{Y} - (\mu_X - \mu_Y)}{s_p\sqrt{\frac{1}{8} + \frac{1}{8}}}$$
will be approximated by a Student t-curve with 14 degrees of freedom, so a 95% confidence interval for $\mu_X - \mu_Y$ is given by
$$\left(\bar{x} - \bar{y} - 2.14\, s_p\sqrt{\frac{1}{8} + \frac{1}{8}},\; \bar{x} - \bar{y} + 2.14\, s_p\sqrt{\frac{1}{8} + \frac{1}{8}}\right)$$
$$= (5.4 - 4.5 - 2.14(0.75)\sqrt{0.25},\; 5.4 - 4.5 + 2.14(0.75)\sqrt{0.25})$$
$$= (0.9 - 0.8,\; 0.9 + 0.8)$$
$$= (0.1, 1.7)$$

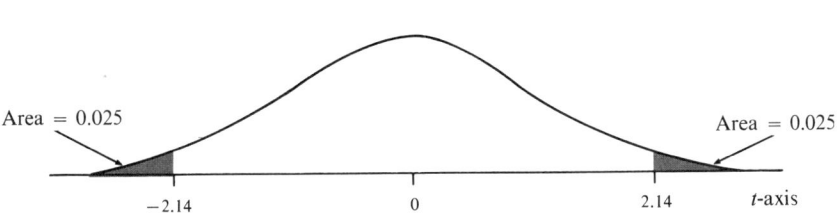

FIGURE 5.13

Comment

The fact that this interval does not include the value 0 means that H: $\mu_X = \mu_Y$ would have been rejected in favor of H: $\mu_X \neq \mu_Y$ at the $P = .05$ level of significance.

Comment

In practice, inference in the two-sample problem generally takes the form of a hypothesis test rather than a confidence interval. This is more a reflection of years of tradition than any superiority of one method over the other. Mathematically, the two approaches are equivalent. The real purpose in developing confidence intervals for $\mu_X - \mu_Y$ is to show how easy it is to adapt the methods of Chapter 4 to other situations.

Question 5.4.2. Do an F-test on the spectropenetration gradients.

Question 5.4.3. How would

$$\text{H:} \quad \mu_X = \mu_Y + 2 \quad \text{versus} \quad \text{A:} \quad \mu_X \neq \mu_Y + 2$$

be tested? *Hint:* Compute $\mu_X - \mu_Y$ when H is true and use the sampling result given at the beginning of this section.

Question 5.4.4. Use the data of Example 1.7.1 to construct a 99% confidence interval for the difference between the average caloric outputs of normal persons (x) and those of persons with Raynaud's syndrome (y).

Note:
$$\sum_{i=1}^{10} x_i = 21.13 \qquad \sum_{i=1}^{10} x_i^2 = 45.87$$

$$\sum_{i=1}^{10} y_i = 6.15 \qquad \sum_{i=1}^{10} y_i^2 = 4.13$$

5.5 SUMMARY

Inference in the two-sample problem follows the same formats previously established for the one-sample problem. Generally, attention is focused on the population means and whether or not they can be assumed equal. However, before testing H: $\mu_X = \mu_Y$, it is necessary to determine the credibility of H: $\sigma_X = \sigma_Y$. If the latter hypothesis *is* true, the appropriate *t*-test for H: $\mu_X = \mu_Y$ involves $n_X + n_Y - 2$ degrees of freedom. If it *is not* true, certain adjustments must be made, including a reduction in the number of degrees of freedom (see Theorem 5.3.1).

The effects that the standard deviations have on the ultimate form of the *t*-test once again underscore the importance of doing a *graphical* analysis prior to a *mathematical* analysis. The first step taken with *any* set of Model Three data should be to plot the two samples on a graph similar to the ones used in Examples 5.2.1, 5.3.1, and 5.3.2. Then, by inspection, it should be clear whether a formal test of H: $\sigma_X = \sigma_Y$ is warranted. Only after a decision is reached about σ_X and σ_Y can we know which approach to follow in testing the equality of μ_X and μ_Y.

The one new concept in this chapter is the *F-distribution*, a mathematical model which describes the behavior of s_X^2/s_Y^2 under the assumption that the population standard deviations are equal. Values of s_X^2/s_Y^2 much smaller or much larger than 1 lead to the rejection of H: $\sigma_X = \sigma_Y$ in favor of A: $\sigma_X \neq \sigma_Y$. Selected critical values for the *F*-test, at the $P = .01$ level of significance, are provided in Appendix III.

Definitions

F-distribution. A mathematical model describing the behavior of s_X^2/s_Y^2 when $\sigma_X = \sigma_Y$ and both P_X and P_Y are bell-shaped.

F-test. A procedure, based on the statistic s_X^2/s_Y^2, for testing the equality of two population standard deviations; in two-sample problems, an *F*-test of H: $\sigma_X = \sigma_Y$ dictates which form of the *t*-test should be used for H: $\mu_X = \mu_Y$.

Pooled standard deviation (s_p). If, on the basis of s_X^2/s_Y^2, the hypothesis H: $\sigma_X = \sigma_Y$ can be accepted, a combined or "pooled" estimate (s_p) is made of $\sigma(=\sigma_X = \sigma_Y)$; in particular,

$$s_p = \sqrt{\frac{(n_X - 1)s_X^2 + (n_Y - 1)s_Y^2}{n_X + n_Y - 2}}$$

Two-sample t-test. A variation of the (one-sample) Student *t*-test first introduced in Chapter 4; used for testing the equality of two population means, H: $\mu_X = \mu_Y$. It has two basic forms, depending on whether the population standard deviations are assumed to be equal or unequal.

Review Exercises

5.1 The effectiveness of charcoal filters has been demonstrated in experiments with protozoa (Weiss, 1968). *Paramecium aurelia* were suspended in a hanging drop inside a smoke chamber. Every 60 seconds, a 6-second puff of smoke was drawn through the chamber. The movements of the paramecia were watched through a stereomicroscope. The variable recorded was the length of time from the start of the experiment to when the last paramecium died. Altogether, the experiment was replicated 12 times. Six of those times the smoke came from a nonfilter cigarette; for the other six, from a cigarette with a charcoal filter,

Survival time (minutes)	
Nonfilter (x_i)	Charcoal filter (y_i)
7	14
8	17
8	19
8	21
9	24
11	37

(a) Graph the data.
(b) Test

$$H: \quad \sigma_X = \sigma_Y \quad \text{versus} \quad A: \quad \sigma_X \neq \sigma_Y$$

at the $P = .01$ level of significance.
(c) Test

$$H: \quad \mu_X = \mu_Y \quad \text{versus} \quad A: \quad \mu_X < \mu_Y$$

at the $P = .05$ level of significance.

5.2 Refer to the data of Example 1.7.2. Let μ_X denote the true average spleen weight of patients with thrombocytopenia for whom a splenectomy would be of no benefit; let μ_Y be similarly defined for patients whose conditions *would* be improved with a splenectomy. Test

$$H: \quad \mu_X = \mu_Y \quad \text{versus} \quad A: \quad \mu_X \neq \mu_Y$$

at the $P = .05$ level of significance. Note that

$$\sum_{i=1}^{5} x_i = 565 \quad \sum_{i=1}^{5} x_i^2 = 76{,}425$$

$$\sum_{i=1}^{14} y_i = 2{,}226 \quad \sum_{i=1}^{14} y_i^2 = 386{,}356$$

5.3 Serotonin is a substance found in the blood that may or may not be related to psychiatric disorders. Also, its concentration may or may not be affected by chronic LSD usage. A two-sample experiment was done to see if any relationship could be established between LSD usage and serotonin formation in an animal population (Diaz and Huttunen, 1971). Twenty-six rats were given a daily oral dose of 20 μg of LSD-25 per kg of body weight. The LSD was dissolved in 1 ml of water. (This particular dosage was thought to be comparable in effect to the dosage a person might take.) A similar procedure was followed with a control group of 25 rats, but their "treatment" consisted of just the water. After 30 days, the animals were sacrificed and the concentrations of serotonin in their brains were measured.

Serotonin concentration (nmole/g)

Control group	LSD group
2.84 ± 0.06 (25)	3.20 ± 0.15 (26)

(a) Define all the relevant parameters and do the appropriate test(s).

(b) Was it necessary that rats in the control group actually be given the 1 ml "dose" of water each day?

5.4 Why wouldn't it be reasonable always to define the pooled standard deviation as the square root of the average of the squared sample standard deviations:

$$s_p = \sqrt{\frac{s_X^2 + s_Y^2}{2}}$$

5.5 One of the "parameters" used in evaluating myocardial function is the end diastolic volume (EDV). Shown below are EDV's recorded for eight persons considered to have normal cardiac function and for six with constrictive pericarditis (Vogel, Horgan, and Strahl, 1971).

End diastolic volume (ml/m²)

Normal (x)	Constrictive pericarditis (y)
62	24
60	56
78	42
62	74
49	44
67	28
80	
48	

(a) Graph the data.

(b) Construct a 95% confidence interval for the difference between the population means that these samples represent.

$$\sum_{i=1}^{8} x_i = 506 \qquad \sum_{i=1}^{8} x_i^2 = 32{,}966$$

$$\sum_{i=1}^{6} y_i = 268 \qquad \sum_{i=1}^{6} y_i^2 = 13{,}672$$

5.6 Test H: $\mu_X = \mu_Y$ against a two-sided alternative for the alpha-wave data of Example 5.3.1. Use the $P = .05$ level of significance.

5.7 In general, if H: $\mu_X = \mu_Y$ is rejected at the P level of significance (in favor of a two-sided alternative), the $100(1 - P)\%$ confidence interval for $\mu_X - \mu_Y$ will not contain 0. Explain why this should be true.

5.8 Out of 31 patients undergoing exploratory surgery for undiagnosed conditions of the lumbar region, a total of 22 were found to have prolapsed, or herniated, discs (Nachemson, 1969). The following are intradiscal pH readings taken on each of the patients.

	Intradiscal pH			
Confirmed prolapse			No prolapse	
6.9	6.9	6.6	7.3	5.7
6.6	6.9	7.4	7.5	7.0
6.8	7.5	7.4	6.2	6.6
7.1	6.7	7.4	6.8	7.2
7.0	7.1	6.8	6.0	
7.0	7.0	7.4		
6.7	6.6	6.7		
7.1				

(a) Graph the data.

(b) State and test an appropriate hypothesis. Define all the parameters in question. State whatever assumptions need to be made. *Note:* If x's and y's are used to denote the pH values associated with the confirmed-prolapse and the no-prolapse groups, respectively, then

$$\sum_{i=1}^{22} x_i = 153.6 \qquad \sum_{i=1}^{22} x_i^2 = 1074.18$$

$$\sum_{i=1}^{9} y_i = 60.3 \qquad \sum_{i=1}^{9} y_i^2 = 407.11$$

5.9 The preening habits of male and female fruit flies (*Drosophila melanogaster*) were the subject of a recent study (Connolly, 1968). The experiment was done in a small chamber that was divided into two parts by a glass partition. Ten flies of one sex were put into one side of the chamber and a single fly of the same sex into the other. (Only flies of a single sex were used so that courtship rituals would not be a factor.) Then, for a three-minute interval, the preening behavior of the single fly was carefully monitored, for both the number of distinct preening actions as well as their duration. Eventually, the entire experiment was done 30 times, 15 times

Average preening time per bout (sec)	
Male (x)	Female (y)
2.3	3.7
1.9	5.4
3.3	2.2
2.9	11.7
2.2	2.8
1.3	2.4
2.2	4.0
2.4	2.8
2.1	2.0
1.2	2.8
2.0	2.4
2.7	2.4
2.3	2.9
1.9	10.7
1.2	3.2

Model Three — The Two-Sample Problem

with male flies and 15 times with female flies. Listed above are the average lengths of time spent by each of the 30 single flies in a preening "bout." Analyze these data. Note that

$$\sum_{i=1}^{15} x_i = 31.9 \qquad \sum_{i=1}^{15} x_i^2 = 72.81$$

$$\sum_{i=1}^{15} y_i = 61.4 \qquad \sum_{i=1}^{15} y_i^2 = 378.52$$

6

MODEL FOUR
The Paired-Data Problem

Chance is nothing; there is no such thing as chance. What we call by that name is the effect which we see of a cause which we do not see.
                                                    Voltaire

6.1 INTRODUCTION

Paired-data problems are similar to two-sample problems in many ways: they both involve two samples, each representing one of two population distributions (P_X and P_Y), and their usual objective is to determine whether or not one of the distributions has shifted in location relative to the other. That is, they both test H: $\mu_X = \mu_Y$. Where the two differ is in the *way* they test H: $\mu_X = \mu_Y$, and in the way the data are collected.

Consider, again, the two-sample t-test of Chapter 5. There the observed location difference *between* the samples, $\bar{x} - \bar{y}$, was compared to the observed variability *within* the samples, s_p (by using the fact that $(\bar{x} - \bar{y})/s_p\sqrt{(1/n_X) + (1/n_Y)}$ has a Student t-distribution with $n_X + n_Y - 2$ degrees of freedom). That means that no matter how large $\bar{x} - \bar{y}$ might be, $s_p\sqrt{(1/n_X) + (1/n_Y)}$ can, itself, be sufficiently large so that the ratio $(\bar{x} - \bar{y})/s_p\sqrt{(1/n_X) + (1/n_Y)}$ will cause H: $\mu_X = \mu_Y$ *not* to be rejected. That is, the denominator can "obscure" the numerator.

Model Four — The Paired-Data Problem

For example, suppose that in a Model Three analysis, $n_X = 8$, $n_Y = 10$, $\bar{x} = 6.3$, $\bar{y} = 4.2$, and that H: $\mu_X = \mu_Y$ is being tested against H: $\mu_X > \mu_Y$ at the $P = .05$ level of significance. For a t-distribution with $16 (= 8 + 10 - 2)$ degrees of freedom,

$$P\{t \geq 1.75\} = .05$$

implying that H will be rejected if

$$\bar{x} - \bar{y} \geq 1.75 \, s_p \sqrt{\frac{1}{n_X} + \frac{1}{n_Y}}$$

But since $\bar{x} - \bar{y}$ is known to equal $6.3 - 4.2 = 2.1$, it also follows that H will be rejected only if

$$s_p \leq \frac{\bar{x} - \bar{y}}{1.75 \sqrt{\frac{1}{n_X} + \frac{1}{n_Y}}} = \frac{2.1}{1.75 \sqrt{\frac{1}{8} + \frac{1}{10}}} = 2.53$$

That is, any amount of "within variability" greater than $s_p = 2.53$ will negate the observed difference in location ($\bar{x} - \bar{y} = 2.1$) in the sense that we can no longer say that that difference is statistically significant at the $P = .05$ level.

To understand the implication of this fully, and to understand how it relates to the paired-data problem, we need to keep in mind what it is that contributes to the numerical value of the x's and the y's and to the numerical value of s_p. One factor, of course, is the treatment effect. But if this were the *only* factor, s_p would be 0; all the individuals receiving treatment T_X would respond alike, as would all the individuals given treatment T_Y. Needless to say, this does not happen, the reason being that there are many factors other than the treatments that influence the measured response. These other sources of variation can be thought of as falling into two groups: (1) those associated with the subjects and (2) those associated with the experimental procedure.

For example, suppose that in a clinical trial Patient 1 is given Pain reliever A and Patient 2, Pain reliever B, with the following results:

Hours of relief

Patient	Pain reliever A	Patient	Pain reliever B
1	4½	2	6

That Patient 1's response (4½ hours) differed from Patient 2's response (6 hours) can be attributed to three sources: (1) the treatment effect — Pain reliever A is not the same, chemically, as Pain reliever B; (2) the subject effect — Patient 1 is physically different from Patient 2; and (3) all other effects — either or both drugs were administered improperly, each patient interpreted "relief" in a different way, etc. The net contribution of this third source of variation is referred to as *experimental error*.

In most experiments it is the treatment effect that is of primary interest. The subject effect and experimental error are simply nuisance factors. The difference between a Model Three analysis and a Model Four analysis centers around the subject effect. As we have just seen, in a two-sample t-test, the treatment effect (as measured by $\bar{x} - \bar{y}$) is compared to the combined influence of the subject effect and the experimental error — namely, s_p. But in a paired-data analysis, the measurements are collected in such a way that the subject effect is greatly reduced, thereby allowing the treatment effect, still estimated by $\bar{x} - \bar{y}$, to be compared to a smaller s_p. All of this is accomplished by grouping the original sample into pairs, and having the members of each pair be as similar as possible.

For instance, suppose a nutrition experiment involving two diets (A and B) is to be done using four subjects:

Subject	Sex	Height	Weight	Present status
A.B.	M	5'10"	190	slightly overweight
C.L.	M	5'8"	210	very overweight
D.S.	M	6'0"	250	very overweight
H.W.	M	5'6"	165	slightly overweight

Even before starting, a reasonable assumption to make is that the amount of weight a person will lose is related to the extent that he is already overweight. Therefore, the two subjects *most* likely to lose weight are C.L. and D.S.; the two *least* likely are A.B. and H.W. Therefore, if this experiment were to be carried out as a Model Four problem, we would pair together the first two (C.L. and D.S.) and the last two (A.B. and H.W.). Then each of the two diets would be assigned to one member in each pair. It follows that the observed difference in the responses between, say, C.L. and D.S., would be due primarily to the treatment effect and to experimental error. The subject effect would not have contributed very much, since C.L. and D.S. are quite similar relative to the variable being measured.

In Section 6.2, a *paired t-test* is introduced for analyzing these "within-pair" differences. Mathematically, the paired t-test is exactly the same as the one-sample t-test of Chapter 4, but the notation is slightly different. In Section 6.3, the problem of titers is considered. As indicated in Review Exercise 1.5, studies evaluating the body's immunological response either to a naturally acquired infection or to a vaccine eventually involve the analysis of antibody counts, or titers. Experiments of this sort can be designed in several ways but often they fall within the domain of Model Four. (Readers not familiar with logarithms should omit this section.)

For physical reasons, not all experiments comparing two treatments can be performed as paired-data problems. But when the opportunity presents itself, it should be weighed carefully. A Model Four analysis is often vastly superior to a Model Three analysis in terms of reaching a clear-cut decision with a minimum of observations.

6.2
A STUDENT t-TEST FOR PAIRED DATA

It is assumed here that the total sample for each analysis has already been paired according to whatever criterion is relevant for the situation at hand. As indicated in Section 1.8, this might have been done on the basis of age, sex, present health status, heredity, or a host of other factors. Or the experiment itself might have been designed as a "before" and "after" study, in which case each individual subject acts as a pair.

But regardless of how the subjects are grouped, two similar observations (x_i and y_i) will be recorded for each of the n pairs — x_i, for example, representing the response of whichever member of the ith pair received treatment T_X. Note that the numerical difference between the two responses for the ith pair — namely, $y_i - x_i \ (= d_i)$ — is a good estimate of the treatment effect, one that is as free as possible of any subject effect.

The primary "target" in paired-data problems, as in two-sample problems, involves the two population means, μ_X and μ_Y. But in Model Four that target is approached somewhat indirectly. Rather than thinking in terms of the population distributions (P_X and P_Y) associated with the two treatments, we will, instead, focus on the population distribution (P_D) associated with the pair *differences*, $y_i - x_i$. When $\mu_X = \mu_Y$, the mean of P_D (denoted μ_D) will be 0, so a (two-sided) test of the treatment effect can be expressed as

$$\text{H:} \quad \mu_D = 0 \quad (\mu_X = \mu_Y)$$

versus

$$\text{A:} \quad \mu_D \neq 0 \quad (\mu_X \neq \mu_Y)$$

In light of our past experience with $\bar{X}$, it would seem reasonable to base a test of H: $\mu_D = 0$ on the observed average difference *within the pairs;* that is, on $\bar{d}$, where

$$\bar{d} = \frac{1}{n} \sum_{i=1}^{n} d_i = \frac{1}{n} \sum_{i=1}^{n} (y_i - x_i)$$

Theorem 6.2.1 defines the *sampling distribution of* $\bar{D}$ and gives the properties of that distribution which are necessary for testing hypotheses about μ_D.

Theorem 6.2.1. Let $\{(x_1, y_1), (x_2, y_2), \ldots, (x_n, y_n)\}$ be the set of responses recorded for the members of n different pairs. Let $(d_1, d_2, \ldots, d_n)$ be the corresponding pair differences, $d_i = y_i - x_i$, and let $\bar{d} = (1/n) \sum_{i=1}^{n} d_i$. If the population mean, μ_D, for the pair differences is 0, the sampling distribution of $\bar{D}$ will have mean equal to 0 and standard deviation (approximately) equal to $s_d/\sqrt{n}$, where

$$s_d = \sqrt{\frac{n \sum_{i=1}^{n} d_i^2 - \left(\sum_{i=1}^{n} d_i\right)^2}{n(n-1)}}$$

Also, if P_X and P_Y are both bell-shaped, the distribution of

$$\frac{\bar{D}}{s_d/\sqrt{n}}$$

will be described by a Student t-curve with $n - 1$ degrees of freedom. When n is greater than 30, the distribution of

$$\frac{\bar{D}}{s_d/\sqrt{n}}$$

is similar to the standard normal.

Except for notation, $\bar{D}/(s_d/\sqrt{n})$ is the same as the statistic $\bar{X}/(s/\sqrt{n})$ that was introduced in Section 4.3. And, as the next two examples show, hypothesis tests for μ_D (Model Four) and hypothesis tests for μ (Model Two) are done in exactly the same way.

EXAMPLE 6.2.1. Drug Therapy for Learning Problems

A double-blind study was set up to evaluate the effectiveness of ethosuximide, a petit-mal anticonvulsant, as a learning "facilitator" (Smith, 1970). The subjects were 10 children ranging in age from 8 to 14, all with a history of learning and behavioral problems. The experiment lasted six weeks. For three of those weeks a child was given a placebo; for the other three weeks, ethosuximide. After each three-week period; each child was given several parts of the Wechsler IQ Test. Listed in the accompanying table are the two verbal IQ scores recorded for each child.

Verbal IQ scores

Child	Placebo (x_i)	Ethosuximide (y_i)
1	97	113
2	106	113
3	106	101
4	95	119
5	102	111
6	111	122
7	115	121
8	104	106
9	90	110
10	96	126

(1) If μ_D denotes the mean of the population distribution associated with differences of the form $y_i - x_i$, the hypotheses to be tested are

H: $\mu_D = 0$ [ethosuximide has *no* effect]

A: $\mu_D \neq 0$ [ethosuximide has *some* effect]

(A two-sided alternative is used here because it is not obvious that if ethosuximide *does* have an effect, that effect will be positive.) Let $P = .05$.

(2) To find $\bar{d}$ and s_d, it is necessary to compute the 10 treatment differences and their squares.

Child	Placebo (x_i)	Ethosuximide (y_i)	$d_i = y_i - x_i$	d_i^2
1	$x_1 = 97$	$y_1 = 113$	$d_1 = 16$	$d_1^2 = 256$
2	$x_2 = 106$	$y_2 = 113$	$d_2 = 7$	$d_2^2 = 49$
3	$x_3 = 106$	$y_3 = 101$	$d_3 = -5$	$d_3^2 = 25$
4	$x_4 = 95$	$y_4 = 119$	$d_4 = 24$	$d_4^2 = 576$
5	$x_5 = 102$	$y_5 = 111$	$d_5 = 9$	$d_5^2 = 81$
6	$x_6 = 111$	$y_6 = 122$	$d_6 = 11$	$d_6^2 = 121$
7	$x_7 = 115$	$y_7 = 121$	$d_7 = 6$	$d_7^2 = 36$
8	$x_8 = 104$	$y_8 = 106$	$d_8 = 2$	$d_8^2 = 4$
9	$x_9 = 90$	$y_9 = 110$	$d_9 = 20$	$d_9^2 = 400$
10	$x_{10} = 96$	$y_{10} = 126$	$d_{10} = 30$	$d_{10}^2 = 900$
			$\sum_{i=1}^{10} d_i = 120$	$\sum_{i=1}^{10} d_i^2 = 2{,}448$

Therefore,

$$\bar{d} = \frac{120}{10} = 12.0$$

and

$$s_d = \sqrt{\frac{10(2448) - (120)^2}{10(9)}} = \sqrt{112} = 10.6$$

(3) If H: $\mu_D = 0$ is true, the sampling distribution of
(4)

$$\frac{\bar{D}}{\frac{s_d}{\sqrt{n}}}$$

is described by a Student t-curve with 9 ($= n - 1$) degrees of freedom. Since

$$P\left\{-2.26 < \frac{\bar{D}}{\frac{s_d}{\sqrt{n}}} < 2.26\right\} = .95$$

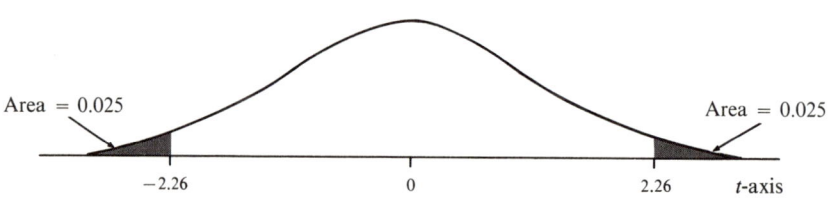

FIGURE 6.1

it follows that the two critical values, D_1' and D_2', for $\bar{d}$ are given by

$$D_1' = -2.26\left(\frac{s_d}{\sqrt{n}}\right) = -2.26\left(\frac{10.6}{\sqrt{10}}\right) = -7.6$$

and

$$D_2' = 2.26\left(\frac{s_d}{\sqrt{n}}\right) = 2.26\left(\frac{10.6}{\sqrt{10}}\right) = 7.6$$

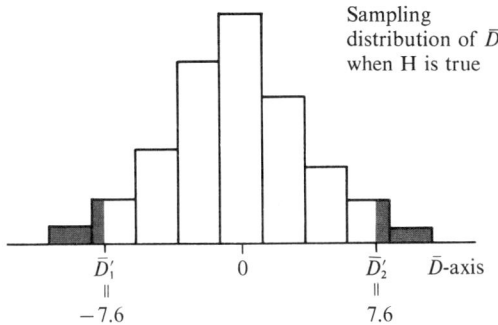

FIGURE 6.2

In Step 2 it was found that $\bar{d} = 12.0$ so our decision, at the $P = .05$ level of significance, is to reject the null hypothesis and conclude that ethosuximide *does* have an effect — in fact, a positive effect.

Question 6.2.1. Construct a 95% confidence interval for μ_D using these same data. (*Hint:* follow the format of Section 4.4).

Question 6.2.2. In this experiment, the *order* in which each child received the two treatments was determined at random. Why would it be a mistake to give all 10 children the placebo for the first three weeks, followed by ethosuximide for the last three weeks?

EXAMPLE 6.2.2. Glaucoma and Cornea Thickness

The glaucomas are serious eye diseases especially prevalent among older people. They are often caused by obstructions that interfere with the circulation of the aqueous humor, the consequence being an increased intraocular pressure (IOP). Exactly what influence, if any, an elevated IOP exerts on other parts of the eye is not entirely known. The relationship between cornea thickness and IOP is examined in the following sample of eight patients with unilateral glaucoma (Ehlers, 1970).

Model Four — The Paired-Data Problem

Cornea thickness (microns)

Patient	Glaucomatous eye (High IOP)	Contralateral eye (Low IOP)
K.H.	488	484
E.L.	478	478
M.J.	480	492
E.M.	426	444
K.F.	440	436
C.M.	410	398
A.T.	458	464
T.J.	460	476

(1) Let μ_D be the true average difference in cornea thickness for persons with unilateral glaucoma. Since there is no indication here of whether an elevated IOP will tend to increase or to decrease cornea thickness, the alternative hypothesis should be two-sided.

$$H: \quad \mu_D = 0 \quad \text{versus} \quad A: \quad \mu_D \neq 0$$

Let $P = .01$.

(2) The sum and the sum of the squares of the differences are calculated in the table.

Patient	High IOP (x_i)	Low IOP (y_i)	$d_i = y_i - x_i$	d_i^2
K.H.	488	484	-4	16
E.L.	478	478	0	0
M.J.	480	492	12	144
E.M.	426	444	18	324
K.F.	440	436	-4	16
C.M.	410	398	-12	144
A.T.	458	464	6	36
T.J.	460	476	16	256
			32	936

It follows that

$$\bar{d} = \frac{32}{8} = 4.0$$

and

$$s_d = \sqrt{\frac{8(936) - (32)^2}{8(7)}} = \sqrt{115.4}$$
$$= 10.7$$

(3) The numbers -3.50 and 3.50 cut off areas of 0.005 in either tail of the
(4) Student t-distribution with 7 degrees of freedom, so

$$P\left\{-3.50 < \frac{\bar{D}}{\frac{s_D}{\sqrt{8}}} < 3.50\right\} = .99$$

making

$$\bar{D}'_1 = -3.50 \frac{s_D}{\sqrt{8}} = -3.50\left(\frac{10.7}{2.83}\right) = -13.2$$

and

$$\bar{D}'_2 = 3.50 \frac{s_D}{\sqrt{8}} = 3.50\left(\frac{10.7}{2.83}\right) = 13.2$$

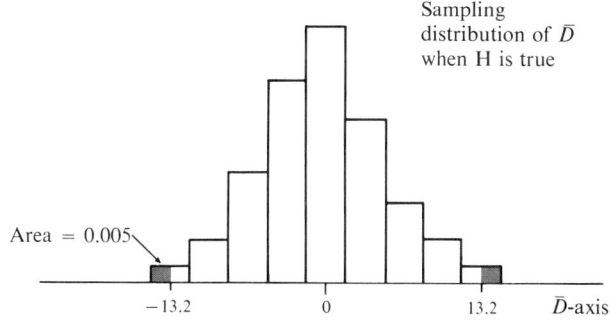

FIGURE 6.3

Since $\bar{d} = 4.0$ lies *between* $\bar{D}'_1$ and $\bar{D}'_2$ we accept H: $\mu_D = 0$. Intraocular pressure has no demonstrable effect on corneal thickness.

Question 6.2.3. Test the same hypothesis at the $P = .05$ level of significance.

Question 6.2.4. How would this same experiment be carried out using a Model Three design? Which approach (Model Three or Model Four) seems preferable?

6.3
TITER DATA: ACUTE AND CONVALESCENT SERA

Certain diseases, particularly in mild cases, have syndromes that are indistinguishable from those of other diseases. Influenza, for example, often follows the same clinical course as the common cold. In these instances a tentative diagnosis can be confirmed only on the basis of serological findings. It was mentioned earlier (Review Exercise 1.5) that individuals exposed to an infectious agent will develop circulating antibodies to the associated antigen. Therefore, a significant increase in the concentration of these antibodies (i.e., a "titer rise") can be taken as evidence of a recent infection.

To be of any use, the antibody level of a patient's blood must be measured twice — once during the early stages of an illness and a second time several weeks later, after the body's immunological system has had sufficient time to respond to the infection. These two blood samples are referred to as *acute* and *convalescent* sera and the antibody concentrations measured are called *pre-* and *posttiters*.

Antibody titers require a special sort of statistical analysis because of the way they are determined in the laboratory. All the data presented up to this point have been recorded on an arithmetic scale, but titers are recorded on a *geometric* scale. The next several paragraphs indicate how this is done and the effect it has on the final analysis.

First, the serum (either acute or convalescent) is divided up into a series of test tubes and mixed with saline solution in such a way that eight or nine different dilutions are reached. For example, the first test tube might contain serum in a 1-to-10 dilution (1 part serum, 9 parts saline), the second tube in a 1-to-20 dilution, the third, in a 1-to-40 dilution, and so on. (The starting dilution varies according to the situation, but each succeeding dilution must be the same multiple of the one before it.)

Into the first test tube a fixed amount of antigen is added. If antibodies are present in the serum in sufficient numbers, they will produce a visible reaction with the antigen (for example, in the form of a precipitate). If that happens, the same amount of antigen is added to the *next* dilution. Possibly, the concentration of antibodies in the serum was high enough initially that the reaction *still* takes place. If so, the same procedure is followed using the next dilution, and so on. Eventually, the serum becomes so diluted that the reaction *does not* take place. The titer of the serum is defined to be the reciprocal of (1 divided by) the weakest dilution for which the reaction is visible. In Figure 6.5, the titer would be recorded as 80.

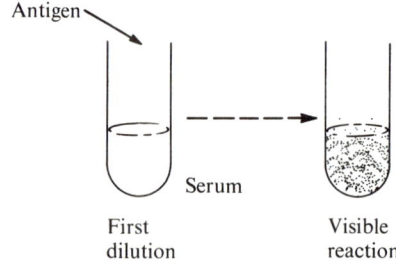

FIGURE 6.4

[6.3] Titer Data: Acute and Convalescent Sera

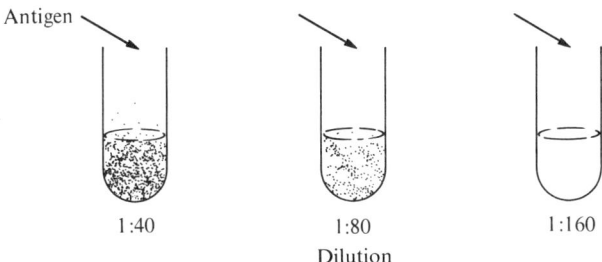

FIGURE 6.5

Because titer values are measured on a geometric scale, and are thereby restricted to certain multiples of one another, certain modifications must be made in calculating an *average* titer. Suppose the titers of four persons to some particular antigen were found to be the following:

Subject	Weakest dilution showing reaction	Titer
C.W.	1:20	$x_1 = 20$
P.H.	1:320	$x_2 = 320$
D.F.	1:40	$x_3 = 40$
R.L.	1:20	$x_4 = 20$

We would define the average titer (or *geometric mean titer*) for these four observations to be that number which, when multiplied by itself four times, gives a product equal to $(x_1)(x_2)(x_3)(x_4) = (20)(320)(40)(20) = 5{,}120{,}000$. Since $(47.6)(47.6)(47.6)(47.6)$ is approximately 5,120,000, the geometric mean titer is 47.6. It is denoted $\bar{x}_{gm}$.

Comment

The number $\bar{x}_{gm}$ is a measure of the location of geometrically scaled numbers in the same sense that $\bar{x}$ was a measure of the location of arithmetically scaled numbers.

Definition 6.3.1 gives the general formula for computing a geometric mean.

Definition 6.3.1. The geometric mean, $\bar{x}_{gm}$ of n titers, $x_1, x_2, \ldots, x_n$, is defined to be the nth root of their product:

$$\bar{x}_{gm} = (x_1 \cdot x_2 \cdot \ldots \cdot x_n)^{1/n}$$

That is, $(x_1 \cdot x_2 \cdot \ldots \cdot x_n)^{1/n}$ is the number which when multiplied by itself n times equals the product $(x_1)(x_2)(\cdots)(x_n)$.

Comment

Logarithms play an important role in the analysis of titer data. Note, for example, that

$$\log \bar{x}_{gm} = \log (x_1 \cdot x_2 \cdot \ldots \cdot x_n)^{1/n}$$
$$= \frac{1}{n} \sum_{i=1}^{n} \log x_i$$

implying that $\bar{x}_{gm}$ is the antilog of the sample mean of the log titers. This, of course, is a much simpler way of calculating $\bar{x}_{gm}$ than that suggested in Definition 6.3.1. In general, any statistical analysis done on titer data should, in fact, be done on the logs of those titers. Example 6.3.1 indicates how this is done.

EXAMPLE 6.3.1. An Influenza Vaccine Trial

Recently volunteers were recruited from a prison population in Atlanta, Georgia, to participate in an influenza vaccine trial (Larsen, 1968). First the pretiter of each volunteer against an A_2 influenza virus was recorded. Then each subject was given one of several experimental vaccines. Several weeks later, his posttiter against the same antigen was measured. The serial dilutions were set up in concentrations of 1:10, 1:20, 1:40, etc. Part of the data for one of the vaccines is shown below.

Subject	Pretiter	Posttiter
1	10	80
2	40	80
3	0	40
4	0	160
5	40	320
6	20	20
7	40	320
8	320	1280
9	10	160

Comment

If no reaction occurs at the lowest dilution, the titer is recorded as 0, but when the titers are replaced by their logs, each 0 titer is thought of as being equal to the number halfway between 0 and the lowest dilution. In this case, 0 titers are given the arbitrary value of 5. These substitutions are necessary because the logarithm of 0 is undefined. (See the table on the facing page.)

Sometimes in studies like this one, the vaccine is considered to be a success if it can be inferred that, in the population, the posttiter to pretiter ratio will be significantly greater than some number, say, 4.

Titer Data: Acute and Convalescent Sera

Subject	Log of pretiter (x_i)	Log of posttiter (y_i)	$d_i = y_i - x_i$	d_i^2
1	1.00000	1.90309	.90309	.81557
2	1.60206	1.90309	.30103	.09062
3	0.69897	1.60206	.90309	.81557
4	0.69897	2.20412	1.50515	2.26548
5	1.60206	2.50515	.90309	.81557
6	1.30103	1.30103	.00000	.00000
7	1.60206	2.50515	.90309	.81557
8	2.50515	3.10721	.60206	.36248
9	1.00000	2.20412	1.20412	1.44990
			7.22472	7.43076

(1) Let μ_D denote the mean of the population distribution associated with the differences between pre- and posttiters. The particular criterion for success just mentioned implies that log (posttiter) — log (pretiter) should be significantly greater than log 4 (= 0.60206). Therefore, the hypotheses to be tested are

$$H: \quad \mu_D = 0.60206 \quad \text{versus} \quad A: \quad \mu_D > 0.60206$$

(2) The sample mean and sample standard deviation (of the logs) are found in the usual way:

$$\bar{d} = \frac{7.22472}{9} = 0.80275$$

and

$$s_D = \sqrt{\frac{9(7.43076) - (7.22472)^2}{9(8)}} = \sqrt{0.20389}$$
$$= 0.45154$$

(3) In order to test the null hypothesis stated in Step (1), we need to generalize
(4) Theorem 6.2.1 slightly. Specifically, if $\mu_D = 0.60206$, the sampling distribution of

$$\frac{\bar{D} - \mu_D}{\frac{s_d}{\sqrt{n}}} = \frac{\bar{D} - 0.60206}{\frac{s_d}{\sqrt{n}}}$$

is described by a Student t-curve with $n - 1$ degrees of freedom (recall Section 5.4). Suppose $P = .05$. For a Student t-curve with 8 (= $n - 1$) degrees of freedom, the value 1.86 cuts off a tail area of 0.05.

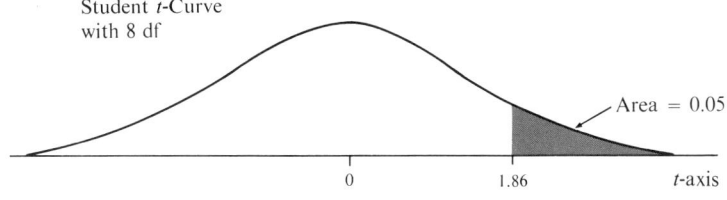

FIGURE 6.6

Therefore,

$$P\left\{\frac{\bar{D} - 0.60206}{\frac{s_d}{\sqrt{n}}} \geq 1.86\right\} = .05$$

which makes

$$\bar{D}' = 0.60206 + 1.86\frac{s_d}{\sqrt{n}} = 0.60206 + 1.86\left(\frac{0.45154}{\sqrt{9}}\right)$$
$$= 0.60206 + 0.27995 = 0.88201$$

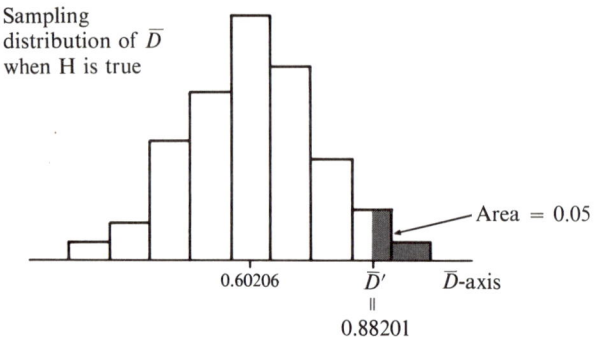

FIGURE 6.7

Since $\bar{d} = 0.80275$, we accept the null hypothesis.

Question 6.3.1. Construct a 95% confidence interval for μ_D. How would this interval be expressed in terms of actual titers?

Question 6.3.2. Would it be necessary to perform this experiment as a double-blind test?

6.4
SUMMARY

In every experiment there are many factors influencing the observed outcome. For example, the amount of weight lost by someone on a crash diet is influenced not only by the diet itself but also by the person's age, sex, present weight, general health condition, mental attitude, amount of daily exercise, and so on. It helps to categorize the effects of all these factors into three groups: those associated with the treatments, those associated with the subjects, and those associated with the experimental procedure. The first is the effect we are looking for; the second and third are simply nuisance factors that make it more difficult to isolate the effects of the first. To some extent, the third factor is beyond our control but the second, the subject effect, is *not;* and it can sometimes be greatly reduced. There are many ways of doing this, but one of the best is to use the paired-data format as described in this chapter.

The analysis of paired data is explained in Section 6.2. The particular method used is the *paired t-test*, which, with the exception of a change in notation, is exactly the same as the one-sample *t*-test introduced in Chapter 4. In Section 6.3 we consider the paired-data problem as it applies to the field of immunology. The only difference here is that the original measurements — the titers — are recorded on a geometric scale, which necessitates that all computations be done on the logs of the titers.

From a practical standpoint, Model Four should always be kept in mind when an experiment involves two treatments. As a general rule of thumb, when the subject variability is expected to influence the measured responses substantially, the paired-data format should be used in preference to the two-sample format, if physically possible.

Definitions

Acute serum. Serum taken from a patient during the initial stages of an infection before the body's immunological system has had time to produce additional antibodies.

Convalescent serum. Serum taken from a patient several weeks after the onset of an illness; presumably, the titer of the antibody related to the antigen of the infectious agent will be increased over its level in the acute serum.

Experimental error. In Model Four, that component of an experimental outcome which is due to all factors other than the treatment effect and the subject effect.

Geometric mean titer ($\bar{x}_{gm}$). Given n titers, the geometric mean titer is defined to be the nth root of their product; geometric means, in general, are used to describe the location of geometrically scaled data.

Posttiter. A titer measured on convalescent serum.

Pretiter. A titer measured on acute serum.

Source of variation. Any factor capable of influencing the observed value of an experimental outcome.

Subject effect. That component of an experimental outcome that may be attributed to the sum total of the characteristics of the sample subject.

Titer. A term used in describing the concentration of a person's (or animal's) circulating antibodies to a specific antigen; titer "rises" can result either from recent exposure to an infectious agent or from the effects of a vaccine. The higher the titer, the greater the capability of the body to fight off the infectious agent.

Treatment effect. That component of an experimental outcome that is directly due to the treatment administered.

Review Exercises

6.1 Research in extra-sensory perception has taken many different directions over the years. Recently, considerable attention has been given to the possibility that hypnosis may be helpful in "bringing out" ESP ability in persons who were not thought to have any. In one experiment 15 college students were each asked to guess the identity of 200 standard ESP cards (see Example 4.5.2) (Casler, 1964).

For 100 of those trials, both the student and the sender were awake; for the other 100, both were hypnotized. The scores are listed below. (If random chance were the only factor involved, the expected number of correct identifications in each 100 trials would be 20.) State and test the appropriate hypothesis.

Number of correct responses (out of 100)

Student	Sender and student in waking state	Sender and student in hypnotic state
1	18	25
2	19	20
3	16	26
4	21	26
5	16	20
6	20	23
7	20	14
8	14	18
9	11	18
10	22	20
11	19	22
12	29	27
13	16	19
14	27	27
15	15	21

6.2 Analyze the bee sting data of Example 1.8.1. Use the $P = .05$ level of significance.

6.3 Using the data of Example 1.8.2, construct a 95% confidence interval for the true average difference in the before and after PEF scores of all manic depressives who might, sometime in the future, be treated with lithium salts.

6.4 Prothrombin times and their importance as a parameter describing blood coagulation were first mentioned in Example 2.6.4. The following data were part of a study that was conducted to determine what effects, if any, *aspirin* has on prothrombin times (Yochem and Roach, 1971). Twelve adult males participated. Their prothrombin times were measured before and three hours after each was given two aspirin tablets (650 mg).

Prothrombin time (seconds)

Subject	Before aspirin	Three hours after aspirin
1	12.3	12.0
2	12.0	12.3
3	12.0	12.5
4	13.0	12.0
5	13.0	13.0
6	12.5	12.5
7	11.3	10.3
8	11.8	11.3
9	11.5	11.5
10	11.0	11.5
11	11.0	11.0
12	11.3	11.5

What can be concluded from these data about the effect of aspirin on prothrombin time?

6.5 How might the experiment described in Review Exercise 6.4 have been done as a Model Three problem? Which way (Model Three or Model Four) seems more reasonable?

6.6 Recall the energy data of Review Exercise 1.12. Test, at the $P = .05$ level of significance, whether or not there are any seasonal differences in energy expenditures for elderly women.

Note: If, for the ith subject, x_i and y_i denote the summer and winter averages, respectively, then

$$\sum_{i=1}^{8} d_i = -1242 \quad \text{and} \quad \sum_{i=1}^{8} d_i^2 = 781{,}164$$

where $d_i = y_i - x_i$.

6.7 One reason cited for the mental deterioration so often seen in the very elderly is the reduction in cerebral blood flow that accompanies the aging process. Addressing itself to this point, a study was recently done in a rest home to see whether cyclandelate, a vasodilator, might be able to stimulate the cerebral circulation and thereby slow down the rate of deterioration (Meyer, 1969). The drug was given to 11 subjects on a daily basis. To measure its physiological effect, radioactive tracers were used to determine each subject's mean circulation time (MCT) at the start of the experiment and four months later when the study was discontinued. (The MCT is the length of time it takes blood to travel from the carotid artery to the jugular vein.)

Mean circulation time (seconds)

Subject	Before (x_i)	After (y_i)
J.B.	15	13
M.B.	12	8
A.B.	12	12.5
M.B.	14	12
J.L.	13	12
S.M.	13	12.5
M.M.	13	12.5
S.McA.	12	14
A.McL.	12.5	12
F.S.	12	11
P.W.	12.5	10

Test the appropriate hypothesis. Use a one-sided alternative.

6.8 Find the two geometric means for the tularemia titers listed in Review Exercise 1.5.

6.9 Why would a two-sample model ever be preferable to a paired-data model?

6.10 Scoliosis is a condition marked by the lateral curvature of the spine. One of its sequellae is an impaired pulmonary function. This contributes to the high mortality rate of persons with this problem. As a possible therapy, it was felt that a regular exercise program might improve the respiration and circulation of scoliosis patients and thereby lengthen their life expectancy. To support this claim, 11 patients (all females, ages 16–27) participated in a study (Bjure, Grimby, and Nachemson, 1969) that called for special exercise sessions to be held three times a week over a period of three months. Before and after measurements were taken on a variety of pulmonary indicators, including forced expiratory volume (see Review Exercise 1.9).

FEV_1 (liters)

Patient	Before	After
1	1.1	1.2
2	2.4	2.3
3	2.2	2.1
4	3.6	3.6
5	2.4	2.6
6	1.9	1.9
7	3.4	3.4
8	3.5	3.6
9	2.1	2.2
10	2.5	2.4
11	1.5	1.3

(a) Graph these data.
(b) Define all the relevant parameters and test the appropriate hypothesis.

7

MODEL FIVE
The Correlation Problem

*'Tis fate that flings the dice,
and as she flings
of Kings makes peasants,
and of peasants Kings.*
                    Dryden

7.1
INTRODUCTION

Like "probability" and "statistics," the word "correlation" has found its way into our everyday vocabulary, and yet its precise meaning is never made very clear. We speak, for example, about the correlations between X-rays and congenital malformations or between coffee drinking and heart attacks, without having any real idea of what those statements mean, quantitatively. In this chapter, the concept of correlation will be examined carefully. Our objective is to learn what it *can* tell us, and, perhaps more importantly, what it *can't*.

The structure of Model Five already been discussed in Section 1.9: two measurements (usually involving two different characteristics) are taken on each member of a random sample of size n. The sample might consist of n expectant mothers hospitalized with suspected preeclampsia and the two measurements might be (1) the duration of her pregnancy and (2) her blood pressure. Or the sample might be n diabetics participating in a study to evaluate the effectiveness of an oral substitute for insulin, with the two measurements being (1) the dosage given and (2) the person's blood sugar level six hours later. Of course, the members of the sample need not be people. In the dental study of Example 2.6.6, the sample members were 21 cities.

But whatever the setting, the basic objective of all correlation problems is to characterize and quantify the relationship between the two characteristics being measured. Suppose $(x_1, y_1), (x_2, y_2), \ldots, (x_n, y_n)$ are the n pairs of observations comprising the sample data. The first step is to plot Y against X. Graphs of this kind are known as *scatterdiagrams* (recall Section 2.6); a few examples are shown in Figure 7.1.

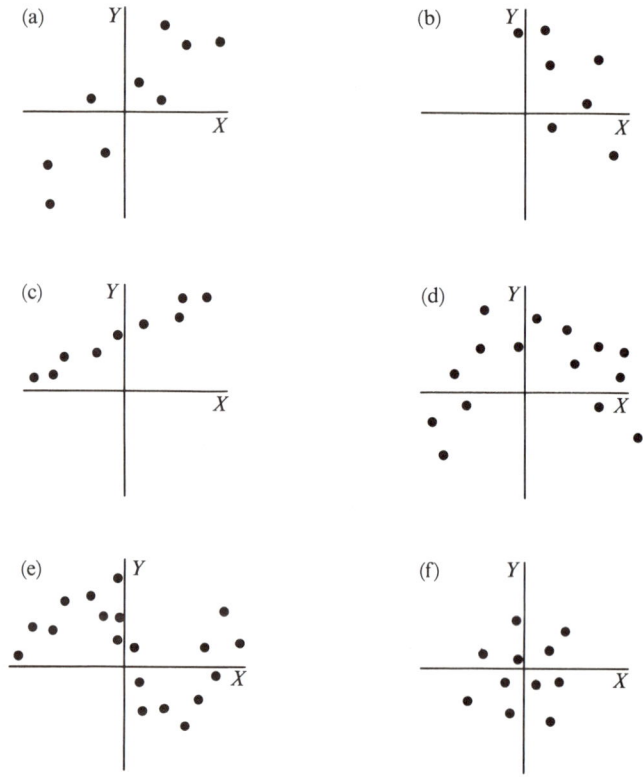

FIGURE 7.1

Figures 7.1(a), 7.1(b), and 7.1(c) are examples of *linear* relationships. In these instances, a straight line of the form $Y = a + bX$ (with a and b suitably chosen) would describe quite well the way Y varies with X. Figures 7.1(d) and 7.1(e) show two *curvilinear* (or nonlinear) relationships. Neither of these could be adequately summarized by a single straight line, no matter where it was located. In Figure 7.1(f) there is *no* apparent relationship between X and Y, linear or otherwise.

In a statistical context, the word "correlation" refers only to linear relationships. If X and Y tend to increase simultaneously (and decrease simultaneously) the correlation is said to be *positive*. If Y tends to increase when X tends to decrease (and vice-versa), the correlation is said to be *negative*. It follows that the points making up Figures 7.1(a) and 7.1(c) are positively correlated while those in Figure 7.1(b) are negatively correlated. (If there is no relationship evident in the data, as in Figure 7.1(f), the variables are said to be *uncorrelated*.)

There are two questions that usually need to be considered when analyzing linearly related data: (1) *which* straight line best fits the points and (2) how *strong* is the correlation between X and Y? All the material in Chapter 7 bears directly on one or both of these two questions.

Comment

While there *are* methods for quantifying nonlinear relationships, none will be considered in this text. Our sole concern here will be with situations such as 7.1(a), 7.1(b), 7.1(c), and 7.1(f).

It may seem that all that must be done to answer the first question is to take a ruler and draw a straight line through the given set of points. That would certainly provide *an* answer, but not *the* answer. What looks like a good fit to one person wouldn't look as good to another. For the sake of uniformity, it is necessary to have an objective criterion for deciding on a "best" straight line — one that everyone would agree on. Section 7.2 presents the criterion that is most often used for this purpose, the *Method of Least Squares*.

Answering the second question (measuring the "strength" of a linear relationship) is another exercise in the *numerical* description of data (such as using $\bar{x}$ and s to quantify location and dispersion). It seems clear that the points in Figure 7.1(c) demonstrate a stronger linear association than the points in Figure 7.1(a). But is it possible to define a statistic whose values will reflect that difference? The answer is yes and the solution, formulated in Section 7.3, is known as the *sample correlation coefficient*. Just as $\bar{x}$ and s have their population counterparts, μ and σ, so does the sample correlation coefficient (which we denote r) have *its* population counterpart, ρ. Hypothesis tests involving ρ are taken up in Section 7.4.

The remainder of Chapter 7 is concerned with the single most important procedure in all of medical statistics, the χ^2 *test*. The purpose of such a test is to establish whether or not the X and Y variables can be considered independent. In this respect, χ^2 tests and tests involving the population correlation coefficient (Section 7.4) are very similar.

7.2
THE LEAST SQUARES LINE

Consider again the data of Review Exercise 1.1 showing the relationship between radiation exposure and cancer mortality for nine Oregon counties. The relationship shown in Figure 7.2 is clearly linear and can be described by a straight line, but it is not obvious which straight line would provide the best description. The purpose of this section is first to define the "best" line and then to show how the equation of that line can be found.

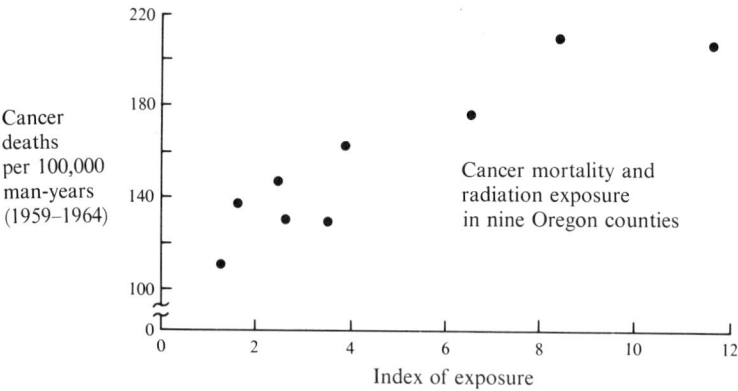

FIGURE 7.2

Comment

Recall from high school algebra that the equation of any straight line will have the form $Y = a + bX$, where a is the *Y-intercept* and b is the *slope*.

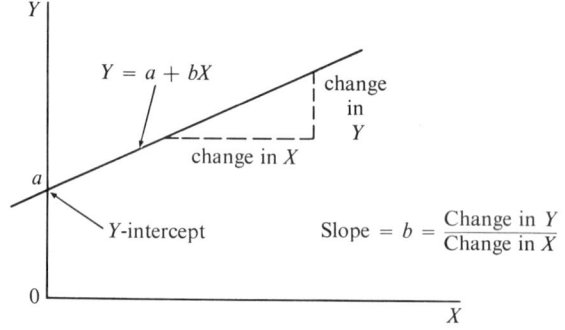

FIGURE 7.3

Values for the Y-intercept and slope of the "best" line will be denoted by the symbols $\hat{a}$ and $\hat{b}$, respectively. But in order to find $\hat{a}$ and $\hat{b}$, we first need to answer a very fundamental question: when does one line fit a set of points better than another line? For example, the two lines $Y = 0.77 + 0.44X$ and $Y = 1.52 + 0.17X$ are shown in Figure 7.4, superimposed over the same set of five points.

Which one more accurately represents the XY-relationship? (The answer is $Y = 0.77 + 0.44X$ for the reasons that follow.)

Consider a set of n points $\{(x_1, y_1), (x_2, y_2), \ldots, (x_n, y_n)\}$ and an arbitrary straight line, $Y = a + bX$. We can measure the extent to which the line fails to "fit" an arbitrary point, (x_i, y_i), by the square of the vertical distance between y_i and $a + bx_i$; that is, by the quantity $[y_i - (a + bx_i)]^2$. If the squared

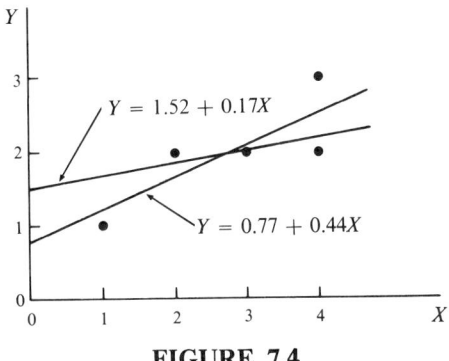

FIGURE 7.4

deviations for each of the n points are added together, the resultant sum, $L = \sum_{i=1}^{n} [y_i - (a + bx_i)]^2$, will be an overall measure of the extent to which the line $Y = a + bX$ fails to fit the data.

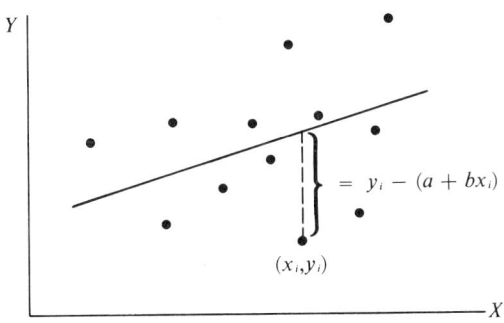

FIGURE 7.5

According to the *least squares criterion*, the best straight line is the one that minimizes the numerical value of L. Formulas for determining the values of a and b that achieve this minimization are provided in the least squares theorem, Theorem 7.2.1.

Theorem 7.2.1. Let $\{(x_1, y_1), (x_2, y_2), \ldots, (x_n, y_n)\}$ be a set of n points. The best straight line, $Y = a + bX$, fitting these points — that is, the line minimizing $\sum_{i=1}^{n} [y_i - (a + bx_i)]^2$ — has slope $\hat{b}$ and y-intercept $\hat{a}$ given by

$$\hat{b} = \frac{n\left(\sum_{i=1}^{n} x_i y_i\right) - \left(\sum_{i=1}^{n} x_i\right)\left(\sum_{i=1}^{n} y_i\right)}{n\left(\sum_{i=1}^{n} x_i^2\right) - \left(\sum_{i=1}^{n} x_i\right)^2}$$

and

$$\hat{a} = \frac{\sum_{i=1}^{n} y_i - \hat{b} \sum_{i=1}^{n} x_i}{n}$$

Comment

The decision to use the sum of the squared deviations, rather than some other function of the X's and Y's, as the criterion for goodness-of-fit was not as arbitrary as it might have appeared. There are some very compelling reasons in support of the least squares criterion but they lie beyond the scope of this text.

Comment

Any straight line whose slope and Y-intercept are calculated using the formulas given in the least squares theorem is called a *least squares line*.

EXAMPLE 7.2.1. Blood Pressure and Heart Weight

The following data were collected on 19 patients with advanced nephritis (Pickering, 1960). The two measurements recorded for each one were (1) heart weight (X) and (2) blood pressure (Y).

Patient	Heart weight (oz.), x_i	Blood pressure (mm Hg), y_i
1	14.3	179
2	14.0	141
3	27.3	197
4	18.2	214
5	15.8	221
6	10.9	115
7	14.0	132
8	14.6	202
9	15.1	197
10	27.2	258
11	10.3	151
12	13.8	175
13	17.0	210
14	8.0	120
15	24.1	192
16	12.7	125
17	16.3	249
18	19.9	235
19	22.1	234

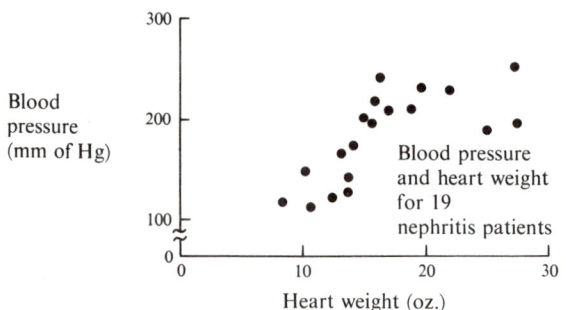

Blood pressure and heart weight for 19 nephritis patients

FIGURE 7.6

Since

$$\sum_{i=1}^{19} x_i = 315.6 \qquad \sum_{i=1}^{19} x_i^2 = 5764.22$$

$$\sum_{i=1}^{19} y_i = 3547 \qquad \sum_{i=1}^{19} x_i y_i = 61{,}963.0$$

and

$$n = 19$$

it follows from the least squares theorem that

$$\hat{b} = \frac{19(61{,}963.0) - (315.6)(3547)}{19(5764.22) - (315.6)^2} = 5.83$$

and

$$\hat{a} = \frac{3547 - (5.83)(315.60)}{19} = 89.8$$

Therefore, the straight line that best fits these data has the equation

$$Y = 89.8 + 5.83X$$

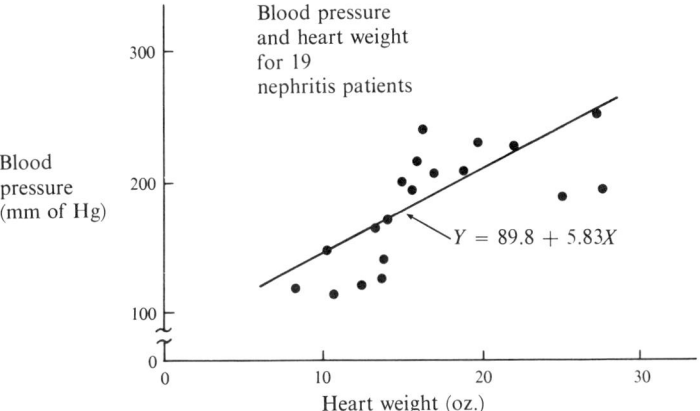

FIGURE 7.7

Question 7.2.1. Suppose it was determined that the heart of a certain nephritis patient (one not connected with the study just described) weighed 22 ounces. Estimate that patient's blood pressure.

The next example shows in specific terms what Theorem 7.2.1 says is true in general.

EXAMPLE 7.2.2. A "Verification" of the Least Squares Theorem

In describing the heart weight–blood pressure data of Example 7.2.1, it was found that the least squares line had the equation $Y = 89.8 + 5.83X$. But suppose some other line was fit to the data — say, $Y = 85.0 + 5.92X$. How would the sum of the squared deviations for the two lines compare?

The accompanying table gives the squared deviations for each of the sample points from each of the fitted lines.

Patient	x_i	y_i	$[y_i - (89.8 + 5.83x_i)]^2$	$[y_i - (85.0 + 5.92x_i)]^2$
1	14.3	179	33.64	88.36
2	14.0	141	924.16	723.61
3	27.3	197	2704.00	2460.16
4	18.2	214	327.61	453.69
5	15.8	221	1528.81	1806.25
6	10.9	115	1466.89	1190.25
7	14.0	132	1552.36	1288.81
8	14.6	202	734.41	936.36
9	15.1	197	368.64	510.76
10	27.2	258	92.16	144.00
11	10.3	151	1.44	25.00
12	13.8	175	23.04	68.89
13	17.0	210	445.21	595.36
14	8.0	120	268.96	153.76
15	24.1	192	1466.89	1274.49
16	12.7	125	1505.44	1239.04
17	16.3	249	4121.64	4556.25
18	19.9	235	852.64	1036.84
19	22.1	234	237.16	331.24
			18655.10	18883.12

Note that the sum of the squared deviations computed around the least squares line, $\sum_{i=1}^{19} [y_i - (89.8 + 5.83x_i)]^2$, equals 18,655.10, which is *less* than the corresponding sum (18,883.12) computed around the line $Y = 85.0 + 5.92X$. Of course, the least squares theorem says that for these particular nineteen points there is *no* straight line whose squared deviations will sum to less than 18655.10.

Question 7.2.2. Would it be possible to fit a line through a set of points by choosing the y-intercept and the slope to be those values of a and b that minimize $\sum_{i=1}^{n} |y_i - (a + bx_i)|$? *Hint:* try to use this criterion to fit a straight line through a sample of just *two* points.

EXAMPLE 7.2.3. A Least Squares Line for the Smoking-CHD Data

From the scatterdiagram shown in Example 1.2.3, it seems clear that the relationship between per capita cigarette consumption (X) and the mortality rate from coronary heart disease (Y) for the $n = 21$ countries represented is essentially linear. To find the straight line that best describes that relationship, we first compute

$$\sum_{i=1}^{21} x_i = 45{,}110 \qquad \sum_{i=1}^{21} x_i^2 = 109{,}957{,}100$$

$$\sum_{i=1}^{21} y_i = 3{,}042.2 \qquad \sum_{i=1}^{21} x_i y_i = 7{,}319{,}602.0$$

Therefore,

$$\hat{b} = \frac{21(7{,}319{,}602.0) - (45{,}110)(3{,}042.2)}{21(109{,}957{,}100) - (45{,}110)^2} = 0.06$$

$$\hat{a} = \frac{3{,}042.2 - (0.06)(45{,}110)}{21} = 16.0$$

and the least squares line is $Y = 16.0 + 0.06X$.

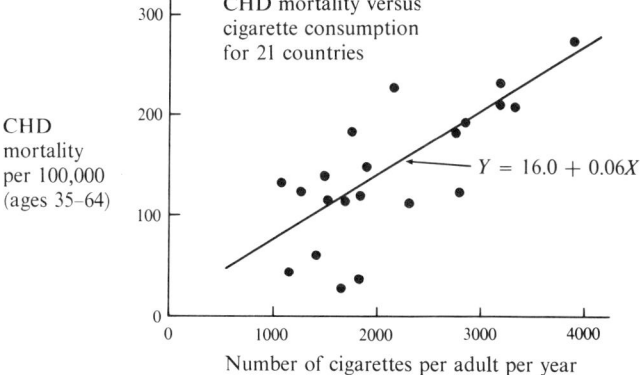

FIGURE 7.8

Question 7.2.3. Find the equation of the best straight line that fits the points $\{(1, 1), (2, 1), (2, 2)\}$. Make a scatterdiagram of the points and draw in the least squares line.

Question 7.2.4. One of the properties of any least squares line is that it goes through the point $(\bar{x}, \bar{y})$. Verify that this is true for the line found in Question 7.2.3.

7.3 THE CORRELATION COEFFICIENT

The introduction to this chapter said that there are two facets of the relationship between a pair of variables that should always be kept in mind. One is the nature of that relationship; in particular, is it linear or nonlinear? The other is its *strength*. If the relationship is linear, its strength can be measured by a statistic known as the *sample correlation coefficient*. In this section we first approach the correlation coefficient from an intuitive standpoint to show *how* it measures the strength of a linear relationship. Then a formula is introduced for simplifying the actual computations that need to be done.

Consider the scatterdiagram in Figure 7.9 which shows a set of n linearly related points and two superimposed straight lines, the least squares line, $Y = \hat{a} + \hat{b}X$; and the horizontal line, $Y = \bar{y}$, where $\bar{y}$ is the average of the Y-coordinates. From Section 7.2, the degree to which the two lines fit the data can be measured by the terms $\sum_{i=1}^{n} [y_i - (\hat{a} + \hat{b}x_i)]^2$ and $\sum_{i=1}^{n} (y_i - \bar{y})^2$. Of course, since $Y = \hat{a} + \hat{b}X$ is the least squares line, it must be true that

$$\sum_{i=1}^{n} [y_i - (\hat{a} + \hat{b}x_i)]^2 \leq \sum_{i=1}^{n} (y_i - \bar{y})^2$$

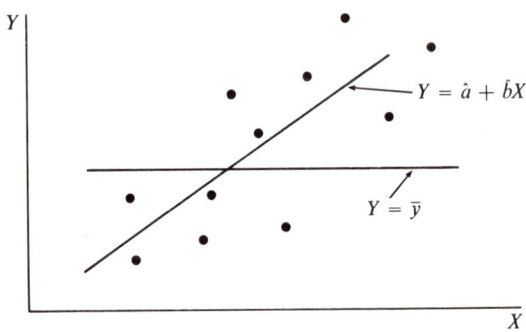

FIGURE 7.9

Notice that the ratio

$$\frac{\sum_{i=1}^{n} [y_i - (\hat{a} + \hat{b}x_i)]^2}{\sum_{i=1}^{n} (y_i - \bar{y})^2}$$

will be close to 0 if the linear relationship between X and Y is nearly perfect (since the numerator, $\sum_{i=1}^{n} [y_i - (\hat{a} + \hat{b}x_i)]^2$, would then be relatively close to 0). Conversely, if the variables are uncorrelated, or nearly so, no straight line will fit the data much better than any other; and the ratio will be close to 1.

With these observations in mind, we define as a measure of the strength of the linear relationship between X and Y the sample correlation coefficient, r, where

$$r = \pm \sqrt{1 - \frac{\sum_{i=1}^{n} [y_i - (\hat{a} + \hat{b}x_i)]^2}{\sum_{i=1}^{n} (y_i - \bar{y})^2}}$$

[7.3] The Correlation Coefficient

Ignore for the moment the $\pm$ sign and the square root sign. Note that the quantity under the square root sign will range numerically from 0 to 1, with values close to 0 describing variables that are essentially uncorrelated and values close to 1 describing those that are highly correlated.

If the slope $\hat{b}$ of the least squares line is positive, the sample correlation coefficient is defined to be

$$r = +\sqrt{1 - \frac{\sum_{i=1}^{n}[y_i - (\hat{a} + \hat{b}x_i)]^2}{\sum_{i=1}^{n}(y_i - \bar{y})^2}}$$

If the slope is negative,

$$r = -\sqrt{1 - \frac{\sum_{i=1}^{n}[y_i - (\hat{a} + \hat{b}x_i)]^2}{\sum_{i=1}^{n}(y_i - \bar{y})^2}}$$

Because of these conventions, sample correlation coefficients always lie in the interval $(-1, 1)$.

Comment

If the slope of the least squares line is 0, it is better not to compute the correlation coefficient. In this one instance, r is no longer a measure of goodness-of-fit and its numerical value (namely, 0) is somewhat misleading.

EXAMPLE 7.3.1. Calculating r (The Long Way)

For the nephritis patients of Example 7.2.1, the least squares line was found to be $Y = 89.8 + 5.83X$. Also, from Example 7.2.2, the corresponding sum of squared deviations was 18,655.10:

$$\sum_{i=1}^{19}[y_i - (89.8 + 5.83x_i)]^2 = 18,655.10$$

Since

$$\bar{y} = \frac{1}{19}\sum_{i=1}^{19} y_i = 186.7$$

the sum of the squared deviations of the y_i's from the line $Y = 186.7$ is given by

$$\sum_{i=1}^{19}(y_i - \bar{y})^2 = 36,422.11$$

Here the slope of the least squares line is positive ($+5.83$), so it follows that

$$r = +\sqrt{1 - \frac{18,655.10}{36,422.11}}$$
$$= \sqrt{1 - 0.51} = \sqrt{0.49}$$
$$= 0.70$$

Question 7.3.1. Compute the sample correlation coefficient for the three points $\{(0, 0), (2, 2), (0, 1)\}$. Also, plot the points on a scatterdiagram and sketch in the least squares line.

The expression

$$r = \pm\sqrt{1 - \frac{\sum_{i=1}^{n}[y_i - (\hat{a} + \hat{b}x_i)]^2}{\sum_{i=1}^{n}(y_i - \bar{y})^2}}$$

should be thought of as a *defining* formula for r, in the same sense that $\sqrt{[1/(n-1)]\sum_{i=1}^{n}(x_i - \bar{x})^2}$ was the defining formula for s. Its sole purpose was to illustrate *how* the correlation coefficient measures the strength of a linear relationship. In practice, though, the value of r is more easily obtained using a special *computing* formula.

Computing formula for r. The sample correlation coefficient r for a set of n linearly-related points, $\{(x_1, y_1), (x_2, y_2), \ldots, (x_n, y_n)\}$ is equal to

$$r = \frac{n\sum_{i=1}^{n} x_i y_i - \left(\sum_{i=1}^{n} x_i\right)\left(\sum_{i=1}^{n} y_i\right)}{\sqrt{n\sum_{i=1}^{n} x_i^2 - \left(\sum_{i=1}^{n} x_i\right)^2}\sqrt{n\sum_{i=1}^{n} y_i^2 - \left(\sum_{i=1}^{n} y_i\right)^2}}$$

The defining formula and the computing formula will always give the same answer. That equality will not be proved formally, but the next example shows it to be true for the nephritis data of Example 7.2.1.

EXAMPLE 7.3.2. Calculating r (The Short Way)

The various sums and sums of squares associated with the heart weight (X) versus blood pressure (Y) data of Example 7.2.1 are

$$\sum_{i=1}^{19} x_i = 315.60 \qquad \sum_{i=1}^{19} x_i^2 = 5764.22$$

$$\sum_{i=1}^{19} y_i = 3547 \qquad \sum_{i=1}^{19} y_i^2 = 698{,}591$$

$$\sum_{i=1}^{19} x_i y_i = 61{,}963.0 \qquad n = 19$$

[7.3] The Correlation Coefficient 239

Substituting these values into the computing formula for r gives

$$r = \frac{19(61{,}963.0) - (315.60)(3547)}{\sqrt{19(5764.22) - (315.60)^2}\sqrt{19(698{,}591) - (3547)^2}}$$

$$= \frac{57{,}863.8}{\sqrt{9916.82}\sqrt{692{,}020}} = 0.70$$

the same answer that was found using the defining formula (Example 7.3.1).

Comment

Besides being simpler, the computing formula has the added feature of determining automatically the proper sign for r. It is not necessary to know whether the slope of the least squares line is positive or negative.

Question 7.3.2. Use the computing formula just described to find the sample correlation coefficient for the three points given in Question 7.3.1.

Except at three particular values (-1, 0, and $+1$), we still do not have a precise interpretation for r. How much stronger, for example, is a linear relationship whose r value is 0.80 than one where r is 0.40? (The obvious answer is 2, but the correct answer, as we will see, is 4.)

Consider the three terms $\sum_{i=1}^{n}(y_i - \bar{y})^2$, $\sum_{i=1}^{n}[y_i - (\hat{a} + \hat{b}x_i)]^2$, and $\sum_{i=1}^{n}(\hat{a} + \hat{b}x_i - \bar{y})^2$, where $Y = \hat{a} + \hat{b}X$ is the least squares line fitting the n points $\{(x_1, y_1), (x_2, y_2), \ldots, (x_n, y_n)\}$ and $\bar{y} = (1/n)\sum_{i=1}^{n} y_i$. For any set of points, it can be proved that

$$\sum_{i=1}^{n}(y_i - \bar{y})^2 = \sum_{i=1}^{n}[y_i - (\hat{a} + \hat{b}x_i)]^2 + \sum_{i=1}^{n}(\hat{a} + \hat{b}x_i - \bar{y})^2$$

The term on the left measures the *total variability* in the sample, that is, the extent to which the n observations are not all the same. The equation says that the total variability can be written as the sum of two parts, with the contributions of the two parts being measured by $\sum_{i=1}^{n}[y_i - (\hat{a} + \hat{b}x_i)]^2$ and $\sum_{i=1}^{n}(\hat{a} + \hat{b}x_i - \bar{y})^2$, respectively.

Note that if all the points fell on a single straight line, that line would be $Y = \hat{a} + \hat{b}X$ and the term $\sum_{i=1}^{n}[y_i - (\hat{a} + \hat{b}x_i)]^2$ would equal 0. But since all the points will *not*, in general, be colinear, we can only conclude that there are *other* factors, in addition to the linear relationship, influencing Y. Clearly, the effect of these other factors — that is, the variability not accounted for by the linear relationship — is measured by the relative magnitude of $\sum_{i=1}^{n}[y_i - (\hat{a} + \hat{b}x_i)]^2$. It follows, then, that the term $\sum_{i=1}^{n}(\hat{a} + \hat{b}x_i - \bar{y})^2$ measures the variability that *is* accounted for by the linear relationship.

Recall the defining formula for r:

$$r = \pm\sqrt{1 - \frac{\sum_{i=1}^{n}[y_i - (\hat{a} + \hat{b}x_i)]^2}{\sum_{i=1}^{n}(y_i - \bar{y})^2}}$$

After converting the expression under the radical sign to a common denominator, we can write

$$r = \pm \sqrt{\frac{\sum_{i=1}^{n}(y_i - \bar{y})^2 - \sum_{i=1}^{n}[y_i - (\hat{a} + \hat{b}x_i)]^2}{\sum_{i=1}^{n}(y_i - \bar{y})^2}}$$

Notice that the numerator equals $\sum_{i=1}^{n}(\hat{a} + \hat{b}x_i - \bar{y})^2$. Therefore,

$$r = \pm \sqrt{\frac{\sum_{i=1}^{n}(\hat{a} + \hat{b}x_i - \bar{y})^2}{\sum_{i=1}^{n}(y_i - \bar{y})^2}}$$

or, equivalently,

$$r^2 = \frac{\sum_{i=1}^{n}(\hat{a} + \hat{b}x_i - \bar{y})^2}{\sum_{i=1}^{n}(y_i - \bar{y})^2}$$

This ratio implies that the quantity r^2 can be thought of as the *proportion* of the total variability in the Y's that can be accounted for by the linear relationship with X. Put another way, if, for a given set of n points, the sample correlation coefficient is equal to, say, 0.50, then only 25% of the variability in the data can be "explained" by the linear dependence that Y shares with X. (This is why a correlation of 0.80 ($r^2 = 0.64$) represents a linear relationship that is *four* times as strong as one whose correlation is 0.40 ($r^2 = 0.16$)).

Question 7.3.3. Numerically verify the equality

$$\sum_{i=1}^{n}(y_i - \bar{y})^2 = \sum_{i=1}^{n}[y_i - (\hat{a} + \hat{b}x_i)]^2 + \sum_{i=1}^{n}(\hat{a} + \hat{b}x_i - \bar{y})^2$$

using the data of Question 7.3.1.

Question 7.3.4. How would the relative strengths of the linear relationships in the smoking-CHD data (Example 7.2.3) and the heart weight–blood pressure data (Example 7.3.2) be described? *Note:* for the data of Example 7.2.3,

$$\sum_{i=1}^{21} y_i^2 = 529{,}321.58$$

7.4 TESTING H: $\rho = 0$

The role that inference has played in Models Two, Three, and Four should suggest to us that r is merely a sample estimate of some population counterpart in the same sense that $\bar{x}$ is an estimate of μ and s is an estimate of σ. For the purposes of this section, we assume that the given set of n points is a random sample from a two-variable (or *bivariate*) normal distribution and that the *true* correlation between X and Y is described by a parameter, ρ.

Comment

The mathematical properties of this particular distribution need not concern us. In terms of appearance, though, it resembles Figure 7.10 (Dixon and Massey, 1957). A random observation from such a distribution is a *pair* of numbers (X_i, Y_i), where the probability that (X_i, Y_i) lies in some *region* of the *XY*-plane is equal to the corresponding *volume* under the given surface. This is completely analogous to the situation for one-dimensional distributions, where the probability that a random observation X_i lies in a given *interval* is equal to the corresponding *area* under a certain curve.

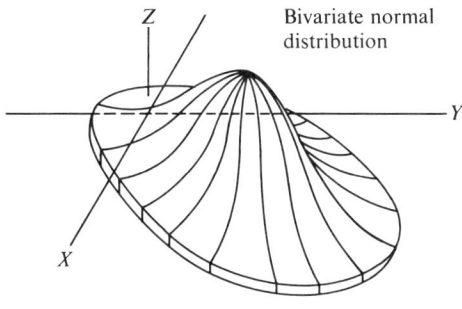

FIGURE 7.10

Like r, ρ can range in value from -1 to $+1$. If, in fact, $\rho = 0$, X and Y are said to be uncorrelated (and independent). When this is the case, knowledge of the X-component of an (x, y) pair is of no help in predicting the value of the Y-component. Since the dependence or independence of X and Y is often the most basic question that needs to be answered in a correlation problem, hypothesis tests for ρ are generally of the form

$$\text{H: } \rho = 0 \quad \text{versus} \quad \text{A: } \rho \neq 0$$

(Of course, depending on the situation at hand, either of the two one-sided alternatives, A: $\rho < 0$ or A: $\rho > 0$, might be more appropriate than A: $\rho \neq 0$.)

Following the patterns already established in Chapters 3, 4, 5, and 6, there are two explanations that can be offered to justify why an observed sample correlation coefficient (r) is not equal to 0:

(1) H: $\rho = 0$ is actually true and the numerical difference between r and ρ (that is, between r and 0) can be accounted for by the sampling variability of r.
(2) H: $\rho = 0$ is false.

To decide between (1) and (2), we will assume H is true and use the properties of the sampling distribution of r (Theorem 7.4.1) to determine the probability of the correlation coefficient being even further away from 0 than the value actually observed. If that probability is quite small — say, less than 0.05 — the null hypothesis will be rejected.

Theorem 7.4.1. Let $\{(x_1, y_1), (x_2, y_2), \ldots, (x_n, y_n)\}$ be a random sample of size n drawn from a bivariate normal distribution. If the population correlation coefficient ρ is 0, the sampling distribution of

$$\frac{r}{\sqrt{\frac{1 - r^2}{n - 2}}}$$

is described by a Student t-curve with $n - 2$ degrees of freedom.

EXAMPLE 7.4.1. Correlation and Future Shock

It was suggested in Example 1.9.1 that a person's health might not be independent of changes in his life style. In particular, the scatterdiagram showing amount of change (SRE) versus illness severity (SIRS) revealed the two to be linearly related with a positive correlation. Does it follow from these data that SRE and SIRS are, in fact, dependent, or is it likely that the two are really independent, with the apparent "trend" being only a product of chance?

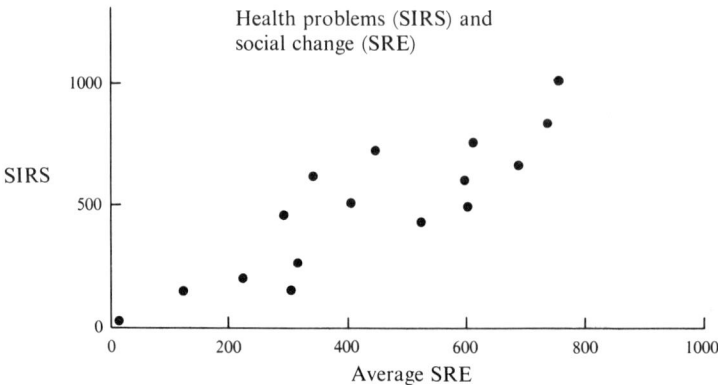

FIGURE 7.11

(1) If the alternative is chosen to be two-sided, the hypotheses to be tested are

$$H: \quad \rho = 0 \quad \text{versus} \quad A: \quad \rho \neq 0$$

where ρ is the true correlation coefficient describing the relationship between SRE and SIRS. Let $P = .05$.

(2) Letting x's and y's denote the SRE and SIRS scores, respectively, we have

$$\sum_{i=1}^{17} x_i = 7973 \qquad \sum_{i=1}^{17} x_i^2 = 4{,}611{,}291$$

$$\sum_{i=1}^{17} y_i = 8517 \qquad \sum_{i=1}^{17} y_i^2 = 5{,}421{,}917$$

$$\sum_{i=1}^{17} x_i y_i = 4{,}759{,}470 \qquad n = 17$$

Therefore,

$$r = \frac{17(4{,}759{,}470) - (7973)(8517)}{\sqrt{17(4{,}611{,}291) - (7973)^2}\sqrt{17(5{,}421{,}917) - (8517)^2}}$$

$$= \frac{13{,}004{,}949}{\sqrt{14{,}823{,}218}\sqrt{19{,}633{,}300}}$$

$$= 0.76$$

(3) Since $n = 17$, the sampling distribution of

$$\frac{r}{\sqrt{\frac{1 - r^2}{15}}}$$

follows a Student t-curve with 15 degrees of freedom (when H is true)

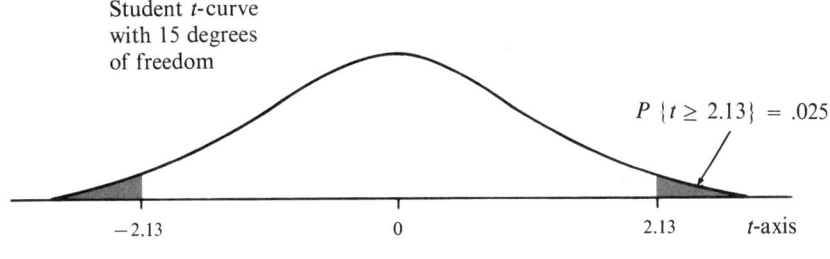

FIGURE 7.12

(4) Since $P\{-2.13 < r/\sqrt{(1 - r^2)/15} < 2.13\} = .95$, the two critical values for r are given by

$$r_1' = -2.13\sqrt{\frac{1 - (0.76)^2}{15}} = -0.36$$

and

$$r_2' = 2.13\sqrt{\frac{1 - (0.76)^2}{15}} = 0.36$$

Therefore, since the observed r (0.76) exceeds r_2 (0.36), the null hypothesis should be rejected.

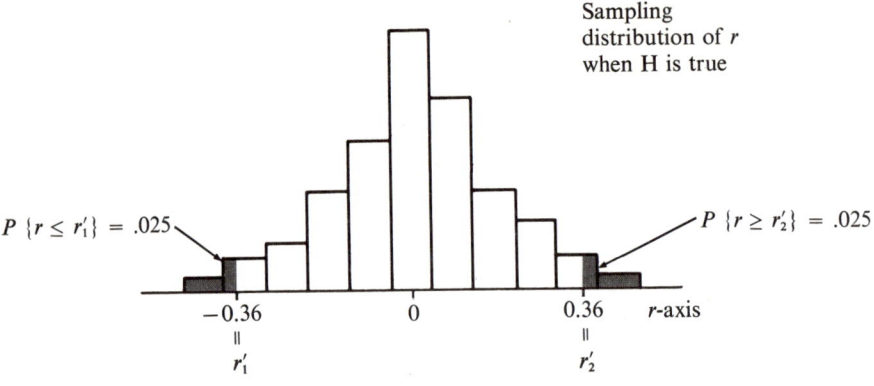

FIGURE 7.13

Question 7.4.1. At the $P = .05$ level of significance, test

$$\text{H:} \quad \rho = 0 \quad \text{versus} \quad \text{A:} \quad \rho > 0$$

for the heart weight–blood pressure data of Example 7.2.1.

No discussion of the merits of correlation coefficients would be complete without the warning that *correlation does not imply causality*. To say that a variable Y is highly correlated (even perfectly correlated) with another variable X is not equivalent to saying that X "causes" Y. It is quite possible for X and Y to have absolutely no physical influence on one another and yet exhibit a strong relationship simply because both are highly dependent on a third variable.

For example, a survey in this country would probably reveal that malnutrition was highly correlated with overcrowdedness; people living in crowded conditions tend to be undernourished. But does this mean that overcrowdedness *causes* malnutrition? Of course not. What causes malnutrition is the inability of individuals to afford sufficient quantities and varieties of food. It just so happens that people in the lower economic classes who are not able to buy enough food are also forced to live in overcrowded conditions. In a case like this, the correlation between overcrowdedness and malnutrition is called *spurious*, no matter how statistically significant it might be.

In any given instance we can never be absolutely certain whether or not an observed correlation is spurious. Only after carefully assessing the overall experimental procedure and collecting whatever additional information might be relevant should any serious consideration be given to the hypothesis that the apparent relationship is, indeed, a reflection of cause and effect. The highly significant correlations linking cigarette smoking and the incidence of cancer, for example, would not in themselves "prove" that cigarettes were harmful. But these correlations coupled with controlled laboratory studies detailing the physiological damage caused by smoke and nicotine make the case against cigarettes hard to refute.

7.5
THE χ^2 TEST: 2 × 2 CONTINGENCY TABLES

One of the first questions that always arises in experiments where the observed responses are pairs (x_i, y_i) of dissimilar measurements is whether or not the two variables are independent. When X and Y are both quantitative, the answer is usually obtained by testing H: $\rho = 0$. If H is accepted, and if the data can be assumed to have come from a bivariate normal distribution, it follows that X and Y are independent. Likewise, if H is rejected, the conclusion is that X and Y are dependent.

Another, often more useful method for establishing the dependence or independence of two variables is the *chi square* (χ^2) *test*. As we will see, this procedure lends itself particularly well to the sort of problems that are common in medical research.

Most typically, the χ^2 test is applied to situations where each of the n sample subjects is categorized according to two *qualitative* criteria. While each of these criteria may have any number of possible "values," we will consider in this section only the case where both are dichotomies. In Section 7.6 the more general form of the test is developed, where the first criterion has R values and the second, C values.

EXAMPLE 7.5.1. Nightmare Frequencies

Over the years, numerous studies have sought to characterize the nightmare sufferer. Out of these has emerged the stereotype of someone with high anxiety, low ego strength, feelings of inadequacy, and poorer than average physical health. But what is not so well-known is whether men fall into this pattern more often than women. To this end, a recent investigation looked at nightmare frequencies for a sample of 160 men and 192 women (Hersen, 1971). Each subject was asked whether he (or she) experienced nightmares "often" (at least once a month) or "seldom" (less than once a month). The findings are displayed in the accompanying *2 × 2 contingency table*.

		Men	Women	
Nightmare frequency	Often	55	60	115
	Seldom	105	132	237
		160	192	352

Question 7.5.1. What two proportions calculated from these data might be used as an indicator of whether or not "sex" and "nightmare frequency" are dependent variables?

For each of the 352 persons included in this study, two observations have been recorded: (1) sex and (2) frequency of nightmares. If these two variables are, in fact, independent, the true proportion (p_{mo}) of *males* having nightmares often should equal the true proportion (p_{fo}) of *females* having nightmares often. Naturally, the sample estimates of these two parameters vary ($55/160 = 0.34$ as compared to $60/192 = 0.31$). The relevant question, though, is whether a difference of 0.03 ($= 0.34 - 0.31$) is large enough to represent an actual effect or small enough to lie within the range of normal sampling variability. This suggests that we should test

$$H: \quad p_{mo} = p_{fo} \quad \text{versus} \quad A: \quad p_{mo} \neq p_{fo}$$

As was the case with hypothesis tests for Models Two, Three, and Four, the problem is to determine the likelihood of the sample data under the assumption that H is true.

Note that *if* H is true, meaning that sex and nightmare frequency are independent, a pooled estimate of the true proportion of persons (whether male or female) having frequent nightmares would be $115/352$, or 32.8%. Applying this proportion to the total number in the first column of the table, it follows that we should "expect" $(115/352) \times 160 = 52.3$ males to have nightmares often.

Similar calculations would show that

(a) The expected number of females having frequent nightmares is $(115/352) \times 160 = 62.7$.

(b) The expected number of males having infrequent nightmares is $(237/352) \times 160 = 107.7$.

(c) The expected number of females having infrequent nightmares is $(237/352) \times 192 = 129.3$.

The next table shows the observed and expected frequencies for each of the four categories.

		Men	Women	
Nightmare frequency	Often	55 (52.3)	60 (62.7)	115
	Seldom	105 (107.7)	132 (129.3)	237
		160	192	352

Comment

It is not necessary to perform the multiplications indicated in (a), (b), and (c). Expected frequencies, like observed frequencies, must add up to their respective row and column totals. For example, having determined that the expected number of males having frequent nightmares is 52.3, it follows that the expected number of females having frequent nightmares is $115 - 52.3 = 62.7$. Likewise, the expected number of males having infrequent nightmares is $160 - 52.3 = 107.7$, and so on. For 2×2 contingency tables, we need to find only *one* expected value directly; the other three can be found by subtraction.

Since the expected frequencies were computed under the assumption that H was true, it seems reasonable that the null hypothesis should be rejected if the discrepancies between the observed and expected frequencies are too large. The statistic used to measure the magnitude of those discrepancies will be

$$\sum \frac{(obs - exp)^2}{exp}$$

where *obs* and *exp* refer to the observed and expected frequencies in a given category (or cell) and the sum ($\sum$) extends over all the cells in the table. For this example,

$$\sum \frac{(obs - exp)^2}{exp} = \frac{(55 - 52.3)^2}{52.3} + \frac{(60 - 62.7)^2}{62.7} + \frac{(105 - 107.7)^2}{107.7}$$
$$+ \frac{(132 - 129.3)^2}{129.3}$$
$$= 0.14 + 0.12 + 0.07 + 0.06$$
$$= 0.39$$

Of course, whether or not a value of 0.39 reflects discrepancies that are too large depends on the sampling distribution of $\sum (obs - exp)^2/exp$.

Theorem 7.5.1. When the rows and columns of a 2×2 contingency table are independent, the sampling distribution of the statistic

$$\sum \frac{(obs - exp)^2}{exp}$$

is described by a χ^2 curve with 1 degree of freedom. (*Note:* For the approximation to be good, none of the expected frequencies should be less than 5.)

Comment

Appendix IV gives areas under χ^2 curves having degrees of freedom anywhere from 1 to 30. In a χ^2 distribution with 1 degree of freedom, for example, 90% of the area under the curve lies to the left of 2.71, 95% to the left of 3.84, and so on. (See Figure 7.14 on the following page.)

Returning to the data of Example 7.5.1, recall that the null hypothesis H: $p_{mo} = p_{fo}$ will be rejected if $\sum (obs - exp)^2/exp$ is too large. Looking at Appendix IV we see that only about 5% of the time will $\sum (obs - exp)^2/exp$

248   Model Five — The Correlation Problem   [7.5]

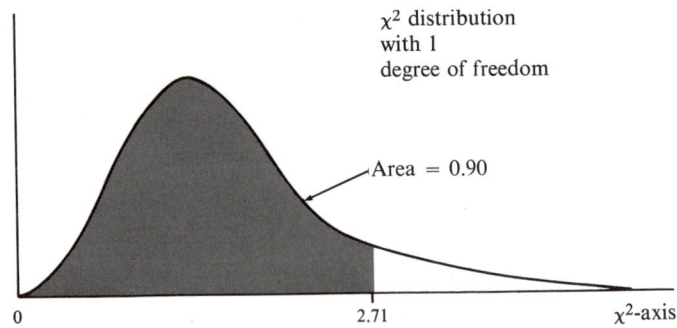

FIGURE 7.14

exceed 3.84 when H is true. Since the computed value of $\sum (obs - exp)^2/exp$ was 0.39, our conclusion, at the $P = .05$ level of significance, would be to *accept* the null hypothesis: males, on the average, have nightmares as often as females.

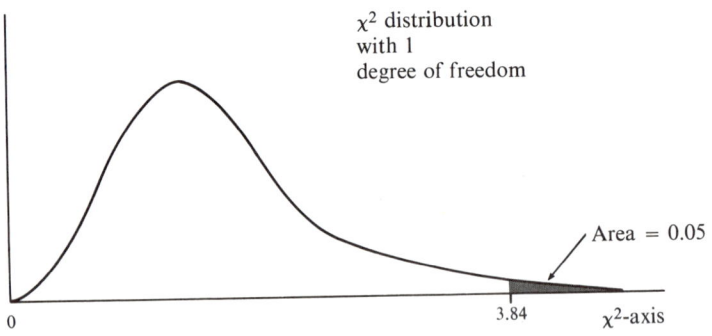

FIGURE 7.15

EXAMPLE 7.5.2. Allergies and Neuropathies

The following data were assembled to see what relationship, if any, could be found between persons with allergies and persons with neuropathies. For the purposes of this study, subjects suffering from conditions such as bronchial asthma or hay fever were considered "allergic." The diagnosis of "neuropath"

		Allergic		
		No	Yes	
Neuropath	Yes	44	58	102
	No	958	220	1178
		1002	278	1280

was something of a catch-all, ranging from people described as "psychopaths" and individuals having a history of mental breakdowns to people who stammer (Leigh and Marley, 1967).

(1) Let p_{NN} and p_{AN} denote the true proportion of (1) nonallergics who are neuropaths and (2) allergics who are neuropaths, respectively. (The sample estimates of p_{NN} and p_{AN} are $44/1002 = 0.04$ and $58/278 = 0.21$.) Our objective is to test

$$\text{H:} \quad p_{NN} = p_{AN} \quad \text{versus} \quad \text{A:} \quad p_{NN} \neq p_{AN}$$

Let $P = .01$.

(2) Following the procedure set out in Example 7.5.1, the expected number of "nonallergic neuropaths" is given by

$$\frac{102}{1280} \times 1002 = 79.8$$

By subtraction, the expected number of allergic neuropaths is $102 - 79.8 = 22.2$. Similarly, the expected number of nonallergics having no neuropathies is $1002 - 79.8 = 922.2$, and the expected number of allergics having no neuropathies is $278 - 22.2 = 255.8$. Therefore,

$$\sum \frac{(obs - exp)^2}{exp} = \frac{(44 - 79.8)^2}{79.8} + \frac{(58 - 22.2)^2}{22.2}$$
$$+ \frac{(958 - 922.2)^2}{922.2} + \frac{(220 - 255.8)^2}{255.8}$$
$$= 16.1 + 57.7 + 1.4 + 5.0$$
$$= 80.2$$

		Allergic		
		No	Yes	
Neuropath	Yes	44 (79.8)	58 (22.2)	102
	No	958 (922.2)	220 (255.8)	1178
		1002	278	1280

(3) By Theorem 7.5.1, the sampling distribution of $\sum (obs - exp)^2/exp$ is
(4) described by a χ^2 distribution with 1 degree of freedom when H: $p_{NN} = p_{AN}$ is true. From Appendix IV, the appropriate critical value, when $P = .01$, is 6.63. It follows, then, that H should be rejected. The proportion of neuropaths is significantly higher among persons *with* allergies than among those *without* allergies.

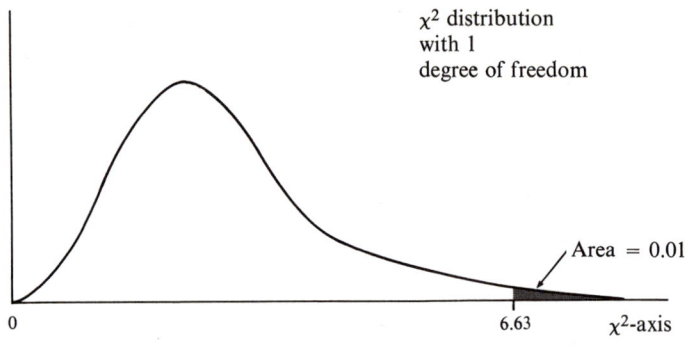

FIGURE 7.16

Question 7.5.2. Do a χ^2 test on the "religion" data of Example 1.9.3. Define carefully the relevant parameters and state your conclusion. Use the $P = .05$ level of significance.

Question 7.5.3. For each of the accompanying 2 × 2 tables, the difference in sample proportions is the same:

$$\left(\frac{200}{1000} - \frac{100}{1000} = \frac{20}{100} - \frac{10}{100}\right)$$

200	100	300
800	900	1700
1000	1000	2000

20	10	30
80	90	170
100	100	200

Which table, if either, will have the higher χ^2 value? Do not do any calculations.

7.6
THE χ^2 TEST: $R \times C$ CONTINGENCY TABLES

With only a few modifications, the χ^2 test described in the previous section can be extended to accommodate contingency tables of *any* size — for example, R rows and C columns. The same statistic, $\sum (obs - exp)^2/exp$, is computed; but the mathematical model that best approximates its sampling distribution is no longer a χ^2 curve with *1* degree of freedom but, rather, a χ^2 curve with $(R - 1)(C - 1)$ degrees of freedom.

EXAMPLE 7.6.1. Drinking and Socioeconomic Status

A while ago, a poll was taken in the state of Washington for the purpose of characterizing drinking habits (Pittman and Snyder, 1962). In one phase of the study, 200 men were asked whether or not they drank. Also, each was placed into one of four socioeconomic strata, the assignment being made on the basis of occupation, education, and family income. ("I" was the highest class; "IV," the lowest.)

		\multicolumn{4}{c}{Socioeconomic class}	
		I	II	III	IV	
Drink	Yes	35	39	52	31	157
	No	12	12	10	9	43
Totals		47	51	62	40	200
(proportions saying "yes")		0.745	0.765	0.839	0.775	

Here, again, the *sample* proportions of drinkers vary from class to class, ranging from 74.5% to 83.9%. What ultimately concerns us, though, is whether the *true* proportions (p_I, p_{II}, p_{III}, p_{IV}) differ, or, equivalently, whether drinking and social class are dependent. Put in the language of hypothesis testing, the problem reduces to

$$H: \quad p_I = p_{II} = p_{III} = p_{IV}$$

versus

$$A: \quad \text{the true proportions are not all equal}$$

If H is true, the best estimate we can give for the true proportion of drinkers (whatever their socioeconomic class) is 157/200, implying that the expected number of drinkers in the upper class is $(157/200) \times 47 = 36.9$. Similarly, the expected numbers of drinkers in the second and third classes are $(157/200) \times 51 = 40.0$ and $(157/200) \times 62 = 48.7$, respectively.

Model Five — The Correlation Problem

	I	II	III	IV	
Drink Yes	35 (36.9)	39 (40.0)	52 (48.7)	31	157
Drink No	12	12	10	9	43
	47	51	62	40	200

Looking at the table and the three expected values already computed, it should be clear that the other five can be obtained by appropriate subtractions. For example, the expected number of lowest class drinkers is $157 - 36.9 - 40.0 - 48.7 = 31.4$; the expected number of highest class nondrinkers is $47 - 36.9 = 10.1$, and so on.

	I	II	III	IV	
Drink Yes	35 (36.9)	39 (40.0)	52 (48.7)	31 (31.4)	157
Drink No	12 (10.1)	12 (11.0)	10 (13.3)	9 (8.6)	43
	47	51	62	40	200

To test the null hypothesis we compute the statistic $\sum (obs - exp)^2/exp$, where the summation now extends over all eight cells:

$$\sum \frac{(obs - exp)^2}{exp} = \frac{(35 - 36.9)^2}{36.9} + \frac{(39 - 40.0)^2}{40.0} + \cdots + \frac{(9 - 8.6)^2}{8.6}$$
$$= 0.10 + 0.02 + \cdots + 0.02$$
$$= 1.63$$

The question of whether or not a value of 1.63 is large enough to warrant the rejection of the null hypothesis is answered in the next theorem.

Theorem 7.6.1. If the rows and columns of an $R \times C$ contingency table are independent, the sampling distribution of

$$\sum \frac{(obs - exp)^2}{exp}$$

is described by a χ^2 curve with $(R - 1)(C - 1)$ degrees of freedom. (*Note:* The approximation is good provided none (or, at the most, very few) of the expected frequencies is less than 5.)

In this example, $(R - 1)(C - 1) = 3$. Also, from Appendix IV, the value from a χ^2 distribution with 3 degrees of freedom that cuts off an area of 0.05 to its right is 7.81. Since the observed χ^2 value (1.63) lies to the left of 7.81, we should accept the null hypothesis (at the $P = .05$ level of significance). The true proportions are equal; the drinking habits of males are not dependent on social class.

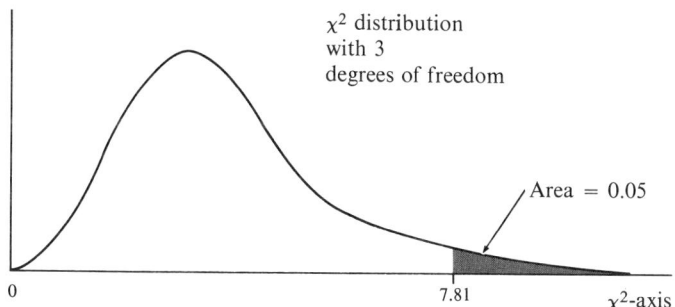

FIGURE 7.17

Question 7.6.1. As part of this same survey, a random sample of 208 women were questioned about *their* drinking habits and similarly assigned to one of four socioeconomic levels. Of the 66 women in class I, 42 drank; of the 56 in class II, 38 drank; of the 57 in class III, 34 drank; and of the 29 in class IV, 6 drank. At the $P = .01$ level of significance, test whether drinking habits and socioeconomic status are independent factors for women.

EXAMPLE 7.6.2. Medication Errors in Five Large Hospitals

During the summer of 1969, audits were made in five large hospitals for the purpose of comparing the frequencies with which their staffs made medication errors (Hynniman et al., 1970). Of particular interest were errors of omission, defined as "any dose determined to be incorrectly not administered to a patient."

		Hospital					
		A	B	C	D	E	
Omission	Yes	54	64	91	116	162	487
	No	1,867	724	1,341	1,163	5,899	10994
		1921	788	1432	1279	6061	11481

(1) Let p_A, p_B, p_C, p_D, and p_E denote the true error rates. Our objective is to test

$$H: \quad p_A = p_B = p_C = p_D = p_E$$

254 Model Five — The Correlation Problem [7.6]

versus

A: true error rates are not all equal

Let .01 be the level of significance.

(2) Under the assumption that H is true, the number of errors of omission that Hospital A would be expected to commit is given by

$$\frac{487}{11{,}481} \times 1{,}921 = 81.4$$

For Hospital B, the corresponding figure is

$$\frac{487}{11{,}481} \times 788 = 33.4$$

Expected values for Hospitals C and D are calculated similarly.

		Hospital A	B	C	D	E	
Omission	Yes	54 (81.4)	64 (33.4)	91 (60.8)	116 (54.2)	162	487
	No	1,867	724	1,341	1,163	5,899	10994
		1921	788	1432	1279	6061	11481

The remaining six expected values can then be found by subtraction.

		Hospital A	B	C	D	E	
Omission	Yes	54 (31.4)	64 (33.4)	91 (60.8)	116 (54.2)	162 (257.2)	487
	No	1,867 (1,839.6)	724 (754.6)	1,341 (1,371.2)	1,163 (1,224.8)	5,899 (5,803.8)	10994
		1921	788	1432	1279	6061	11481

Therefore,

$$\sum \frac{(obs - exp)^2}{exp} = \frac{(54 - 81.4)^2}{81.4} + \frac{(64 - 33.4)^2}{33.4} + \cdots$$
$$+ \frac{(5{,}899 - 5{,}803.8)^2}{5{,}803.8}$$
$$= 9.22 + 28.03 + \cdots + 1.56$$
$$= 165.02$$

[7.6] The χ^2 Test: $R \times C$ Contingency Tables 255

(3) The χ^2 curve that approximates the sampling distribution of
(4) $\sum (obs - exp)^2/exp$ has $(R - 1)(C - 1) = (2 - 1)(5 - 1) = 4$ degrees of freedom. From Appendix IV, the corresponding $P = .01$ critical value would be 13.3.

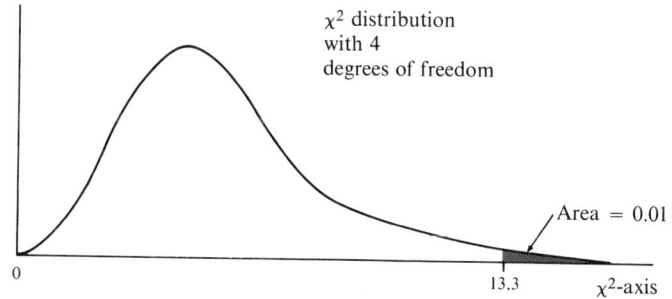

FIGURE 7.18

Our conclusion in this case is obvious: reject H, because the observed differences in error rates are far too great to be attributed to chance.

Question 7.6.2. By rejecting H in this example, have we, at the same time, rejected the hypothesis that $p_B = p_D$?

The final example in this section shows the analysis of an $R \times C$ contingency table where R is greater than 2. The only real difference between this problem and the two preceding ones is in the formation of the null hypothesis.

EXAMPLE 7.6.3. Schizophrenia — Is it Inherited?

Hebephrenia, catatonia, and paranoia are three mental disorders related to schizophrenia. The following data were collected to see what influence, if any, heredity has in determining the *type* of schizophrenic a person is likely to become (Rosenthal, 1970). The subjects were 160 children and young adults with mental disorders who also had a relative with a diagnosed mental condition. A summary of the findings is shown in the accompanying 3×3 table.

		Diagnosis of index case			
		Hebephrenia	Catatonia	Paranoia	
	Hebephrenia	49	6	5	60
Diagnosis of relative	Catatonia	10	31	10	51
	Paranoia	21	15	13	49
		80	52	28	160

Model Five — The Correlation Problem

The question to be answered by these data is whether the mental states of the index cases are independent of the conditions of their relatives. To be more specific, let p_H, p_C, and p_P be the true proportions of hebephrenic, catatonic, and paranoic children, respectively, who have relatives with hebephrenia. The sample estimates of p_H, p_C, p_P are $49/80$ ($= 0.61$), $6/52$ ($= 0.12$), and $5/28$ ($= 0.18$). Likewise, let q_H, q_C, and q_P be the true proportions of hebephrenic, catatonic, and paranoic children who have relatives with catatonia. These proportions are estimated by $10/80$ ($= 0.12$), $31/52$ ($= 0.60$), and $10/28$ ($=0.36$). Let r_H, r_C, and r_P be similarly defined for children whose relatives have paranoia.

The formal statement of our test would be

$$H: \quad p_H = p_C = p_P$$
$$q_H = q_C = q_P$$
$$r_H = r_C = r_P$$

versus

A: at least one of the null hypothesis equalities is false

Assuming H to be true, the expected number of hebephrenic children having hebephrenic relatives is $(60/160) \times 80 = 30.0$. Similarly, the expected number of catatonic children with hebephrenic relatives is $(60/160) \times 52 = 19.5$. Likewise, the expected values for the two left-most cells in the *second* row of the table are $(51/160) \times 80 = 25.5$ and $(51/160) \times 52 = 16.6$, respectively. Note that once these four numbers have been computed, the other five expected frequencies can be obtained by subtraction.

		Diagnosis of index case			
		Hebephrenia	Catatonia	Paranoia	
Diagnosis of relative	Hebephrenia	49 (30.0)	6 (19.5)	5 (10.5)	60
	Catatonia	10 (25.5)	31 (16.6)	10 (8.9)	51
	Paranoia	21 (24.5)	15 (15.9)	13 (8.6)	49
		80	52	28	160

Here the sampling distribution of $\sum (obs - exp)^2/exp$ is approximated by a χ^2 curve with $4 = [(3-1)(3-1)]$ degrees of freedom, so it follows from Appendix IV that H should be rejected at the $P = .05$ level of significance if $\sum (obs - exp)^2/exp > 9.49$. But,

$$\sum \frac{(obs - exp)^2}{exp} = \frac{(49 - 30.0)^2}{30.0} + \frac{(6 - 19.5)^2}{19.5} + \cdots + \frac{(13 - 8.6)^2}{8.6}$$
$$= 12.03 + 9.35 + \cdots + 2.25$$
$$= 79.11$$

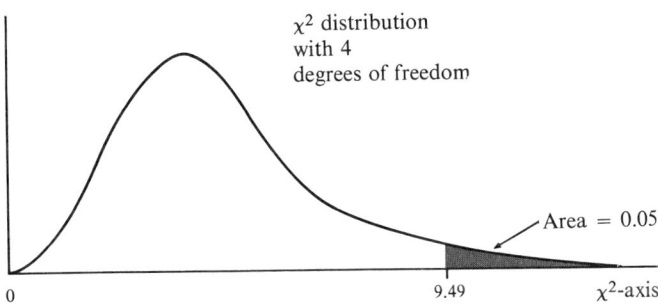

FIGURE 7.19

Therefore, we must reject H and conclude that there is some factor *other* than chance that must be accounting for the observed pattern of schizophrenic types among relatives. In particular, there is a strong tendency for the *same* type to reappear in a given "family," as evidenced by the fact that the observed frequencies greatly exceed the expected frequencies along the diagonal of the contingency table.

Question 7.6.3. How might these data be reduced from a 3 × 3 table to a 2 × 2 table and still include all 160 subjects?

7.7 SUMMARY

In a Model Five problem, two observations, x_i and y_i, are recorded for each of the members in the sample. Typically, the two traits being measured will be dissimilar, and $x_i - y_i$ will have no meaning. But in this case that does not matter, because the purpose of a correlation analysis is to characterize the *relationship* between X and Y (as opposed to, say, comparing μ_X and μ_Y).

If X and Y are both *quantitative*, a scatterdiagram should be drawn before anything more mathematical is even considered. If the relationship proves to be linear, we might then find the *least squares line* (Section 7.2) and/or compute the *sample correlation coefficient* (Section 7.3). (The least squares line, in addition to summarizing the way in which X and Y are related, is essential should it become necessary to predict the value of Y given a particular value of X. The correlation coefficient is important when the situation demands that the strength of one linear relationship be compared to that of another.)

The *independence* of X and Y can be established by testing H: $\rho = 0$, where ρ is the population correlation coefficient. Section 7.4 explains how such a test is carried out and how its results are to be interpreted. Of course, if the scatterdiagram shows a very strong XY-relationship, any formal test of H: $\rho = 0$ would belabor the obvious.

If the two variables are *qualitative*, the χ^2 test becomes the appropriate technique for testing independence (Sections 7.5 and 7.6). This is actually a more useful technique than it might at first appear for the simple reason that any quantitative variable can always be reduced to one that is qualitative. Blood pressures, for example, do not have to be measured in terms of millimeters of mercury; in some instances, it may be quite adequate to record them, qualitatively, as low, normal, or high. Because of its generality, and because the independence of two variables is often an extremely important question, the χ^2 test is the most frequently used analysis in medical statistics.

Definitions

Chi square test (χ^2). A procedure for testing whether either of two factors has any influence over the other. If not, the two are said to be *independent*. It compares observed and expected frequencies with the statistic $\Sigma \, (obs - exp)^2/exp$.

Contingency table. A table having R rows and C columns, where each row corresponds to a level of one factor and each column to a level of the other factor; entries in the body of the table are the frequencies with which each factor combination occurred.

Correlation. A term referring to the linear relationship between two variables; if the variables tend to increase simultaneously the correlation is said to be *positive;* if one tends to increase when the other decreases, the correlation is said to be *negative.*

Least squares line. A straight line whose slope and Y-intercept are determined by the method of least squares.

Method of least squares. A technique for fitting a straight line, $Y = a + bX$, through a set of points $\{(x_1, y_1), (x_2, y_2), \ldots, (x_n, y_n)\}$; the coefficients, a and b, are chosen so that the sum of the squared vertical distances from the n points to the line is minimized.

Sample correlation coefficient (r). The statistic for measuring the *strength* of the linear relationship between two variables; estimates ρ, the population correlation coefficient.

Review Exercises

7.1 One way to gauge the overall success of heart transplantation is to look at the three-month survival rate — that is, the proportion of recipients who lived for at least three months after their operation. The table below lists the number of transplants performed and the three-month survival rates for three different time periods (Brim et al., 1970).

	Dec., 1967–May, 1968	June, 1968–Nov., 1968	Dec., 1968–May, 1969
Number of transplants	19	78	35
3-month survival rate	16%	38%	23%

(a) Use a χ^2 test to determine whether "date of operation" and "success of operation" are independent. (Remember that the χ^2 test can be used only on frequencies, and not on rates.)

(b) What might account for the fact that the survival rate has not steadily improved with time?

7.2 In a study designed to see whether a controlled diet could retard the process of arteriosclerosis, a total of 846 randomly chosen persons were followed over an eight-year period (Brunner et al., 1972). Half were instructed to eat only certain foods; the other half could eat whatever they wanted. At the end of eight years, 66 persons in the diet group were found to have died of either myocardial infarction or cerebral infarction, as compared to 93 deaths of a similar nature in the control group. What inference can be drawn? Be as quantitative as possible.

7.3 Do a χ^2 test on the rubella–birth defects data of Example 1.9.4. Use the $P = .01$ level of significance.

7.4 The following data are estimates of the total lung capacity for 25 persons. Two values were determined for each; both were obtained solely on the basis of standard chest roentgenograms (Harris, Pratt, and Kilburn, 1971).

	Total lung capacity (liters)	
Patient	Planimeter method (x)	Barnhard method (y)
R.S.	6.25	6.49
W.M.	5.57	5.33
J.B.	7.25	6.92
K.T.	6.86	7.08
J.A.	6.23	7.11
S.V.	5.22	5.05
R.T.	6.70	6.62
H.B.	6.37	6.09
C.D.	6.48	7.29
R.B.	7.70	8.20
B.G.	8.19	8.45
K.K.	6.98	6.49
V.G.	5.72	6.30
R.W.	7.15	7.12
W.G.	6.55	6.16
W.P.	5.11	4.40
R.H.	5.81	6.25
H.A.	7.85	7.56
L.H.	5.99	6.17
H.L.	7.68	7.63
M.R.	5.15	4.42
E.M.	6.31	5.26
E.G.	3.76	3.26
M.J.	5.07	4.58
A.M.	6.01	5.42

(a) Plot the data and find the least squares line. Note:

$$\sum_{i=1}^{25} x_i = 157.96 \qquad \sum_{i=1}^{25} x_i^2 = 1023.7124$$

$$\sum_{i=1}^{25} y_i = 155.65 \qquad \sum_{i=1}^{25} y_i^2 = 1007.7919$$

$$\sum_{i=1}^{25} x_i y_i = 1012.6751$$

(b) If a person's total lung capacity according to the planimeter method was 5.70 liters, what estimate would we expect from the Barnhard method?

(c) Verify that the least squares line goes through the point $(\bar{x}, \bar{y})$.

7.5 Find the least squares line for the radiation exposure–cancer mortality data of Review Exercise 1.1. If X represents the exposure index and Y, the mortality rate, then

$$\sum_{i=1}^{9} x_i = 41.56 \qquad \sum_{i=1}^{9} x_i^2 = 289.4222$$

$$\sum_{i=1}^{9} y_i = 1416.1 \qquad \sum_{i=1}^{9} y_i^2 = 232{,}498.97$$

$$\sum_{i=1}^{9} x_i y_i = 7439.37$$

7.6 Compute the correlation coefficient for the radiation data of Review Exercise 1.1. Also, at the $P = .05$ level of significance, test

$$H: \rho = 0 \quad \text{versus} \quad A: \rho > 0$$

(See Review Exercise 7.5.)

7.7 High blood pressure is known to be one of the major contributors to coronary heart disease. The purpose of the following study was to see whether or not there was a significant relationship between the blood pressures of children and those of their fathers. (If such a relationship *did* exist, it might be possible to use one group to screen for high risk individuals in the other group.) The subjects were 92 eleventh graders, 47 males and 45 females, and their fathers. Blood pressures for both the children and the fathers were categorized as belonging to either the lower, middle, or upper third of their respective distributions (Ibrahim et al., 1968).

		Child's blood pressure		
		Lower third	Middle third	Upper third
Father's blood pressure	Lower third	14	11	8
	Middle third	11	11	9
	Upper third	6	10	12

Test whether or not the blood pressures of children can be considered to be independent of the blood pressures of their fathers. Use the $P = .05$ level of significance.

7.8 Compare the suicide rates for male and female members of the American Chemical Society (Review Exercise 1.4). Use the $P = .05$ level of significance.

7.9 Test the effectiveness of carbolic acid as a wound disinfectant, using Lister's amputation data as given in Review Exercise 1.13.

7.10 The question of whether or not birth order is related to delinquency was examined in a large-scale study using a high school population (Nye, 1958). A total of 1154 girls in public high school were given a questionnaire which measured the degree to which each had exhibited delinquent behavior, in terms of criminal acts, "immoral" conduct, etc. Some 111 were thought to have shown, on the basis of the questionnaire, definite delinquent tendencies. Each girl in the sample was also asked to indicate her birth order as being either (1) the oldest, (2) in between, (3) the youngest, or (4) an only child.

		Oldest	In between	Youngest	Only child
Delinquent	Yes	24	29	35	23
tendencies	No	450	312	211	70
Totals		474	341	246	93

Analyze these data. Define all the relevant parameters.

8

MODEL SIX
The *k*-Sample Problem

*Chance is always powerful.
Let your hook be always cast;
in the pool where you least expect it,
there will be a fish.*
                                    Ovid

8.1
INTRODUCTION

Making a comparison is often the primary reason for doing an experiment. Does Treatment 1 elicit a more favorable response than Treatment 2? Do persons living under Condition X behave differently from those living under Condition Y? or Condition Z? Can surfaces sprayed with Disinfectant A maintain lower bacterial counts than ones sprayed with Disinfectants B, C, or D? These are all very reasonable questions; and what they suggest is that statistical methods, if they are to be of any real value to a researcher, must be capable of making many different kinds of comparisons, in a variety of experimental settings.

Of course, much of what we have covered has already touched on this very problem. Both the two-sample model and the paired-data model are concerned almost exclusively with testing the effects of one treatment (or condition) against those of another. And even the one-sample model and the correlation model are sometimes used to make comparisons. Unfortunately, all of these procedures are rather limited — by the *number* of treatments they can accommodate. In fact, two is the upper limit. But with the k-sample model described in this chapter, an experimenter has the capability of comparing *any* number of treatments, all at the same time.

Actually, the *structure* of a k-sample problem contains nothing that is fundamentally new. There are k populations being considered, and each is represented by a sample. The sizes of the samples do not have to be the same but, for obvious reasons, all the measurements must be similar (in the sense of Section 1.7). The major restriction of Model Six is that each of the k samples must be *independent*. That is, none of the responses in the ith sample should have any influence on, or be correlated with, any of the responses in the jth sample. In this sense, the k-sample problem is a direct extension of the two-sample problem.

Comment

The k-sample model is actually much more general than it might appear to be from this chapter. With certain modifications, it can be used to analyze extremely complex experiments, ones where the factors are all interrelated. But here our attention will be restricted to the simplest type of k-sample problem, the kind that was illustrated in Examples 1.10.1 and 1.10.2.

Despite its similarity to the two-sample problem, Model Six requires a somewhat different system of notation. The subscript idea of Chapter 1 can still be used but a second index needs to be added. This means that an arbitrary observation will no longer be written as x_i, but rather, as x_{ij}. The details of this new notation, and the reasons it is necessary, are the subjects of Section 8.2.

In Section 8.3, a procedure is developed for testing the hypothesis that the means of k populations are all equal; that is, for testing H: $\mu_1 = \mu_2 = \cdots = \mu_k$. (This is the usual objective in a k-sample problem.) Then, in Section 8.4, a series of computing formulas are introduced that simplify the calculations indicated in Section 8.3.

8.2 DOUBLE SUBSCRIPT NOTATION

The subscript notation introduced in Chapter 1 has been perfectly adequate up to now but it is not quite general enough to cope with the k-sample problem. When there were only two sets of measurements to be considered, as in Models Three, Four, and Five, it was always possible to denote the first set as $x_1, x_2, \ldots, x_n$ and the second as $y_1, y_2, \ldots, y_n$. But what would happen if the number of treatment groups was much larger than two? Clearly, using a different letter to represent each set of measurements would soon become unworkably cumbersome. A far better solution is a method of indexing known as *double subscript notation*.

For example, suppose an experiment involving $k = 3$ treatment groups has produced the following eight observations:

Double Subscript Notation

	Treatment group	
1	2	3
16	9	14
21	17	15
14		8

We will let the symbol x_{ij} denote the jth observation in the ith treatment group. Here the j simply refers to the *order* in which the observation appears (within the ith group). Therefore, 16 would become x_{11}, 21 would be x_{12}, 9 would be x_{21}, and so on.

	Treatment group	
1	2	3
16 (= x_{11})	9 (= x_{21})	14 (= x_{31})
21 (= x_{12})	17 (= x_{22})	15 (= x_{32})
14 (= x_{13})		8 (= x_{33})

Also, n_i will denote the number of individuals receiving treatment i and N will denote the total sample size. Therefore,

$$\sum_{i=1}^{k} n_i = N$$

In this example, $k = 3$, $n_1 = 3$, $n_2 = 2$, $n_3 = 3$, and $N = 8$.

For reasons explained in the next section, it will also be helpful to have a special notation for (1) the sum and the mean of the ith sample and (2) the sum and the mean for the *entire* sample. The symbols $T_1.$ and $\bar{x}_1.$ will denote the sum and the mean of the ith sample. That is,

$$T_i. = \sum_{j=1}^{n_i} x_{ij} \quad \text{and} \quad \bar{x}_i. = \frac{1}{n_i} \sum_{j=1}^{n_i} x_{ij}$$

For these data,

$$T_1. = 16 + 21 + 14 = 51$$
$$\bar{x}_1. = \frac{1}{3}(16 + 21 + 14) = 17.0$$
$$T_2. = 9 + 17 = 26$$
$$\bar{x}_2. = \frac{1}{2}(9 + 17) = 13.0$$
$$T_3. = 14 + 15 + 8 = 37$$
$$\bar{x}_3. = \frac{1}{3}(14 + 15 + 8) = 12.3$$

Comment

The purpose of dots in subscript notation is to indicate that a particular index has already been summed. For example, $T_3.$ refers to the sum of terms such as

x_{3j}, over all possible values of j. Likewise, $T..$, as defined in the next paragraph, denotes the sum of terms like x_{ij} over all possible values of i and j.

To denote the sum of *all* the observations in a k-sample problem we need to have *two* sigma signs, one indicating summation over i, and the other, summation over j. To see how this is done, note that the overall total, or "grand sum," can be broken down into the sum *between* the groups of the sums *within* the groups. That is,

$$\text{Grand sum} = (\text{sum of 1}^{\text{st}}\text{ group}) + (\text{sum of 2}^{\text{nd}}\text{ group})$$
$$+ \cdots + (\text{sum of } k^{\text{th}} \text{ group})$$
$$= \sum_{j=1}^{n_1} x_{1j} + \sum_{j=1}^{n_2} x_{2j} + \cdots + \sum_{j=1}^{n_k} x_{kj}$$
$$= \text{sum "over" the } k \text{ values for } i \text{ of } \sum_{j=1}^{n_i} x_{ij}$$

This last expression can be written with a second sigma sign so that

$$\text{Grand sum} = \sum_{i=1}^{k} \sum_{j=1}^{n_i} x_{ij}$$

Using the symbol $T..$ to designate the grand sum,

$$T.. = \sum_{i=1}^{k} \sum_{j=1}^{n_i} x_{ij}$$
$$= (16 + 21 + 14) + (9 + 17) + (14 + 15 + 8)$$
$$= 51 + 26 + 37$$
$$= 114$$

Having developed a notation for the grand sum, it remains a simple matter to write a formula for the grand mean. Specifically,

$$\bar{x}.. = \text{grand mean} = \frac{1}{N} \sum_{i=1}^{k} \sum_{j=1}^{n_i} x_{ij}$$

or, equivalently,

$$\bar{x}.. = \frac{1}{N} \sum_{i=1}^{k} T_{i.} = \frac{T..}{N}$$

For the eight measurements listed,

$$\bar{x}.. = \frac{1}{8}(114) = 14.2$$

Question 8.2.1. For the data in the table, evaluate the designated expressions.

Treatment group			
1	2	3	4
2	3	1	2
0	1	4	1
	1	2	5
	2		

(a) $\sum_{i=1}^{4} \sum_{j=1}^{n_i} x_{ij}$

(b) $\sum_{j=1}^{3} x_{3j}$

(c) $\bar{x}_2.$

(d) $\bar{x}..$

(e) $\sum_{j=1}^{2} (x_{1j} - \bar{x}_1.)^2$

Question 8.2.2. Write a general formula for the sample standard deviation of the observations in the ith treatment group.

Question 8.2.3. Explain the difference between

$$\sum_{i=1}^{k} \sum_{j=1}^{n_i} x_{ij}^2 \quad \text{and} \quad \left(\sum_{i=1}^{k} \sum_{j=1}^{n_i} x_{ij} \right)^2$$

Question 8.2.4. Show that another way of writing the grand mean is

$$\bar{x}.. = \frac{1}{N} \sum_{i=1}^{k} n_i \bar{x}_i.$$

8.3
HYPOTHESIS TESTING IN THE k-SAMPLE PROBLEM

Analyzing a k-sample problem is considerably more difficult than doing a t-test or a χ^2 test; the computations are lengthier, and the statistical reasoning is more abstract. For this reason, the procedure that is used, a technique known as the *analysis of variance*, will be developed over the next *two* sections. Here the objective is to formulate the appropriate null hypothesis and indicate, on intuitive grounds, how it might be tested. Then in Section 8.4 we will show how the analysis of variance is actually done in practice.

Imagine an experiment designed to compare the "cure" times associated with four different counseling techniques. Cure times will be measured in terms of the number of patient–counselor sessions that are needed to resolve the patient's problem. Suppose that a total of $N \,(= 12)$ patients, all with the same condition, are randomly allocated into four groups, with the n_1 persons in the first group receiving Therapy 1; the n_2 in the second group, Therapy 2; and so on. (In the discussion that follows, all the n_i's will be assumed equal and will be denoted by the symbol n, but the same method applies when the sample sizes are unequal.) When the study is over, the data might look like the accompanying table.

Number of sessions required
Therapy

1	2	3	4
$6\,(= x_{11})$	$12\,(= x_{21})$	$6\,(= x_{31})$	$4\,(= x_{41})$
$8\,(= x_{12})$	$13\,(= x_{22})$	$7\,(= x_{32})$	$6\,(= x_{42})$
$11\,(= x_{13})$	$10\,(= x_{23})$	$4\,(= x_{33})$	$9\,(= x_{43})$
$\bar{x}_1. = 8.3$	$\bar{x}_2. = 11.7$	$\bar{x}_3. = 5.7$	$\bar{x}_4. = 6.3$

$\bar{x}.. = 8.0$

Probably the first question this experiment should answer is whether or not the treatments being considered will elicit, in the long run, the same *average* response. We know, of course, that the *sample* averages — in this case, $\bar{x}_1.$, $\bar{x}_2.$, $\bar{x}_3.$, and $\bar{x}_4.$ — will not all be the same; the relevant question, though, is whether it can be concluded that the *population* averages — μ_1, μ_2, μ_3, and μ_4 — are not all the same. This suggests that we do a hypothesis test, where the alternatives are

$$H: \quad \mu_1 = \mu_2 = \mu_3 = \mu_4$$

versus

$$A: \quad \text{not all the } \mu_i\text{'s are equal}$$

Intuitively, if the sample averages are sufficiently close to one another, the null hypothesis will be accepted; if not, it will be rejected.

Deciding what is "close" in a situation like this is accomplished in what may seem to be a very roundabout way. In fact, we will measure the closeness of the sample means by looking at a ratio of sample variances (see the Comment following Definition 3.5.1.) This is why the method is known as the analysis of *variance* even though the hypothesis being tested involves means.

As always, a good way to begin *any* analysis, whatever the model, is by displaying the data graphically. In this case, the most appropriate format would be the kind that was used for Model Three. A typical example is Figure 8.1, showing the individual cure times (x_{ij}), the treatment means ($\bar{x}_i.$), and the grand mean ($\bar{x}..$).

Looking at the graph, it seems plausible that testing the null hypothesis that $\mu_1 = \mu_2 = \mu_3 = \mu_4$ could be accomplished by comparing the variability *between* the groups (as reflected in the differences among the $\bar{x}_i.$'s) to the variabil-

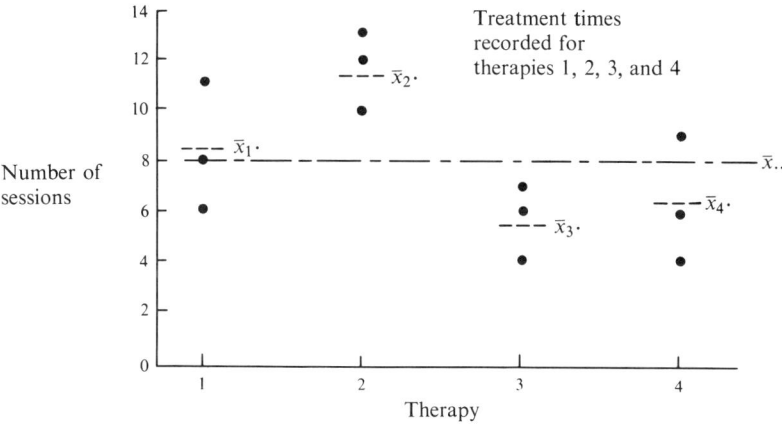

FIGURE 8.1

ity *within* the groups (as reflected in the differences of the x_{ij}'s from their respective $\bar{x}_i.$'s). Specifically, if the former is too large relative to the latter, we reject the null hypothesis. The rest of Section 8.3 shows how this basic idea is translated into a precise mathematical formulation.

Comment

The rationale that is being suggested here is nothing new. In Model Three the null hypothesis that $\mu_X = \mu_Y$ was also tested by comparing the between-treatment variability (as measured by $\bar{x} - \bar{y}$) to the within-treatment variability (as measured by s_p).

To begin, recall from Question 8.2.2 that the sample standard deviation for the ith treatment group can be written as

$$s_i = \sqrt{\frac{1}{n_i - 1} \sum_{j=1}^{n_i} (x_{ij} - \bar{x}_i.)^2}$$

Therefore,

$$s_1 = \sqrt{\frac{1}{2}\{(6 - 8.3)^2 + (8 - 8.3)^2 + (11 - 8.3)^2\}}$$
$$= \sqrt{\frac{1}{2}(12.67)} = \sqrt{6.3}$$
$$= 2.5$$

Similarly,

$$s_2 = \sqrt{\frac{1}{2}\{(12 - 11.7)^2 + (13 - 11.7)^2 + (10 - 11.7)^2\}}$$
$$= \sqrt{2.3} = 1.5$$

$$s_3 = \sqrt{\frac{1}{2}\{(6-5.7)^2 + (7-5.7)^2 + (4-5.7)^2\}}$$
$$= \sqrt{2.3} = 1.5$$

and

$$s_4 = \sqrt{\frac{1}{2}\{(4-6.3)^2 + (6-6.3)^2 + (9-6.3)^2\}}$$
$$= \sqrt{6.3} = 2.5$$

Back in Chapter 5, two sample variances (s_X^2 and s_Y^2, based on n_X and n_Y observations, respectively) were combined to form a pooled standard deviation, s_p, where

$$s_p = \sqrt{\frac{(n_X - 1)s_X^2 + (n_Y - 1)s_Y^2}{n_X + n_Y - 2}}$$

This same rationale can be used in Model Six to pool k sample variances. Here the appropriate formula, by analogy, would be

$$\sqrt{\frac{(n_1 - 1)s_1^2 + (n_2 - 1)s_2^2 + \cdots + (n_k - 1)s_k^2}{n_1 + n_2 + \cdots + n_k - k}}$$

or, using sigma notation

$$\sqrt{\frac{\sum_{i=1}^{k}(n_i - 1)s_i^2}{N - k}} = \sqrt{\frac{\sum_{i=1}^{k}\sum_{j=1}^{n_i}(x_{ij} - \bar{x}_{i\cdot})^2}{N - k}}$$

For the therapy data, the pooled standard deviation becomes

$$\sqrt{\frac{2(2.5)^2 + 2(1.5)^2 + 2(1.5)^2 + 2(2.5)^2}{12 - 4}} = \sqrt{\frac{34.4}{8}} = 2.1$$

Recall that in the two-sample problem, it was assumed that the X and Y populations had the same standard deviation, σ. Furthermore, σ was estimated by the pooled standard deviation, s_p. Here we assume that all k populations have the same standard deviation: $\sigma_1 = \sigma_2 = \cdots = \sigma_k \ (= \sigma)$. It follows that this "new" σ can be estimated by the "new" pooled standard deviation

$$\sqrt{\frac{\sum_{i=1}^{k}(n_i - 1)s_i^2}{N - k}}$$

Because of the way it is formed, this is referred to as the within-treatment estimate of σ, and is written $\hat{\sigma}$ (within).

As we will soon see, the procedure for testing H: $\mu_1 = \mu_2 = \cdots = \mu_k$ hinges on finding *two* "independent" estimates for the parameter σ. We already have one, $\hat{\sigma}$ (within). A second can be found from the $\bar{x}_{i\cdot}$'s. Note that if the null hypothesis is true, and $\mu_1 = \mu_2 = \cdots = \mu_k$, the quantity

$$\sqrt{\frac{\sum_{i=1}^{k}(\bar{x}_{i\cdot} - \bar{x}_{\cdot\cdot})^2}{k-1}}$$

will estimate the standard deviation of the sample means, $\sigma/\sqrt{n}$. Therefore,

$$\sqrt{n}\sqrt{\frac{\sum_{i=1}^{k}(\bar{x}_{i\cdot} - \bar{x}_{\cdot\cdot})^2}{k-1}} = \sqrt{\frac{n\sum_{i=1}^{k}(\bar{x}_{i\cdot} - \bar{x}_{\cdot\cdot})^2}{k-1}}$$

should estimate σ. For obvious reasons, this is called the between-treatment estimate of σ, and we write it $\hat{\sigma}$ (between). For the sample data,

$$\hat{\sigma}\text{ (between)} = \sqrt{\frac{3}{3}\{(8.3 - 8.0)^2 + (11.7 - 8.0)^2 + (5.7 - 8.0)^2 + (6.3 - 8.0)^2\}}$$

$$= \sqrt{\frac{3}{3}\{21.96\}} = 4.7$$

Actually, our interest will focus on the *squares* of these two estimates for σ. Of course, since both $\hat{\sigma}^2$ (within) and $\hat{\sigma}^2$ (between) are statistics, each has an associated sampling distribution. It can be shown mathematically that, *if H is true*, the means of these two sampling distributions are the same; they both equal σ^2. But if the null hypothesis is *not* true, the mean of the between-treatment estimate will be inflated by virtue of the differences between the μ_i's. These same differences, though, will leave the mean of the $\hat{\sigma}^2$ (within) distribution unaffected. It follows that the *ratio* of these two variances can be used to assess the credibility of the null hypothesis.

All of this implies that we should test

H: $\mu_1 = \mu_2 = \cdots = \mu_k$ versus   A: not all the μ_i's are equal

by computing

$$\frac{\hat{\sigma}^2 \text{ (between)}}{\hat{\sigma}^2 \text{ (within)}} = \frac{\dfrac{n\sum_{i=1}^{k}(\bar{x}_{i\cdot} - \bar{x}_{\cdot\cdot})^2}{k-1}}{\dfrac{\sum_{i=1}^{k}\sum_{j=1}^{n}(x_{ij} - \bar{x}_{i\cdot})^2}{N-k}}$$

$$= \frac{n(N-k)\sum_{i=1}^{k}(\bar{x}_{i\cdot} - \bar{x}_{\cdot\cdot})^2}{(k-1)\sum_{i=1}^{k}\sum_{j=1}^{n}(x_{ij} - \bar{x}_{i\cdot})^2}$$

If this ratio is too much larger than 1, we should reject the null hypothesis.

Of course, in order to formulate a precise decision rule, it is necessary to know the sampling distribution of the test statistic — in this case, the sampling distribution of

$$\frac{n(N-k)\sum_{i=1}^{k}(\bar{x}_{i.}-\bar{x}_{..})^2}{(k-1)\sum_{i=1}^{k}\sum_{j=1}^{n}(x_{ij}-\bar{x}_{i.})^2}$$

> **Theorem 8.3.1.** Suppose each of k treatments is represented by a random sample of size n. Also suppose the k response distributions associated with the treatments are all bell-shaped and have the same standard deviation. Then, if H: $\mu_1 = \mu_2 = \cdots = \mu_k$ is true, the sampling distribution of
>
> $$\frac{n(N-k)\sum_{i=1}^{k}(\bar{x}_{i.}-\bar{x}_{..})^2}{(k-1)\sum_{i=1}^{k}\sum_{j=1}^{n}(x_{ij}-\bar{x}_{i.})^2}$$
>
> is described by an F-distribution with $k-1$ and $N-k$ degrees of freedom, where N is the total sample size.
>
> If the sample sizes are not all equal, the same conclusion holds, but the test statistic is written
>
> $$\frac{(N-k)\sum_{i=1}^{k}n_i(\bar{x}_{i.}-\bar{x}_{..})^2}{(k-1)\sum_{i=1}^{k}\sum_{j=1}^{n_i}(x_{ij}-\bar{x}_{i.})^2}$$

Comment

For the sake of generality, we will write the test statistic for H: $\mu_1 = \mu_2 = \cdots = \mu_k$ in the *second* form given in Theorem 8.3.1; that is, as

$$\frac{(N-k)\sum_{i=1}^{k}n_i(\bar{x}_{i.}-\bar{x}_{..})^2}{(k-1)\sum_{i=1}^{k}\sum_{j=1}^{n_i}(x_{ij}-\bar{x}_{i.})^2}$$

When all the n_i's are equal (to n), this second form reduces to the first.

Since the mean of the $\hat{\sigma}^2$ (between) distribution will be *larger* than σ^2 when the μ_i's are not all equal, Theorem 8.3.1 implies that H: $\mu_1 = \mu_2 = \cdots = \mu_k$ should be rejected at, say, the $P = .05$ level of significance if

$$\frac{(N-k)\sum_{i=1}^{k}n_i(\bar{x}_{i.}-\bar{x}_{..})^2}{(k-1)\sum_{i=1}^{k}\sum_{j=1}^{n_i}(x_{ij}-\bar{x}_{i.})^2} \geq F'$$

where

$$P\{F \geq F'\} = 0.05$$

Comment

Values of F' for $P = .05$ and $P = .01$ and for various values of $k - 1$ and $N - k$ are provided in Appendix V.

For this example, $k - 1 = 3$, and $N - k = 9$, so that $F' = 3.86$. But

$$\frac{\hat{\sigma}^2 \text{ (between)}}{\hat{\sigma}^2 \text{ (within)}} = \frac{(4.7)^2}{(2.1)^2} = 5.0$$

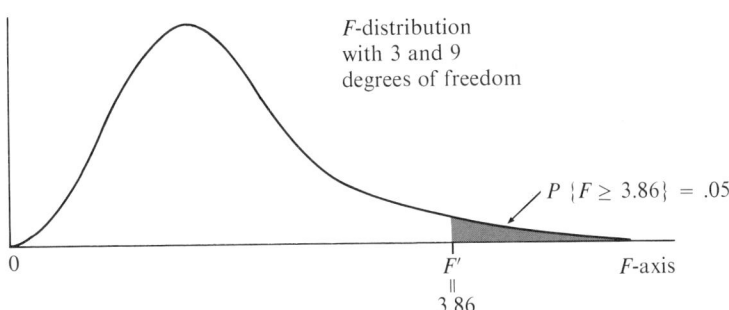

FIGURE 8.2

which lies to the *right* of F'. Therefore, at the $P = .05$ level of significance, we reject H, and conclude that there *is* reason to believe that the treatments are not all equally effective.

EXAMPLE 8.3.1. Mental Problems

Recall the data of Example 1.10.1 showing average daily admissions to the emergency room of a mental hospital before, during, and after the full moon. Let the parameter μ_1 denote the true average daily admissions that could be expected at this hospital *prior* to a full moon; let μ_2 and μ_3 be similarly defined for the periods *during* and *after* the full moon, respectively.

Here the relevant question is whether μ_2 is greater than μ_1 or μ_3, as the data would suggest. The format of the hypothesis test, though, would be

$$\text{H:} \quad \mu_1 = \mu_2 = \mu_3 \quad \text{versus} \quad \text{A:} \quad \text{not all the } \mu_i\text{'s are equal}$$

For these data,

$$\bar{x}_{1.} = \frac{1}{12} \sum_{j=1}^{12} x_{1j} = \frac{1}{12}\{6.4 + 7.1 + \cdots + 15.8\}$$
$$= \frac{131.0}{12} = 10.9$$

Similarly,

$$\bar{x}_{2.} = \frac{160.0}{12} = 13.3$$

and
$$\bar{x}_3. = \frac{137.5}{12} = 11.4$$

Also,
$$\bar{x}.. = \frac{1}{36}\sum_{i=1}^{3}\sum_{j=1}^{12} x_{ij} = \frac{1}{36}\{6.4 + 7.1 + \cdots + 14.5\}$$
$$= \frac{428.5}{36} = 11.9$$

Therefore,
$$\sum_{i=1}^{3} n_i(\bar{x}_i. - \bar{x}..)^2 = 12(10.9 - 11.9)^2 + 12(13.3 - 11.9)^2$$
$$+ 12(11.4 - 11.9)^2$$
$$= 38.52$$

making the numerator of the F-ratio equal to
$$(36 - 3)\sum_{i=1}^{3} n_i(\bar{x}_i. - \bar{x}..)^2 = (33)(38.52) = 1271.16$$

To compute the denominator, note that
$$\sum_{j=1}^{12} (x_{1j} - \bar{x}_1.)^2 = (6.4 - 10.9)^2 + \cdots + (15.8 - 10.9)^2$$
$$= 144.14$$

Likewise,
$$\sum_{j=1}^{12} (x_{2j} - \bar{x}_2.)^2 = (5.0 - 13.3)^2 + \cdots + (20.0 - 13.3)^2$$
$$= 332.68$$

and
$$\sum_{j=1}^{12} (x_{3j} - \bar{x}_3.)^2 = (5.8 - 11.4)^2 + \cdots + (14.5 - 11.4)^2$$
$$= 106.39$$

Therefore,
$$\sum_{i=1}^{3}\sum_{j=1}^{12} (x_{ij} - \bar{x}_i.)^2 = 144.14 + 332.68 + 106.39$$
$$= 583.21$$

in which case the denominator of the test statistic becomes
$$(3 - 1)\sum_{i=1}^{3}\sum_{j=1}^{12} (x_{ij} - \bar{x}_i.)^2 = (2)(583.21) = 1166.42$$

[8.3] Hypothesis Testing in the k-Sample Problem

Diving the numerator sum by the denominator sum gives a variance ratio of

$$\frac{1271.16}{1166.42} = 1.09$$

Suppose it was decided to test H: $\mu_1 = \mu_2 = \mu_3$ at the $P = .05$ level of significance. Since the sampling distribution of

$$\frac{(36-3) \sum_{i=1}^{3} (\bar{x}_{i.} - \bar{x}_{..})^2}{(3-1) \sum_{i=1}^{3} \sum_{j=1}^{12} (x_{ij} - \bar{x}_{i.})^2}$$

will be described by an F-distribution with 2 and 33 degrees of freedom, it follows from Appendix V that F' will be somewhere between 3.23 and 3.32. (The particular curve with 2 and 33 degrees of freedom is not included in Appendix V.) In this case, not knowing the exact value of F' does not matter because the observed ratio (1.09) lies far to the left of either 3.23 or 3.32. Therefore, we should accept the null hypothesis.

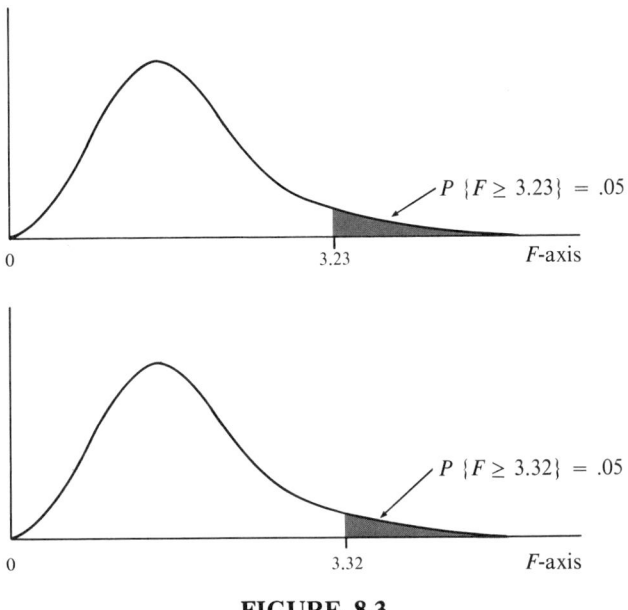

FIGURE 8.3

Question 8.3.1. Analyze the data of Example 5.2.1 according to the procedure presented in this section.

8.4
COMPUTING FORMULAS FOR THE ANALYSIS OF VARIANCE

The analysis of variance, as described in Section 8.3, is not the way H: $\mu_1 = \mu_2 = \cdots = \mu_k$ is tested in practice. The principles are the same, but there are easier formulas, from the standpoint of computation, for evaluating the numerator and denominator of the F-ratio than

$$(N - k) \sum_{i=1}^{k} n_i(\bar{x}_i. - \bar{x}..)^2 \quad \text{and} \quad (k - 1) \sum_{i=1}^{k} \sum_{j=1}^{n_i} (x_{ij} - \bar{x}_i.)^2$$

Usually, the calculations for a Model Six problem are presented in what is known as an *analysis of variance table*. For the kind of k-sample problem being considered here, the format of an analysis of variance (or, ANOVA) table is always the same: it has three rows and five columns.

ANOVA Table

Source of variation	df	SS	MS	F
Between treatments				
Within treatments				
Total				

In explaining how this table is filled in, and what the various entries mean, we should probably begin by focussing on the first and the third columns. (These two are considered together because the number that will eventually appear in the SS ("sum of squares") column *quantifies* what appears in the first column.)

First, the word "Total." In the k-sample model, as in all the models previously encountered, the sample observations are not all the same; they vary. By definition, the *extent* that they vary (that is, their "total variation") is measured in terms of the sum of the squares of the x_{ij}'s from the grand mean. Specifically,

$$\text{Total variation} = \sum_{i=1}^{k} \sum_{j=1}^{n_i} (x_{ij} - \bar{x}..)^2$$

The expression on the right is called the "total sum of squares" and is written SS (total). This is the number that will appear in the third row of the column marked SS.

The other words in the first column are meant to signify that the total variation in a set of data is the sum of *two* components: (1) variation due to the treatments and (2) variation due to everything *other* than the treatments:

$$\text{Total variation} = \begin{matrix} \text{Between-treatment variation} \\ + \text{ Within-treatment variation} \end{matrix}$$

By analogy with the way the term on the left was measured, the sums of squares reflecting between-treatment variation and within-treatment variation are given by

$$SS\text{ (between)} = \sum_{i=1}^{k}\sum_{j=1}^{n_i}(\bar{x}_{i.} - \bar{x}_{..})^2$$

and

$$SS\text{ (within)} = \sum_{i=1}^{k}\sum_{j=1}^{n_i}(x_{ij} - \bar{x}_{i.})^2$$

Numerically,

$$SS\text{ (total)} = SS\text{ (between)} + SS\text{ (within)}$$

Therefore,

$$\sum_{i=1}^{k}\sum_{j=1}^{n_i}(x_{ij} - \bar{x}_{..})^2 = \sum_{i=1}^{k}\sum_{j=1}^{n_i}(\bar{x}_{i.} - \bar{x}_{..})^2 + \sum_{i=1}^{k}\sum_{j=1}^{n_i}(x_{ij} - \bar{x}_{i.})^2$$

These three sums are entered in their appropriate places in this analysis of variance table.

ANOVA Table

Source of variation	df	SS	MS	F
Between treatments		$\sum\sum(\bar{x}_{i.} - \bar{x}_{..})^2$		
Within treatments		$\sum\sum(x_{ij} - \bar{x}_{i.})^2$		
Total		$\sum\sum(x_{ij} - \bar{x}_{..})^2$		

Comment

To simplify the notation in analysis of variance tables, sigma signs will usually be shown without subscripts. The intended range of summation in these cases will be over all possible values of i and j.

The second and fourth columns in the ANOVA table refer to degrees of freedom and mean square, respectively. The entries in the *df* column, from top to bottom, will always be $k - 1$, $N - k$, and $N - 1$. Here, also, the last entry is the sum of the first two:

$$N - 1 = (k - 1) + (N - k)$$

The numbers that appear in the *MS* column are the quotients formed by dividing the number in the *SS* column by the corresponding number in the *df* column:

$$MS\text{(between)} = \frac{\sum_{i=1}^{k}\sum_{j=1}^{n_i}(\bar{x}_{i.} - \bar{x}_{..})^2}{k - 1}$$

$$MS\text{(within)} = \frac{\sum_{i=1}^{k}\sum_{j=1}^{n_i}(x_{ij} - \bar{x}_{i.})^2}{N - k}$$

Nothing is entered for *MS* (total).

Model Six — The k-Sample Problem

ANOVA Table

Source of variation	df	SS	MS	F
Between treatments	$k - 1$	$\sum\sum (\bar{x}_{i.} - \bar{x}_{..})^2$	$SS/(k-1)$	
Within treatments	$N - k$	$\sum\sum (x_{ij} - \bar{x}_{i.})^2$	$SS/(N-k)$	
Total	$N - 1$	$\sum\sum (x_{ij} - \bar{x}_{..})^2$		

Only one number is entered in the F column, the ratio

$$MS \text{ (between)}/MS \text{ (within)}$$

Numerically, this is the same quantity that was used as the test statistic in Section 8.3. That is,

$$\frac{MS(\text{between})}{MS(\text{within})} = \frac{(N - k) \sum_{i=1}^{k} n_i(\bar{x}_{i.} - \bar{x}_{..})^2}{(k - 1) \sum_{i=1}^{k} \sum_{j=1}^{n_i} (x_{ij} - \bar{x}_{i.})^2}$$

This means that if H: $\mu_1 = \mu_2 = \cdots = \mu_k$ is true, the sampling distribution of MS (between)/MS (within) is described by an F-curve with $k - 1$ and $N - k$ degrees of freedom, and that H should be rejected at, say, the $P = .05$ level of significance if

$$\frac{MS(\text{between})}{MS(\text{within})} \geq F' \quad \text{where} \quad P\{F \geq F'\} = .05$$

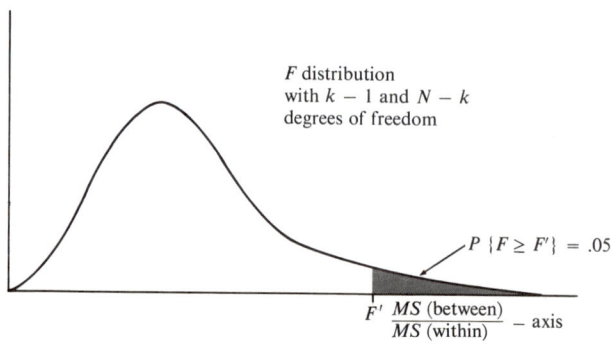

FIGURE 8.4

So far, none of this is really any different from what was done in Section 8.3. The notation has been changed, and the table format allows the computations to be presented in a more orderly way, but the formulas are basically the same. However, there is still one modification that needs to be made. "Computing" formulas will be substituted for the three "defining" formulas that now appear in the SS column. These will make the sum of squares calculations much easier.

First, we define a number c, where

$$c = \frac{\left(\sum_{i=1}^{k} \sum_{j=1}^{n_i} x_{ij}\right)^2}{N}$$

Then, using only the usual summation rules, the original formulas for SS (total) and SS (between) can be reduced to

$$SS(\text{total}) = \sum_{i=1}^{k} \sum_{j=1}^{n_i} x_{ij}^2 - c \quad \text{and} \quad SS(\text{between}) = \sum_{i=1}^{k} \frac{T_{i\cdot}^2}{n_i} - c$$

Furthermore, since the first two entries in the SS column always sum to the third, it follows that

$$SS(\text{within}) = SS(\text{total}) - SS(\text{between})$$

It may not be obvious, but these formulas are really much simpler to use than the ones given earlier, particularly if a desk calculator is available.

Replacing the three previous entries in the SS column with their respective computing formulas leaves the analysis of variance table in the form shown below.

ANOVA Table

Source of variation	df	SS*	MS	F
Between treatments	$k - 1$	$\sum_{i=1}^{k} \frac{T_{i\cdot}^2}{n_i} - c$	$SS/(k-1)$	$\dfrac{MS(\text{between})}{MS(\text{within})}$
Within treatments	$N - k$	$SS(\text{total}) - SS(\text{between})$	$SS/(N-k)$	
Total	$N - 1$	$\sum \sum x_{ij}^2 - c$		

$$*c = \frac{\left(\sum_{i=1}^{k} \sum_{j=1}^{n_i} x_{ij}\right)^2}{N}$$

The next two examples show how these various computations are done.

EXAMPLE 8.4.1. ANOVA Calculations

Consider again the admissions data of Example 8.3.1.

Average daily admissions

Before full moon	During full moon	After full moon
6.4	5.0	5.8
7.1	13.0	9.2
6.5	14.0	7.9
8.6	12.0	7.7
8.1	6.0	11.0
10.4	9.0	12.9
11.5	13.0	13.5
13.8	16.0	13.1
15.4	25.0	15.8
15.7	13.0	13.3
11.7	14.0	12.8
15.8	20.0	14.5
$T_1. = 131.0$	$T_2. = 160.0$	$T_3. = 137.5$
$n_1 = 12$	$n_2 = 12$	$n_3 = 12$
	$T.. = 428.5$	

Here the sources of variation are between phases, within phases, and total. Since

$$\left(\sum_{i=1}^{3}\sum_{j=1}^{12} x_{ij}\right)^2 = (428.5)^2 = 183{,}612.25$$

the number c is equal to

$$c = \frac{183{,}612.25}{36} = 5100.34$$

Therefore,

$$SS(\text{total}) = (6.4)^2 + \cdots + (14.5)^2 - 5100.34$$
$$= 621.75$$

and

$$SS(\text{between}) = \frac{(131.0)^2}{12} + \frac{(160.0)^2}{12} + \frac{(137.5)}{12} - 5100.34$$
$$= 38.59$$

so that

$$SS(\text{within}) = 621.75 - 38.59 = 583.16$$

Since $k = 3$ and $N = 36$, the three entries in the df column are $2\ (= k - 1)$, $33\ (= N - k)$, and $35\ (= N - 1)$.

ANOVA Table

Source of variation	df	SS	MS	F
Between phases	2	38.59		
Within phases	33	583.16		
Total	35	621.75		

Dividing the first two sums of squares by their respective degrees of freedom gives the two entries in the MS column:

$$MS(\text{between}) = \frac{38.59}{2} = 19.30$$

and

$$MS(\text{within}) = \frac{583.16}{33} = 17.67$$

making the F ratio equal to

$$\frac{19.30}{17.67} = 1.09$$

which is the same value calculated in Example 8.3.1.

ANOVA Table

Source of variation	df	SS	MS	F
Between phases	2	38.59	19.30	1.09
Within phases	33	583.16	17.67	
Total	35	621.75		

Since MS (between)/MS (within) has an F-distribution with 2 and 33 degrees of freedom when H: $\mu_1 = \mu_2 = \mu_3$ is true, the $P = .05$ critical value lies somewhere between 3.32 and 3.23 (see p. 277). Therefore, we accept the null hypothesis.

Question 8.4.1. Is it possible that the F-ratio, for a given set of data, will be less than 1?

EXAMPLE 8.4.2. Comparing Exercise Programs for the Newborn

In Example 1.10.2, an experiment was described that compared the effectiveness of four different exercise programs. The subjects were 23 infants and the measured response was the age at which each of them first walked alone.

Age when first walked alone (months)

	Group A	Group B	Group C	Group D
	9.00	11.00	11.50	13.25
	9.50	10.00	12.00	11.50
	9.75	10.00	9.00	12.00
	10.00	11.75	11.50	13.50
	13.00	10.50	13.25	11.50
	9.50	15.00	13.00	
T_i.:	60.75	68.25	70.25	61.75
	$n_1 = 6$	$n_2 = 6$	$n_3 = 6$	$n_4 = 5$

Let μ_1 be the true average "first walking time" that could be expected among infants assigned to Group A; let μ_2 be similarly defined for Group B, and so on. Then the hypotheses to be tested are

$$\text{H:} \quad \mu_1 = \mu_2 = \mu_3 = \mu_4$$

versus

$$\text{A:} \quad \text{not all the } \mu_i\text{'s are equal}$$

Let $P = .05$ be the level of significance.

The first step in *any* analysis of variance is to compute $\sum_{i=1}^{k} \sum_{j=1}^{n_i} x_{ij}$ and $\sum_{i=1}^{k} \sum_{j=1}^{n_i} x_{ij}^2$. (With a desk calculator, these sums can be obtained simultaneously.) For these data,

$$\sum_{i=1}^{4} \sum_{j=1}^{n_i} x_{ij} = 261.0 \quad \text{and} \quad \sum_{i=1}^{4} \sum_{j=1}^{n_i} x_{ij}^2 = 3020.25$$

Therefore,

$$c = \frac{(261.0)^2}{23} = 2961.78$$

which makes

$$SS(\text{total}) = 3020.25 - 2961.78 = 58.47$$

$$SS(\text{between}) = \frac{(60.75)^2}{6} + \frac{(68.25)^2}{6} + \frac{(70.25)^2}{6} + \frac{(61.75)^2}{5}$$
$$- 2961.78 = 14.77$$

and

$$SS(\text{within}) = SS(\text{total}) - SS(\text{between})$$
$$= 58.47 - 14.77 = 43.70$$

At this point, the first three columns of the analysis of variance table can be filled in:

ANOVA Table

Source of variation	df	SS	MS	F
Between programs	3	14.77		
Within programs	19	43.70		
Total	22	58.47		

Also,

$$MS(\text{between}) = \frac{14.77}{3} = 4.92$$

and

$$MS(\text{within}) = \frac{43.70}{19} = 2.30$$

making the F-ratio

$$\frac{4.92}{2.3} = 2.14$$

ANOVA Table

Source of variation	df	SS	MS	F
Between programs	3	14.77	4.92	2.14
Within programs	19	43.70	2.30	
Total	22	58.47		

If H: $\mu_1 = \mu_2 = \mu_3 = \mu_4$ is true, the sampling distribution of MS (between)/MS (within) will be described by an F-distribution with 3 and 19 degrees of freedom. From Appendix V, the value cutting off a right-hand tail area of 0.05 under that particular curve is 3.13. Therefore, H is accepted. We cannot conclude at the $P = .05$ level of significance that the average first walking times associated with these four exercise programs are not all the same.

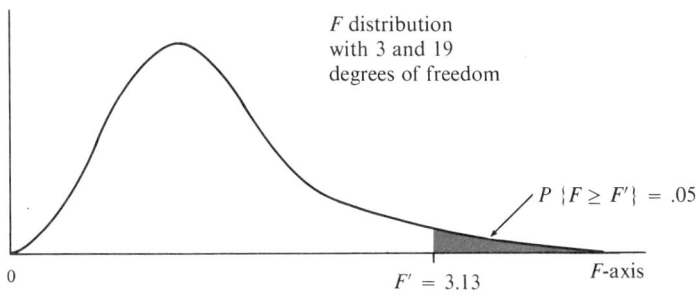

FIGURE 8.5

Question 8.4.2. What are some of the factors that might contribute to the "within program" variability?

8.5 SUMMARY

Chapter 8 has served as an introduction to a very broad and powerful technique in statistical inference known as the *analysis of variance*. Here the method was applied to one particular kind of problem — testing whether the location parameters associated with k different response distributions are all the same. In every instance, the question to be answered reduced to a test of

$$H: \quad \mu_1 = \mu_2 = \cdots = \mu_k$$

versus

$$A: \quad \text{not all } \mu_i\text{'s are equal}$$

The transition from two populations to k populations added complexity to the final analysis at several different levels. First, the subscript notation that was introduced in Chapter 1 and used effectively ever since was no longer adequate. In Section 8.2 the necessary modification was made: single subscripts (x_i) were replaced with double subscripts (x_{ij}), which meant that the single sigma sign ($\sum$) had to be replaced with a double sigma sign ($\sum\sum$).

Another change involved the form of the test statistic. In Models Two, Three, Four, and, to some extent, Five, testing hypotheses about location parameters (or correlation coefficients) required either the normal distribution or the t-distribution. But in Model Six, means are tested by comparing variances — and the particular "variance ratio" that is used as the test statistic

$$\frac{\hat{\sigma}^2(\text{between})}{\hat{\sigma}^2(\text{within})} = \frac{MS(\text{between})}{MS(\text{within})}$$

has an *F-distribution*. More specifically, values of

$$\frac{MS(\text{between})}{MS(\text{within})} = \frac{(N-k)\sum_{i=1}^{k} n_i(\bar{x}_i. - \bar{x}..)^2}{(k-1)\sum_{i=1}^{k}\sum_{j=1}^{n_i}(x_{ij} - \bar{x}_i.)^2}$$

in the extreme right-hand tail of an F-distribution with $k-1$ and $N-k$ degrees of freedom, where k is the number of treatments and N is the total sample size, lead to the rejection of H: $\mu_1 = \mu_2 = \cdots = \mu_k$. Exact cutoff points, F', for the $P = .05$ and $P = .01$ levels of significance are tabulated in Appendix V.

Section 8.3 presented a series of computing formulas for simplifying the calculation of MS (between) and MS (within). Usually the intermediate steps in these calculations are displayed in an *analysis of variance table*. This particular format serves two purposes, especially in more complicated k-sample problems: (1) it helps the person *doing* the analysis to organize what are often very lengthy computations, and (2) it provides the person *reading* the analysis with all the relevant information about the way the experiment was designed and how the results are to be interpreted.

Definitions

Analysis of variance (ANOVA). The name given to certain procedures for testing hypotheses of the form H: $\mu_1 = \mu_2 = \cdots = \mu_k$; when H is true, the test statistic, a ratio of variance estimates, has an F-distribution.

Between-treatment variation. The variation in a set of Model Six data that can be attributed to the k treatments; measured by the quantity

$$\sum_{i=1}^{k} n_i(\bar{x}_{i.} - \bar{x}_{..})^2$$

Mean square (MS). The sum of squares for a particular source of variation divided by the number of degrees of freedom associated with that source; a variance estimate.

Source of variation. In k-sample problems, the total variation in a set of data can be attributed to two sources: (1) the treatments and (2) everything other than the treatments.

Sum of squares (SS). A way of measuring variation in k-sample problems; separate sums of squares are calculated for (1) total variation, (2) between-treatment variation, and (3) within-treatment variation.

Total variation. The net influence on the response variable of all the factors in an experiment; measured by the quantity

$$\sum_{i=1}^{k} \sum_{j=1}^{n_i} (x_{ij} - \bar{x}_{..})^2$$

Within-treatment variation. The variation in a set of Model Six data that can be attributed to all factors other than the treatments; measured by the quantity

$$\sum_{i=1}^{k} \sum_{j=1}^{n_i} (x_{ij} - \bar{x}_{i.})^2$$

Review Exercises

8.1 Of the many pesticides that leave residues capable of killing wildlife, dieldrin is the second-most prevalent. The following data were collected as part of an experiment to characterize the mechanism of dieldrin poisoning (Stickel, Stickel, and Spann, 1969). The subjects were Japanese quail. A total of 33 of the birds were equally divided into three groups: the first group was fed a diet that included 250 ppm of dieldrin; the second group, 50 ppm; and the third, 10 ppm. Listed below are the concentrations of dieldrin residues found in the brains of the 17 quail that died.

Brain residues (ppm of dieldrin)
Dosage (ppm of dieldrin)

250	50	10
7.01	6.23	19.52
12.69	12.55	32.03
9.99	22.56	21.91
23.00	19.48	21.61
11.03	31.29	
19.33	24.90	
32.94		

(a) Graph the data.

(b) Let μ_1, μ_2, and μ_3 be the true average brain residues associated with these three diets under these particular conditions. Test

$$H: \quad \mu_1 = \mu_2 = \mu_3 \quad \text{vs.} \quad A: \quad \text{not all the } \mu_i\text{'s are equal}$$

at the $P = .05$ level of significance. Note that

$$\sum_{i=1}^{3}\sum_{j=1}^{n_i} x_{ij} = 328.07 \quad \text{and} \quad \sum_{i=1}^{3}\sum_{j=1}^{n_i} x_{ij}^2 = 7457.1347$$

(c) Other data related to this experiment revealed a strong relationship between dosage level and life span. Birds fed higher concentrations of dieldrin tended to die sooner. What does this fact, together with the conclusion of part (b), suggest about the mechanism of dieldrin poisoning?

8.2 Verify the computing formula for SS(between). That is, prove that

$$\sum_{i=1}^{k} n_i(\bar{x}_{i.} - \bar{x}_{..})^2 = \sum_{i=1}^{k} \frac{T_{i.}^2}{n_i} - c$$

where

$$c = \frac{\left(\sum_{i=1}^{k}\sum_{j=1}^{n_i} x_{ij}\right)^2}{n}$$

8.3 In a field trial comparing three live attenuated rubella vaccines, it was found that 419 of the school-age subjects were initially seronegative (Kehrer and Isaacson,

1971). That is, their pretiter to the rubella virus was less than 10. The table below shows the posttiters for these same children. (The convalescent sera were collected 35 to 45 days after the data of vaccination.)

		Vaccine		
		Cendehill	HPV-77 + 12	HPV-77 + 5
	<10	3	5	5
	10	1	1	1
	20	15	13	18
Posttiter	40	56	40	39
	80	52	53	40
	160	20	28	14
	320	2	6	6
	640+	1	0	0

Use the analysis of variance to test whether these three vaccines are equally effective (in terms of the posttiters of persons initially seronegative.) Let $P = .05$ be the level of significance. *Hint:* Do all calculations on the *logs* of the posttiters, and not on the posttiters themselves.

8.4 There are several ways of measuring, indirectly, a person's total lung capacity (TLC). One of these is Barnhard's ellipsoid method, which requires nothing but two chest X-rays, a front view and a side view. Recently, an experiment was done to see how "reproducible" this method really is (Reger and Jacobs, 1970). A total of 11 sets of X-rays were shown to five nonmedical personnel, all of whom had been taught the Barnhard method. Each of the subjects made three independent estimates on the 11 sets of X-rays. The results for four of the 11 are shown below.

		Estimated TLC (liters) Observer				
		1	2	3	4	5
		6.06	6.12	5.92	5.55	6.02
	1	6.34	5.99	6.21	5.62	6.59
		5.64	6.15	6.05	5.61	6.48
		6.50	6.08	5.56	5.85	6.66
	2	6.94	6.43	5.41	6.43	6.41
X-ray		6.87	6.23	5.81	6.50	6.88
set		6.46	5.53	5.64	5.88	6.08
	3	6.35	5.57	5.40	5.78	5.98
		6.13	5.86	5.12	6.05	6.39
		8.24	7.44	7.39	7.60	7.75
	4	8.50	7.42	7.39	7.42	8.28
		7.71	7.34	7.45	7.79	7.31

Let x_{ijk} denote the kth estimate made on the jth X-ray by the ith observer. For these data, i ranges from 1 to 5; j, from 1 to 4; and k, from 1 to 3. The number 6.06 in the upper left-hand corner would be written x_{111}; 6.34 would be x_{112}; the last entry in the first column, 7.71, would be x_{143}; in the second column, 6.12 would be x_{211}, and so on.

(a) Using the same conventions that were introduced for *double* subscript notation, evaluate the following expressions:
  (1) x_{342}
  (2) $\bar{x}_{22\cdot}$
  (3) $\bar{x}_{3\cdot\cdot}$
  (4) $\sum_{k=1}^{3} (x_{23k} - \bar{x}_{23\cdot})^2$
  (5) $T_{14\cdot}$

(b) Write expressions for the following quantities:
  (1) $SS(\text{total})$
  (2) s_{ij}

8.5 Construct an analysis of variance table for the therapy example of Section 8.3. Verify that the F-ratio is 5.0.

8.6 Use the analysis of variance on the cardiac data given in Review Exercise 5.5. Let $P = .05$ be the level of significance.

8.7 The ages and the mercury levels of 12 walleyed pike caught in Lake Erie were graphed in Review Exercise 1.3. The exact values for those mercury concentrations are listed below.

Mercury levels (ppm) in walleyed pike

Young of the year	Yearlings	Two years and older
.60	.75	1.03
.64	.92	.67
.62	.93	.78
.44	.75	.98

Define the parameters in question and test an appropriate hypothesis.

BIBLIOGRAPHY

Abse, Dannie, *Medicine on Trial* (Crown, 1967), p. 263. © 1967 Aldus Books Limited, London. Used by permission of Crown Publishers, Inc.

Anderson, Carl, *Community Health* (Mosby, 1969), p. 63.

Barclay, George, *Techniques of Population Analysis* (Wiley, 1958), p. 195.

Barnicot, N. A. and Brothwell, D. R., "The Evaluation of Metrical Data in the Comparison of Ancient and Modern Bones," in *Medical Biology and Etruscan Origins*, G. E. W. Wolstenholme and Cecilia M. O'Connor, eds. (Little, Brown, 1959), p. 136.

Bartels, Heinz, *Methods in Pulmonary Physiology* (Hafner, 1963), p. 73. Copyright © 1959 Springer-Verlag.

Benjamin, Bernard, *Demographic Analysis* (Praeger, 1969), pp. 14–15.

Biggs, Rosemary, *Prothrombin Deficiency* (Thomas, 1951), p. 15.

Bjure, J., Grimby, G., and Nachemson, A., "The Effect of Physical Training in Girls with Idiopathic Scoliosis," *Acta Orthopaedica Scandinavia*, **40,** 1969, 328.

Blackman, S. and Catalina, D. "The Moon and the Emergency Room," *PERCEPTUAL AND MOTOR SKILLS*, 1973, **37,** 624–26. Reprinted with permission of author and publisher.

Brim, Orville G., Jr., et al. (ed.), *The Dying Patient* (Russell Sage Foundation, 1970), p. 107.

Brummer, D., et al., "Diet," in *Advances in Experimental Medicine and Biology*, *16B*, Stewart Wolf, ed. (Plenum Press, 1972), p. 116.

Buchanan, T. M., Brooks, G. F., and Brachman, P. S., "The Tularemia Skin Test," *Annals of Internal Medicine*, **74,** 1971, 336–43.

Carter, C. C., "Multifactorial Genetic Disease," *Hospital Practice*, **5,** 1970, 45–49.

Casler, Lawrence, "The Effects of Hypnosis on GESP," *Journal of Parapsychology*, **28,** 1964, 126–34.

Center for Disease Control, Epidemic Intelligence Service Course Notes (unpubl., 1968).

Connolly, Kevin, "The Social Facilitation of Preening Behaviour in *Drosophila Melanogaster*," *Animal Behavior*, **16**, 1968, 385–91.

Diaz, Jose Luis and Huttunen, Matti O., "Persistent Increase in Brain Serotonin Turnover after Chronic Administration of LSD in the Rat," *Science*, **174**, October 1, 1971, 62–63. Copyright 1971 by the American Association for the Advancement of Science.

Diem, Konrad (ed.), *Scientific Tables*, 6th ed. (Geigy, 1962).

Dixon, Wilfrid J. and Massey, Frank J., Jr., *Introduction to Statistical Analysis*, 2nd ed. (McGraw-Hill, 1957), p. 199. Copyright © 1957 by McGraw-Hill Book Company.

Doster, Daphine D., "Utilization of Available 'Nurse Power' in Public Health," *American Journal of Public Health*, **60**, 1970, 25–37.

Ehlers, Niels, "On Corneal Thickness and Intraocular Pressure. II," *Acta Ophthalmologica*, **48**, 1970, 1108.

Fadeley, Robert Cunningham, "Oregon Malignancy Pattern Physiographically Related to Hanford Washington Radioisotope Storage," *Journal of Environmental Health*, **27**, 1965, 883–97.

Fichtler, H., Zimmerman, R. R., and Moore, R. T., "Comparison of Self-Esteem of Prison and Non-prison Groups," PERCEPTUAL AND MOTOR SKILLS, 1973, **36**, 39–44. Reprinted with permission of author and publisher.

Fieve, Ronald R., Platman, Stanley R., and Fleiss, Joseph L., "A Clinical Trial of Methysergide and Lithium in Mania," in *Lithium and Psychiatry Journal Articles*, David J. Kupfer, ed. (Medical Examination Publishing Co., 1971), p. 42.

Fishbein, Morris, *Birth Defects* (Lippincott, 1962), p. 177.

Free, J. B., "The Stimuli Releasing the Stinging Response of Honeybees," *Animal Behavior*, **9**, 1961, 193.

Furuhata, Tanemoto and Yamamoto, Katsuichi, *Forensic Odontology* (Thomas, 1967), p. 84.

Gendreau, Paul, et al., "Changes in EEG Alpha Frequency and Evoked Response Latency During Solitary Confinement," *Journal of Abnormal Psychology*, **79**, 1972, 54–59. Copyright 1972 by the American Psychological Association. Reprinted by permission.

Gerber, Robert C., et al., "Kinetics of Aurothiomalate in Serum and Synovial Fluid," *Arthritis and Rheumatism*, **15**, 1972, 626.

Getz, Steven, *Environment and the Deaf Child* (Thomas, 1953), p. 66.

Götz, K. O. and Götz, K., "Introversion-Extraversion and Neuroticism in Gifted and Ungifted Art Students," PERCEPTUAL AND MOTOR SKILLS, 1973, **36**, 675–78. Reprinted with permission of author and publisher.

Graham, Saxon, "Social Factors in Relation to the Chronic Illnesses," in *Handbook of Medical Sociology*, Howard Freeman, Sol Levine, and Leo G. Reeder, eds. (Prentice-Hall, 1963), p. 69.

Graw, Robert G., Jr. and Santos, George W., "Bone Marrow Transplantation in Patients with Leukemia," *Transplantation*, **11**, 1971, 198. Copyright © 1971 The Williams & Wilkins Co., Baltimore.

Griffin, Donald R., Webster, Frederic A., and Michael, Charles R., "The Echolocation of Flying Insects by Bats," *Animal Behavior*, **8,** 1960, 148.

Hall, Carrie E., Cooney, Marion K., and Fox, John P., "The Seattle Virus Watch Program. I. Infection and Illness Experience of Virus Watch Families During a Community-wide Epidemic of Echovirus Type 30 Aseptic Meningitis," *American Journal of Public Health*, **60,** 1970, 1456–65.

Hansel, C. E. M., *ESP: A Scientific Evaluation* (Scribner, 1966), pp. 86–89.

Harris, Thomas Reginald, Pratt, Philip Chase, and Kilburn, Kaye Hatch, "Total Lung Capacity Measured by Roentgenograms," *American Journal of Medicine*, **50,** 1971, 759.

Hersen, Michel, "Personality Characteristics of Nightmare Sufferers," *Journal of Nervous and Mental Diseases*, **153,** 1971, 29–31. Copyright © 1971 The Williams & Wilkins Co., Baltimore.

Hollingsworth, Thomas Henry, *Historical Demography* (Cornell University Press, 1969), p. 18. Copyright © 1969 by T. H. Hollingsworth.

Holton, Susan Chapin, "The Woman Physician: A Study of Role Conflict," *American Medical Women's Association Journal*, **24,** 1969, 639.

Holtzman, Richard B., "Natural Content of RaD (Pb^{210}) and RaF (Po^{210}) in the Human Body," in *Radioactivity in Man*, George R. Meneely and Shirley Motter Linde, eds. (Thomas, 1965), p. 439.

Hon, Edward H. G., "Direct Monitoring of the Fetal Heart," *Hospital Practice*, **5,** 1970, 91–97.

Horvath, Frank S. and Reid, John E., "The Reliability of Polygraph Examiner Diagnosis of Truth and Deception," *Journal of Criminal Law, Criminology, and Police Science*, **62,** 1971, 276–81. Reprinted by special permission of the Journal of Criminal Law, Criminology, & Police Science. Copyright © 1971 by Northwestern University School of Law, Vol. 62, No. 2.

Hutt, Max L. and Gibby, Robert Gwyn, *Patterns of Abnormal Behavior* (Allyn & Bacon, 1957), p. 379.

Hynniman, Clifford E., et al., "A Comparison of Medication Errors Under the University of Kentucky Unit Dose System and Traditional Drug Distribution Systems in Four Hospitals," *American Journal of Hospital Pharmacy*, **27,** 1970, 807.

Ibrahim, Michel A., et al., "Coronary Heart Disease: Screening by Familial Aggregation," *Archives of Environmental Health*, **16,** 1968, 235–40. Copyright 1968, American Medical Association.

James, Andrew and Moncada, Robert, "Many Set Color TV Lounges Show Highest Radiation," *Journal of Environmental Health*, **31,** 1969, 359–60.

Jones, Jack Colvard and Pilitt, Dana Richard, "Blood-feeding Behavior of Adult *Aedes Aegypti* Mosquitoes," *Biological Bulletin*, **145,** 1973, 127–39.

Kehrer, Anthony F. and Isaacson, Peter, "A Comparative Evaluation of Three Live, Attenuated Rubella Virus Vaccines," *American Journal of Public Health*, **61,** 1971, 153.

Kronoveter, Kenneth J. and Somerville, Gordon W., "Airplane Cockpit Noise Levels and Pilot Hearing Sensitivity," *Archives of Environmental Health*, **20,** 1970, 498. Copyright 1970, American Medical Association.

Bibliography

Ladd, Everett Carll, Jr. and Lipset, S. M., "Politics of Academic Natural Scientists and Engineers," *Science*, **176,** June 9, 1972, 1091–1100. Copyright 1972 by the American Association for the Advancement of Science.

Langmuir, Alexander, "The Surveillance of Communicable Diseases of National Importance," *New England Journal of Medicine*, **268,** 1963, 182–91.

Larsen, Richard J., unpubl. data, 1968.

Lawrence, Joseph J. and Maxwell, Milton A., "Drinking and Socioeconomic Status," in *Society, Culture, and Drinking Patterns*, David J. Pittman and Charles R. Snyder, eds. (Wiley, 1962), p. 143.

Leigh, Denis and Marley, Edward, *Bronchial Asthma* (Pergamon Press, 1967), p. 178. Reprinted with permission.

Li, Frederick P., "Suicide Among Chemists," *Archives of Environmental Health*, **19,** 1969, 519.

Lindgren, Henry Clay, Byrne, Donn, and Petrinovich, Lewis, *Psychology: An Introduction to a Behavioral Science* (Wiley, 1966), p. 315.

Lipp, Martin R., Benson, Samuel G., and Allen, Patricia S., "Marijuana Use by Nurses and Nursing Students," *American Journal of Nursing*, **71,** 1971, 2339–41.

Lottenbach, K., "Vasomotor Tone and Vascular Response to Local Cold in Primary Raynaud's Disease," *Angiology*, **22,** 1971, 4–8.

Lowell, Anthony, Edwards, Lydia B., and Palmer, Carroll E., *Tuberculosis* (Harvard University Press, 1969), p. 19. Copyright © 1969 by the President and Fellows of Harvard College.

McFarland, Ross A., "Review of Experimental Findings in Sensory and Mental Functions," in *Biomedicine of High Terrestrial Elevations*, A. H. Hegnauer, ed. (USARIEM, 1969), p. 258.

"Medical News," *Journal of the American Medical Association*, **219,** 1972, 981.

Meyer, John (ed.), *Research on the Cerebral Circulation* (Thomas, 1969), p. 110.

Minkoff, Eli C., "A Fossil Baboon from Angola, with a Note on *Australopithecus*," *Journal of Paleontology*, **46,** 1972, 836–44.

Morton, William E., "Hypertension and Drinking Water Constituents in Colorado," *American Journal of Public Health*, **61,** 1971, 1371–78.

Mulcahy, Risteard, McGilvray, J. W., and Hickey, Noel, "Cigarette Smoking Related to Geographic Variations in Coronary Heart Disease Mortality and to Expectation of Life in the Two Sexes," *American Journal of Public Health*, **60,** 1970, 1516.

Nachemson, Alf, "Intradiscal Measurements of pH in Patients with Lumbar Rhizopathies," *Acta Orthopaedica Scandinavia*, **40,** 1969, 28–31.

Nash, Harvey, *Alcohol and Caffeine* (Thomas, 1962), p. 96.

Nicholes, Paul S., "Bacteria in Laundered Fabrics," *American Journal of Public Health*, **60,** 1970, 2177.

Nye, Francis Iven, *Family Relationships and Delinquent Behavior* (Wiley, 1958), p. 37.

Orringer, Eugene, et al., "Splenectomy in Chronic Thrombocytopenic Purpura," *Journal of Chronic Diseases*, **23,** 1970, 117–22.

Bibliography 295

Petersen, William, *Population*, 2nd ed. (Macmillan, 1969), p. 66. Copyright © William Petersen 1969.

Phillips, David P., "Deathday and Birthday: An Unexpected Connection," in *Statistics: A Guide to the Unknown*, Judith M. Tanur et al., ed. (Holden-Day, 1972), pp. 52-65.

Pickering, Sir George, "The Quantitative Approach to Disease," in *Ciba Foundation: Significant Trends in Medical Research* (Little, Brown, 1960), pp. 278-91.

Pillay, K. K. S., et al., "Mercury Pollution of Lake Erie Ecosphere," *Environmental Research*, **5,** 1972, 172-81.

Reger, Robert B. and Jacobs, Andrew C., "Analysis of Components of Variation," *Archives of Environmental Health*, **21,** 1970, 780. Copyright 1970, American Medical Association.

Resnick, Richard B., Fink, Max, and Freedman, Alfred M., "A Cyclazocine Typology in Opiate Dependence," *American Journal of Psychiatry*, 1970, Vol. **126,** pp. 1256-60. Copyright 1970, the American Psychiatric Association.

Riis, Jacob A., *How the Other Half Lives* (Dover, 1971), p. 54.

Rosenthal, David, *Genetic Theory and Abnormal Behavior* (McGraw-Hill, 1970), p. 139. Copyright © 1970 by McGraw-Hill Book Company.

Rumke, C. L. and de Jonge, H., "Design, Statistical Analysis and Interpretation," in *Evaluation of Drug Activities — Pharmacometrics*, Desmond Laurence, ed. (Academic Press, 1964), p. 62.

Salvosa, Carmencita B., Payne, Philip R., and Wheeler, Erica F., "Energy Expenditure of Elderly People Living Alone or in Local Authority Homes," *American Journal of Clinical Nutrition*, **24,** 1971, 1468.

Schaps, Eric and Sanders, Clinton R., "Purposes, Patterns, and Protection in a Campus Drug Using Community," *Journal of Health and Social Behavior*, **11,** 1970, 139.

Sever, John L., "Viral Teratogens: A Status Report," *Hospital Practice*, **5,** 1970, 75-78.

Shahidi, Syed A., et al., "Celery Implicated in High Bacteria Count Salads," *Journal of Environmental Health*, **32,** 1970, 669.

Shore, Neil S., Greene, Reginald, and Kazemi, Homayoun, "Lung Dysfunction in Workers Exposed to *Bacillus subtilis* Enzyme," *Environmental Research*, **4,** 1971, 512-19.

Smith, W. Lynn, "Facilitating Verbal-Symbolic Functions in Children with Learning Problems and 14-6 Positive Spike EEG Patterns with Ethosuximide (Zarontin)," in *Drugs and Cerebral Function*, Wallace Smith, ed. (Thomas, 1970), p. 125.

Steiner, Paul E., *Disease in the Civil War* (Thomas, 1968), p. 9.

Stickel, W. H., Stickel, L. F., and Spann, J. W., "Tissue Residues of Dieldrin in Relation to Mortality in Birds and Mammals," in *Chemical Fallout*, Morton W. Miller and George G. Berg, eds. (Thomas, 1969), pp. 178-79.

Susser, M. W. and Watson, W., *Sociology in Medicine* (Oxford University Press, 1971).

Szalontai, S. and Timaffy, M., "Involutional Thrombopathy," in *Age with a Future*. P. From Hansen, ed. (F. A. Davis, 1964), p. 345.

Treuhaft, Paul S. and McCarty, Daniel J., "Synovial Fluid pH, Lactate, Oxygen and Carbon Dioxide Partial Pressure in Various Joint Diseases," *Arthritis and Rheumatism*, **14**, 1971, 476-77.

Vidins, Eva I., Fox, Jo Ann E., and Beck, Ivan T., "Transmural Potential Difference (PD) in the Body of the Esophagus in Patients with Esophagitis, Barrett's Epithelium and Carcinoma of the Esophagus," *American Journal of Digestive Diseases*, **16**, 1971, 991-99.

Vincent, Pauline, "Factors Influencing Patient Noncompliance: A Theoretical Approach," *Nursing Research*, **20**, 1971, 514.

Vogel, John H. K., Horgan, John A., and Strahl, Cheryl L., "Left Ventricular Dysfunction in Chronic Constrictive Pericarditis," *Chest*, **59**, 1971, 489.

Walter, William G. and Stober, Angie, "Microbial Air Sampling in a Carpeted Hospital," *Journal of Environmental Health*, **30**, 1968, 405. Copyright 1968 by the American Association for the Advancement of Science.

Weil, Andrew T., Zinberg, Norman E., and Nelsen, Judith M., "Clinical and Psychological Effects of Marihuana in Man," *Science*, **162**, 1968, 1234-42.

Weiss, William, "Cigarette Smoke Gas Phase and *Paramecium* Survival," *Archives of Environmental Health*, **17**, 1968, 63. Copyright 1968, American Medical Association.

Werner, Martha, Stabenau, James R., and Pollin, William, "Thematic Apperception Test Method for the Differentiation of Families of Schizophrenics, Delinquents and 'Normals'," *Journal of Abnormal Psychology*, **75**, 1970, 139-45. Copyright 1970 by the American Psychological Association. Reprinted by permission.

Winslow, Charles, *The Conquest of Epidemic Disease* (Princeton, 1943), p. 303.

World Health Organization, *Fluorides and Human Health* (WHO, 1970), p. 276.

Wyler, Allen R., Masuda, Ninoru, and Holmes, Thomas H., "Magnitude of Life Events and Seriousness of Illness," *Psychosomatic Medicine*, **33**, 1971, 115-22.

Yochem, Donald E. and Roach, Darrell E., "Aspirin: Effect on Thrombus Formation Time and Prothrombin Time of Human Subjects," *Angiology*, **27**, 1971, 72.

Zelazo, Philip R., Zelazo, Nancy Ann, and Kolb, Sarah, " 'Walking' in the Newborn," *Science*, **176**, 1972, 314-15. Copyright 1972 by the American Association for the Advancement of Science.

APPENDIX I

Areas Under the Standard Normal Curve

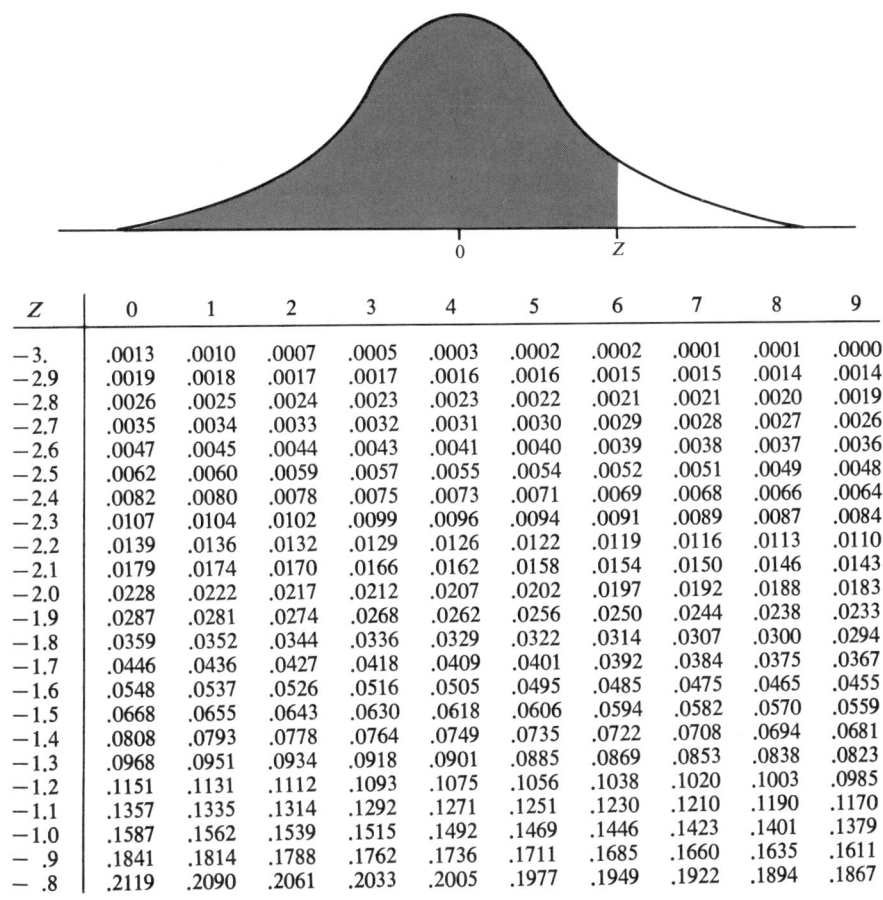

Z	0	1	2	3	4	5	6	7	8	9
−3.	.0013	.0010	.0007	.0005	.0003	.0002	.0002	.0001	.0001	.0000
−2.9	.0019	.0018	.0017	.0017	.0016	.0016	.0015	.0015	.0014	.0014
−2.8	.0026	.0025	.0024	.0023	.0023	.0022	.0021	.0021	.0020	.0019
−2.7	.0035	.0034	.0033	.0032	.0031	.0030	.0029	.0028	.0027	.0026
−2.6	.0047	.0045	.0044	.0043	.0041	.0040	.0039	.0038	.0037	.0036
−2.5	.0062	.0060	.0059	.0057	.0055	.0054	.0052	.0051	.0049	.0048
−2.4	.0082	.0080	.0078	.0075	.0073	.0071	.0069	.0068	.0066	.0064
−2.3	.0107	.0104	.0102	.0099	.0096	.0094	.0091	.0089	.0087	.0084
−2.2	.0139	.0136	.0132	.0129	.0126	.0122	.0119	.0116	.0113	.0110
−2.1	.0179	.0174	.0170	.0166	.0162	.0158	.0154	.0150	.0146	.0143
−2.0	.0228	.0222	.0217	.0212	.0207	.0202	.0197	.0192	.0188	.0183
−1.9	.0287	.0281	.0274	.0268	.0262	.0256	.0250	.0244	.0238	.0233
−1.8	.0359	.0352	.0344	.0336	.0329	.0322	.0314	.0307	.0300	.0294
−1.7	.0446	.0436	.0427	.0418	.0409	.0401	.0392	.0384	.0375	.0367
−1.6	.0548	.0537	.0526	.0516	.0505	.0495	.0485	.0475	.0465	.0455
−1.5	.0668	.0655	.0643	.0630	.0618	.0606	.0594	.0582	.0570	.0559
−1.4	.0808	.0793	.0778	.0764	.0749	.0735	.0722	.0708	.0694	.0681
−1.3	.0968	.0951	.0934	.0918	.0901	.0885	.0869	.0853	.0838	.0823
−1.2	.1151	.1131	.1112	.1093	.1075	.1056	.1038	.1020	.1003	.0985
−1.1	.1357	.1335	.1314	.1292	.1271	.1251	.1230	.1210	.1190	.1170
−1.0	.1587	.1562	.1539	.1515	.1492	.1469	.1446	.1423	.1401	.1379
− .9	.1841	.1814	.1788	.1762	.1736	.1711	.1685	.1660	.1635	.1611
− .8	.2119	.2090	.2061	.2033	.2005	.1977	.1949	.1922	.1894	.1867

Appendix I

z	0	1	2	3	4	5	6	7	8	9
−.7	.2420	.2389	.2358	.2327	.2297	.2266	.2236	.2206	.2177	.2148
−.6	.2743	.2709	.2676	.2643	.2611	.2578	.2546	.2514	.2483	.2451
−.5	.3085	.3050	.3015	.2981	.2946	.2912	.2877	.2843	.2810	.2776
−.4	.3446	.3409	.3372	.3336	.3300	.3264	.3228	.3192	.3156	.3121
−.3	.3821	.3783	.3745	.3707	.3669	.3632	.3594	.3557	.3520	.3483
−.2	.4207	.4168	.4129	.4090	.4052	.4013	.3974	.3936	.3897	.3859
−.1	.4602	.4562	.4522	.4483	.4443	.4404	.4364	.4325	.4286	.4247
−.0	.5000	.4960	.4920	.4880	.4840	.4801	.4761	.4721	.4681	.4641
.0	.5000	.5040	.5080	.5120	.5160	.5199	.5239	.5279	.5319	.5359
.1	.5398	.5438	.5478	.5517	.5557	.5596	.5636	.5675	.5714	.5753
.2	.5793	.5832	.5871	.5910	.5948	.5987	.6026	.6064	.6103	.6141
.3	.6179	.6217	.6255	.6293	.6331	.6368	.6406	.6443	.6480	.6517
.4	.6554	.6591	.6628	.6664	.6700	.6736	.6772	.6808	.6844	.6879
.5	.6915	.6950	.6985	.7019	.7054	.7088	.7123	.7157	.7190	.7224
.6	.7257	.7291	.7324	.7357	.7389	.7422	.7454	.7486	.7517	.7549
.7	.7580	.7611	.7642	.7673	.7703	.7734	.7764	.7794	.7823	.7852
.8	.7881	.7910	.7939	.7967	.7995	.8023	.8051	.8078	.8106	.8133
.9	.8159	.8186	.8212	.8238	.8264	.8289	.8315	.8340	.8365	.8389
1.0	.8413	.8438	.8461	.8485	.8508	.8531	.8554	.8577	.8599	.8621
1.1	.8643	.8665	.8686	.8708	.8729	.8749	.8770	.8790	.8810	.8830
1.2	.8849	.8869	.8888	.8907	.8925	.8944	.8962	.8980	.8997	.9015
1.3	.9032	.9049	.9066	.9082	.9099	.9115	.9131	.9147	.9162	.9177
1.4	.9192	.9207	.9222	.9236	.9251	.9265	.9278	.9292	.9306	.9319
1.5	.9332	.9345	.9357	.9370	.9382	.9394	.9406	.9418	.9430	.9441
1.6	.9452	.9463	.9474	.9484	.9495	.9505	.9515	.9525	.9535	.9545
1.7	.9554	.9564	.9573	.9582	.9591	.9599	.9608	.9616	.9625	.9633
1.8	.9641	.9648	.9656	.9664	.9671	.9678	.9686	.9693	.9700	.9706
1.9	.9713	.9719	.9726	.9732	.9738	.9744	.9750	.9756	.9762	.9767
2.0	.9772	.9778	.9783	.9788	.9793	.9798	.9803	.9808	.9812	.9817
2.1	.9821	.9826	.9830	.9834	.9838	.9842	.9846	.9850	.9854	.9857
2.2	.9861	.9864	.9868	.9871	.9874	.9878	.9881	.9884	.9887	.9890
2.3	.9893	.9896	.9898	.9901	.9904	.9906	.9909	.9911	.9913	.9916
2.4	.9918	.9920	.9922	.9925	.9927	.9929	.9931	.9932	.9934	.9936
2.5	.9938	.9940	.9941	.9943	.9945	.9946	.9948	.9949	.9951	.9952
2.6	.9953	.9955	.9956	.9957	.9959	.9960	.9961	.9962	.9963	.9964
2.7	.9965	.9966	.9967	.9968	.9969	.9970	.9971	.9972	.9973	.9974
2.8	.9974	.9975	.9976	.9977	.9977	.9978	.9979	.9979	.9980	.9981
2.9	.9981	.9982	.9982	.9983	.9984	.9984	.9985	.9985	.9986	.9986
3.	.9987	.9990	.9993	.9995	.9997	.9998	.9998	.9999	.9999	1.0000

APPENDIX II

Areas Under the Student t-Curve

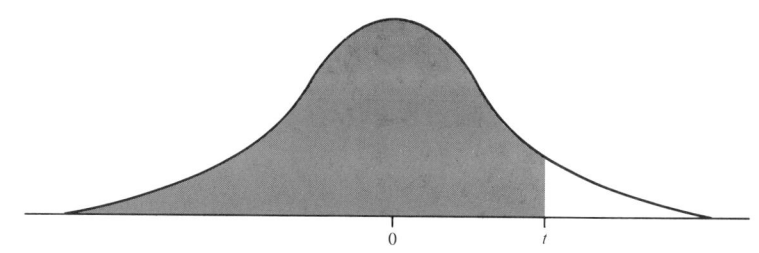

Areas to the left of t

df	.70	.80	.90	.95	.975	.99	.995
1	.73	1.38	3.08	6.31	12.71	31.82	63.66
2	.62	1.06	1.89	2.92	4.30	6.96	9.92
3	.58	.98	1.64	2.35	3.18	4.54	5.84
4	.57	.94	1.53	2.13	2.78	3.75	4.60
5	.56	.92	1.48	2.01	2.57	3.36	4.03
6	.55	.91	1.44	1.94	2.45	3.14	3.71
7	.55	.90	1.42	1.90	2.36	3.00	3.50
8	.55	.89	1.40	1.86	2.31	2.90	3.36
9	.54	.88	1.38	1.83	2.26	2.82	3.25
10	.54	.88	1.37	1.81	2.23	2.76	3.17
11	.54	.88	1.36	1.80	2.20	2.72	3.11
12	.54	.87	1.36	1.78	2.18	2.68	3.06
13	.54	.87	1.35	1.77	2.16	2.65	3.01
14	.54	.87	1.34	1.76	2.14	2.62	2.98
15	.54	.87	1.34	1.75	2.13	2.60	2.95
16	.54	.86	1.34	1.75	2.12	2.58	2.92
17	.53	.86	1.33	1.74	2.11	2.57	2.90
18	.53	.86	1.33	1.73	2.10	2.55	2.88
19	.53	.86	1.33	1.73	2.09	2.54	2.86
20	.53	.86	1.32	1.72	2.09	2.53	2.84
21	.53	.86	1.32	1.72	2.08	2.52	2.83
22	.53	.86	1.32	1.72	2.07	2.51	2.82

df	.70	.80	.90	.95	.975	.99	.995
23	.53	.86	1.32	1.71	2.07	2.50	2.81
24	.53	.86	1.32	1.71	2.06	2.49	2.80
25	.53	.86	1.32	1.71	2.06	2.48	2.79
26	.53	.86	1.32	1.71	2.06	2.48	2.78
27	.53	.86	1.31	1.70	2.05	2.47	2.77
28	.53	.86	1.31	1.70	2.05	2.47	2.76
29	.53	.85	1.31	1.70	2.04	2.46	2.76
30+	.52	.84	1.28	1.64	1.96	2.33	2.58

APPENDIX III

Critical Values for the F-Test

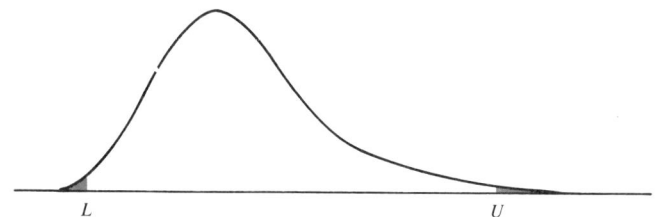

D \ N	1 L	1 U	2 L	2 U	3 L	3 U	4 L	4 U	5 L	5 U
1	.0⁴62	162²	.02⁵1	200²	.018	216²	.032	225²	.044	231²
2	.0⁴50	198	.02⁵0	199	.020	199	.038	199	.055	199
3	.0⁴46	55.6	.02⁵0	49.8	.021	47.5	.041	46.2	.060	45.4
4	.0⁴44	31.3	.02⁵0	26.3	.022	24.3	.043	23.2	.064	22.5
5	.0⁴43	22.8	.02⁵0	18.3	.022	16.5	.045	15.6	.067	14.9
6	.0⁴43	18.6	.02⁵0	14.5	.022	12.9	.045	12.0	.069	11.5
7	0⁴42	16.2	.02⁵0	12.4	.023	10.9	.046	10.0	.070	9.52
8	.0⁴42	14.7	.02⁵0	11.0	.023	9.60	.047	8.81	.072	8.30
9	.0²42	13.6	.02⁵0	10.1	.023	8.72	.047	7.96	.073	7.47
10	.0⁴41	12.8	.02⁵0	9.43	.023	8.08	.048	7.34	.073	6.87
11	.0⁴40	12.2	.02⁵0	8.91	.023	7.60	.048	6.88	.074	6.42
12	.0⁴39	11.8	.02⁵0	8.51	.023	7.23	.048	6.52	.075	6.07
15	.0⁴39	10.8	.02⁵0	7.70	.023	6.48	.049	5.80	.076	5.37
20	.0⁴39	9.94	.02⁵0	6.99	.023	5.82	.050	5.17	.077	4.76
24	.0⁴40	9.55	.02⁵0	6.66	.023	5.52	.050	4.89	.078	4.49
30	.0⁴40	9.18	.02⁵0	6.35	.024	5.24	.050	4.62	.079	4.23
40	.0⁴40	8.83	.02⁵0	6.07	.024	4.98	.051	4.37	.080	3.99
60	.0⁴40	8.49	.02⁵0	5.80	.024	4.73	.051	4.14	.081	3.76
120	.0⁴39	8.18	.02⁵0	5.54	.024	4.50	.051	3.92	.081	3.55
∞	.0⁴39	7.88	.02⁵0	5.30	.024	4.28	.052	3.72	.082	3.35

Note: $.0^462 = .000062$ $162^2 = 16200$, etc.

Appendix III

D \ N	6		7		8		9		10	
	L	U	L	U	L	U	L	U	L	U
1	.054	234[2]	.062	237[2]	.068	239[2]	.073	241[2]	.078	242[2]
2	.069	199	.081	199	.091	199	.099	199	.106	199
3	.077	44.8	.092	44.4	.104	44.1	.115	43.9	.124	43.7
4	.083	22.0	.100	21.6	.114	21.4	.126	21.1	.137	21.0
5	.087	14.5	.105	14.2	.120	14.0	.134	13.8	.146	13.6
6	.090	11.1	.109	10.8	.126	10.6	.140	10.4	.153	10.2
7	.093	9.16	.113	8.89	.130	8.68	.145	8.51	.159	8.38
8	.095	7.95	.115	7.69	.133	7.50	.149	7.34	.164	7.21
9	.096	7.13	.117	6.88	.136	6.69	.153	6.54	.168	6.42
10	.098	6.54	.119	6.30	.139	6.12	.156	5.97	.171	5.85
11	.099	6.10	.121	5.86	.141	5.68	.158	5.54	.174	5.42
12	.100	5.76	.122	5.52	.143	5.35	.161	5.20	.177	5.09
15	.102	5.07	.125	4.85	.147	4.67	.166	4.54	.183	4.42
20	.104	4.47	.129	4.26	.151	4.09	.171	3.96	.190	3.85
24	.106	4.20	.131	3.99	.154	3.83	.175	3.69	.193	3.59
30	.107	3.95	.133	3.74	.156	3.58	.178	3.45	.197	3.34
40	.108	3.71	.135	3.51	.159	3.35	.181	3.22	.201	3.12
60	.110	3.49	.137	3.29	.162	3.13	.185	3.01	.206	2.90
120	.111	3.28	.139	3.09	.165	2.93	.189	2.81	.211	2.71
∞	.113	3.09	.141	2.90	.168	2.74	.193	2.62	.216	2.52

D \ N	11		12		15		20		24	
	L	U	L	U	L	U	L	U	L	U
1	.082	243[2]	.085	244[2]	.093	246[2]	.101	248[2]	.105	249[2]
2	.112	199	.118	199	.130	199	.143	199	.150	199
3	.132	43.5	.138	43.4	.154	43.1	.172	42.8	.181	42.6
4	.145	20.8	.153	20.7	.172	20.4	.193	20.2	.204	20.0
5	.156	13.5	.165	13.4	.186	13.1	.210	12.9	.223	12.8
6	.164	10.1	.174	10.0	.197	9.81	.224	9.59	.238	9.47
7	.171	8.27	.181	8.18	.206	7.97	.235	7.75	.251	7.65
8	.176	7.10	.187	7.01	.214	6.81	.244	6.61	.261	6.50
9	.181	6.31	.192	6.23	.220	6.03	.253	5.83	.271	5.73
10	.185	5.75	.197	5.66	.226	5.47	.260	5.27	.279	5.14
11	.188	5.32	.200	5.24	.231	5.05	.266	4.86	.286	4.76
12	.191	4.99	.204	4.91	.235	4.72	.272	4.53	.292	4.43
15	.198	4.33	.212	4.25	.246	4.07	.286	3.88	.308	3.79
20	.206	3.76	.221	3.68	.258	3.50	.301	3.32	.327	3.22
24	.210	3.50	.226	3.42	.264	3.25	.310	3.06	.337	2.97
30	.215	3.25	.231	3.18	.271	3.01	.320	2.82	.349	2.73
40	.220	3.03	.237	2.95	.279	2.78	.331	2.60	.362	2.50
60	.225	2.82	.243	2.74	.287	2.57	.343	2.39	.376	2.29
120	.230	2.62	.249	2.54	.297	2.37	.356	2.19	.393	2.09
∞	.236	2.43	.256	2.36	.307	2.19	ε72.	2.00	.412	1.90

Appendix III

N / D	30 L	30 U	40 L	40 U	60 L	60 U	120 L	120 U	∞ L	∞ U
1	.109	250^2	.113	251^2	.118	253^2	.122	254^2	.127	255^2
2	.157	199	.165	199	.173	199	.181	199	.189	200
3	.191	42.5	.201	42.3	.211	42.1	.222	42.0	.234	41.8
4	.216	19.9	.229	19.8	.242	19.6	.255	19.5	.269	19.3
5	.237	12.7	.251	12.5	.266	12.4	.282	12.3	.299	12.2
6	.253	9.36	.269	9.24	.286	9.12	.304	9.00	.324	8.88
7	.267	7.53	.285	7.42	.304	7.31	.324	7.19	.345	7.08
8	.279	6.40	.299	6.29	.319	6.18	.341	6.06	.364	5.95
9	.290	5.62	.310	5.52	.332	5.41	.356	5.30	.382	5.19
10	.299	5.07	.321	4.97	.344	4.86	.370	4.75	.397	4.64
11	.308	4.65	.330	4.55	.355	4.45	.382	4.34	.412	4.23
12	.315	4.33	.339	4.23	.365	4.12	.393	4.01	.424	3.90
15	.333	3.69	.360	3.59	.389	3.48	.422	3.37	.457	3.26
20	.354	3.12	.385	3.02	.419	2.92	.457	2.81	.500	2.69
24	.367	2.87	.400	2.77	.437	2.66	.479	2.55	.527	2.43
30	.381	2.63	.416	2.52	.457	2.42	.504	2.30	.559	2.18
40	.396	2.40	.436	2.30	.481	2.18	.534	2.06	.599	1.93
60	.414	2.19	.458	2.08	.510	1.96	.572	1.83	.652	1.69
120	.434	1.98	.484	1.87	.545	1.75	.623	1.61	.733	1.43
∞	.460	1.79	.518	1.67	.592	1.53	.699	1.36	1.00	1.00

APPENDIX IV

Areas Under the χ^2 Curve

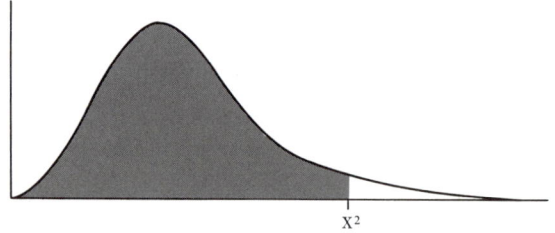

Areas to the left of X^2

df	.90	.95	.975	.99	.995
1	2.71	3.84	5.02	6.63	7.88
2	4.61	5.99	7.38	9.21	10.6
3	6.25	7.81	9.35	11.3	12.8
4	7.78	9.49	11.1	13.3	14.9
5	9.24	11.1	12.8	15.1	16.7
6	10.6	12.6	14.4	16.8	18.5
7	12.0	14.1	16.0	18.5	20.3
8	13.4	15.5	17.5	20.1	22.0
9	14.7	16.9	19.0	21.7	23.6
10	16.0	18.3	20.5	23.2	25.2
11	17.3	19.7	21.9	24.7	26.8
12	18.5	21.0	23.3	26.2	28.3
13	19.8	22.4	24.7	27.7	29.8
14	21.1	23.7	26.1	29.1	31.3
15	22.3	25.0	27.5	30.6	32.8
16	23.5	26.3	28.8	32.0	34.3
17	24.8	27.6	30.2	33.4	35.7
18	26.0	28.9	31.5	34.8	37.2
19	27.2	30.1	32.9	36.2	38.6
20	28.4	31.4	34.2	37.6	40.0
21	29.6	32.7	35.5	38.9	41.4
22	30.8	33.9	36.8	40.3	42.8

df	.90	.95	.975	.99	.995
23	32.0	35.2	38.1	41.6	44.2
24	33.2	36.4	39.4	43.0	45.6
25	34.4	37.7	40.6	44.3	46.9
26	35.6	38.9	41.9	45.6	48.3
27	36.7	40.1	43.2	47.0	49.6
28	37.9	41.3	44.5	48.3	51.0
29	39.1	42.6	45.7	49.6	52.3
30	40.3	43.8	47.0	50.9	53.7

APPENDIX V

Critical Values for the Analysis of Variance ($P = .05$ and $P = .01$ Levels of Significance)

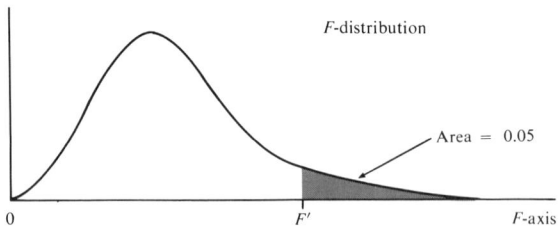

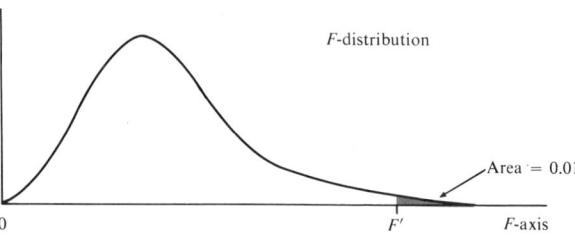

$P = .05$ Critical Values for the Analysis of Variance (The F-Distribution)

Degrees of freedom for numerator

	1	2	3	4	5	6	7	8	9	10	12	15	20	24	30	40	60	120	∞
1	161	200	216	225	230	234	237	239	241	242	244	246	248	249	250	251	252	253	254
2	18.5	19.0	19.2	19.2	19.3	19.3	19.4	19.4	19.4	19.4	19.4	19.4	19.4	19.5	19.5	19.5	19.5	19.5	19.5
3	10.1	9.55	9.28	9.12	9.01	8.94	8.89	8.85	8.81	8.79	8.74	8.70	8.66	8.64	8.62	8.59	8.57	8.55	8.53
4	7.71	6.94	6.59	6.39	6.26	6.16	6.09	6.04	6.00	5.96	5.91	5.86	5.80	5.77	5.75	5.72	5.69	5.66	5.63
5	6.61	5.79	5.41	5.19	5.05	4.95	4.88	4.82	4.77	4.74	4.68	4.62	4.56	4.53	4.50	4.46	4.43	4.40	4.37
6	5.99	5.14	4.76	4.53	4.39	4.28	4.21	4.15	4.10	4.06	4.00	3.94	3.87	3.84	3.81	3.77	3.74	3.70	3.67
7	5.59	4.74	4.35	4.12	3.97	3.87	3.79	3.73	3.68	3.64	3.57	3.51	3.44	3.41	3.38	3.34	3.30	3.27	3.23
8	5.32	4.46	4.07	3.84	3.69	3.58	3.50	3.44	3.39	3.35	3.28	3.22	3.15	3.12	3.08	3.04	3.01	2.97	2.93
9	5.12	4.26	3.86	3.63	3.48	3.37	3.29	3.23	3.18	3.14	3.07	3.01	2.94	2.90	2.86	2.83	2.79	2.75	2.71
10	4.96	4.10	3.71	3.48	3.33	3.22	3.14	3.07	3.02	2.98	2.91	2.85	2.77	2.74	2.70	2.66	2.62	2.58	2.54
11	4.84	3.98	3.59	3.36	3.20	3.09	3.01	2.95	2.90	2.85	2.79	2.72	2.65	2.61	2.57	2.53	2.49	2.45	2.40
12	4.75	3.89	3.49	3.26	3.11	3.00	2.91	2.85	2.80	2.75	2.69	2.62	2.54	2.51	2.47	2.43	2.38	2.34	2.30
13	4.67	3.81	3.41	3.18	3.03	2.92	2.83	2.77	2.71	2.67	2.60	2.53	2.46	2.42	2.38	2.34	2.30	2.25	2.21
14	4.60	3.74	3.34	3.11	2.96	2.85	2.76	2.70	2.65	2.60	2.53	2.46	2.39	2.35	2.31	2.27	2.22	2.18	2.13
15	4.54	3.68	3.29	3.06	2.90	2.79	2.71	2.64	2.59	2.54	2.48	2.40	2.33	2.29	2.25	2.20	2.16	2.11	2.07
16	4.49	3.63	3.24	3.01	2.85	2.74	2.66	2.59	2.54	2.49	2.42	2.35	2.28	2.24	2.19	2.15	2.11	2.06	2.01
17	4.45	3.59	3.20	2.96	2.81	2.70	2.61	2.55	2.49	2.45	2.38	2.31	2.23	2.19	2.15	2.10	2.06	2.01	1.96
18	4.41	3.55	3.16	2.93	2.77	2.66	2.58	2.51	2.46	2.41	2.34	2.27	2.19	2.15	2.11	2.06	2.02	1.97	1.92
19	4.38	3.52	3.13	2.90	2.74	2.63	2.54	2.48	2.42	2.38	2.31	2.23	2.16	2.11	2.07	2.03	1.98	1.93	1.88
20	4.35	3.49	3.10	2.87	2.71	2.60	2.51	2.45	2.39	2.35	2.28	2.20	2.12	2.08	2.04	1.99	1.95	1.90	1.84
21	4.32	3.47	3.07	2.84	2.68	2.57	2.49	2.42	2.37	2.32	2.25	2.18	2.10	2.05	2.01	1.96	1.92	1.87	1.81
22	4.30	3.44	3.05	2.82	2.66	2.55	2.46	2.40	2.34	2.30	2.23	2.15	2.07	2.03	1.98	1.94	1.89	1.84	1.78
23	4.28	3.42	3.03	2.80	2.64	2.53	2.44	2.37	2.32	2.27	2.20	2.13	2.05	2.01	1.96	1.91	1.86	1.81	1.76
24	4.26	3.40	3.01	2.78	2.62	2.51	2.42	2.36	2.30	2.25	2.18	2.11	2.03	1.98	1.94	1.89	1.84	1.79	1.73
25	4.24	3.39	2.99	2.76	2.60	2.49	2.40	2.34	2.28	2.24	2.16	2.09	2.01	1.96	1.92	1.87	1.82	1.77	1.71
30	4.17	3.32	2.92	2.69	2.53	2.42	2.33	2.27	2.21	2.16	2.09	2.01	1.93	1.89	1.84	1.79	1.74	1.68	1.62
40	4.08	3.23	2.84	2.61	2.45	2.34	2.25	2.18	2.12	2.08	2.00	1.92	1.84	1.79	1.74	1.69	1.64	1.58	1.51
60	4.00	3.15	2.76	2.53	2.37	2.25	2.17	2.10	2.04	1.99	1.92	1.84	1.75	1.70	1.65	1.59	1.53	1.47	1.39
120	3.92	3.07	2.68	2.45	2.29	2.18	2.09	2.02	1.96	1.91	1.83	1.75	1.66	1.61	1.55	1.50	1.43	1.35	1.25
∞	3.84	3.00	2.60	2.37	2.21	2.10	2.01	1.94	1.88	1.83	1.75	1.67	1.57	1.52	1.46	1.39	1.32	1.22	1.00

Degrees of freedom for denominator

$P = .01$ Critical Values for the Analysis of Variance (The F-Distribution)

Degrees of freedom for numerator

	1	2	3	4	5	6	7	8	9	10	12	15	20	24	30	40	60	120	∞
1	4052	5000	5403	5625	5764	5859	5928	5982	6023	6056	6106	6157	6209	6235	6261	6287	6313	6339	6366
2	98.5	99.0	99.2	99.2	99.3	99.3	99.4	99.4	99.4	99.4	99.4	99.4	99.4	99.5	99.5	99.5	99.5	99.5	99.5
3	34.1	30.8	29.5	28.7	28.2	27.9	27.7	27.5	27.3	27.2	27.1	26.9	26.7	26.6	26.5	26.4	26.3	26.2	26.1
4	21.2	18.0	16.7	16.0	15.5	15.2	15.0	14.8	14.7	14.5	14.4	14.2	14.0	13.9	13.8	13.7	13.7	13.6	13.5
5	16.3	13.3	12.1	11.4	11.0	10.7	10.5	10.3	10.2	10.1	9.89	9.72	9.55	9.47	9.38	9.29	9.20	9.11	9.02
6	13.7	10.9	9.78	9.15	8.75	8.47	8.26	8.10	7.98	7.87	7.72	7.56	7.40	7.31	7.23	7.14	7.06	6.97	6.88
7	12.2	9.55	8.45	7.85	7.46	7.19	6.99	6.84	6.72	6.62	6.47	6.31	6.16	6.07	5.99	5.91	5.82	5.74	5.65
8	11.3	8.65	7.59	7.01	6.63	6.37	6.18	6.03	5.91	5.81	5.67	5.52	5.36	5.28	5.20	5.12	5.03	4.95	4.86
9	10.6	8.02	6.99	6.42	6.06	5.80	5.61	5.47	5.35	5.26	5.11	4.96	4.81	4.73	4.65	4.57	4.48	4.40	4.31
10	10.0	7.56	6.55	5.99	5.64	5.39	5.20	5.06	4.94	4.85	4.71	4.56	4.41	4.33	4.25	4.17	4.08	4.00	3.91
11	9.65	7.21	6.22	5.67	5.32	5.07	4.89	4.74	4.63	4.54	4.40	4.25	4.10	4.02	3.94	3.86	3.78	3.69	3.60
12	9.33	6.93	5.95	5.41	5.06	4.82	4.64	4.50	4.39	4.30	4.16	4.01	3.86	3.78	3.70	3.62	3.54	3.45	3.36
13	9.07	6.70	5.74	5.21	4.86	4.62	4.44	4.30	4.19	4.10	3.96	3.82	3.66	3.59	3.51	3.43	3.34	3.25	3.17
14	8.86	6.51	5.56	5.04	4.70	4.46	4.28	4.14	4.03	3.94	3.80	3.66	3.51	3.43	3.35	3.27	3.18	3.09	3.00
15	8.68	6.36	5.42	4.89	4.56	4.32	4.14	4.00	3.89	3.80	3.67	3.52	3.37	3.29	3.21	3.13	3.05	2.96	2.87
16	8.53	6.23	5.29	4.77	4.44	4.20	4.03	3.89	3.78	3.69	3.55	3.41	3.26	3.18	3.10	3.02	2.93	2.84	2.75
17	8.40	6.11	5.19	4.67	4.34	4.10	3.93	3.79	3.68	3.59	3.46	3.31	3.16	3.08	3.00	2.92	2.83	2.75	2.65
18	8.29	6.01	5.09	4.58	4.25	4.01	3.84	3.71	3.60	3.51	3.37	3.23	3.08	3.00	2.92	2.84	2.75	2.66	2.57
19	8.19	5.93	5.01	4.50	4.17	3.94	3.77	3.63	3.52	3.43	3.30	3.15	3.00	2.92	2.84	2.76	2.67	2.58	2.49
20	8.10	5.85	4.94	4.43	4.10	3.87	3.70	3.56	3.46	3.37	3.23	3.09	2.94	2.86	2.78	2.69	2.61	2.52	2.42
21	8.02	5.78	4.87	4.37	4.04	3.81	3.64	3.51	3.40	3.31	3.17	3.03	2.88	2.80	2.72	2.64	2.55	2.46	2.36
22	7.95	5.72	4.82	4.31	3.99	3.76	3.59	3.45	3.35	3.26	3.12	2.98	2.83	2.75	2.67	2.58	2.50	2.40	2.31
23	7.88	5.66	4.76	4.26	3.94	3.71	3.54	3.41	3.30	3.21	3.07	2.93	2.78	2.70	2.62	2.54	2.45	2.35	2.26
24	7.82	5.61	4.72	4.22	3.90	3.67	3.50	3.36	3.26	3.17	3.03	2.89	2.74	2.66	2.58	2.49	2.40	2.31	2.21
25	7.77	5.57	4.68	4.18	3.86	3.63	3.46	3.32	3.22	3.13	2.99	2.85	2.70	2.62	2.53	2.45	2.36	2.27	2.17
30	7.56	5.39	4.51	4.02	3.70	3.47	3.30	3.17	3.07	2.98	2.84	2.70	2.55	2.47	2.39	2.30	2.21	2.11	2.01
40	7.31	5.18	4.31	3.83	3.51	3.29	3.12	2.99	2.89	2.80	2.66	2.52	2.37	2.29	2.20	2.11	2.02	1.92	1.80
60	7.08	4.98	4.13	3.65	3.34	3.12	2.95	2.82	2.72	2.63	2.50	2.35	2.20	2.12	2.03	1.94	1.84	1.73	1.60
120	6.85	4.79	3.95	3.48	3.17	2.96	2.79	2.66	2.56	2.47	2.34	2.19	2.03	1.95	1.86	1.76	1.66	1.53	1.38
∞	6.63	4.61	3.78	3.32	3.02	2.80	2.64	2.51	2.41	2.32	2.18	2.04	1.88	1.79	1.70	1.59	1.47	1.32	1.00

Degrees of freedom for denominator

APPENDIX VI

Answers to Selected Questions and Review Exercises

CHAPTER 1

Questions

1.5.1 No. The vertical axis expresses the suicide frequency as a *rate* — per 100,000 white males or per 100,000 black males. Since there were almost eight times as many whites as blacks in 1965, there were approximately 16 times as many white male suicides as black male suicides.

1.5.3 The number of single persons, ages 14 and over, is not the same for each of the four regions. Therefore, it would be incorrect to compute an overall U.S. average with the expression

$$\frac{109.9 + 122.7 + 124.5 + 149.1}{4}$$

1.6.1 Each location could be designated as being either "safe" or "unsafe," depending on whether the original measurement fell below or above the limit set by the National Council on Radiation Protection.

1.6.2 Probably not. In a nonlaboratory environment, a person's movements would reduce the bite duration.

1.7.1   The subjects in the control group should be approximately the same age as the patients with Raynaud's syndrome and their overall health profiles should be similar.

1.7.2   If it was determined that a patient with thrombocytopenia had a small spleen, then it might be wise to elect something other than a splenectomy as a mode of treatment.

1.8.2   Definitely. In this particular experiment, the staff might want lithium to appear effective and their evaluations would be biased accordingly. Furthermore, the psychological reactions of the patients, if they knew their behavior was being monitored at a certain time, might mask the physiological effects of the treatment.

1.9.1   There might be a third variable that is actually the cause of the apparent relationship between the first two. For example, a person who is very nervous and insecure may tend to develop more serious illnesses and change his lifestyle more frequently than someone who is *not* nervous and insecure. If this were the case, both the SRE and SIRS measurements would be effects, and neither would be a cause of the other.

1.9.2   Heavy users will be discovered no matter how hard they try to cover up; light users will probably go undetected if they use just a minimum of secrecy. But those who are moderate users are in the most vulnerable position and would be expected to exercise the most caution.

1.9.4 $143/(59 + 143) = 0.71 = 71\%$.

1.10.1 No attempt was made to "preselect" individuals who were, say, heavy users or moderate users.

1.10.2 Perhaps the apparent increase in admissions when the moon was full was due simply to chance; and, if similar data were collected for another year, a completely different pattern would emerge.

1.10.3 As a group the parents involved in this study were probably more concerned about their children than "typical" parents would be (just by virtue of the fact that they were interested enough to volunteer for the experiment). It shouldn't be surprising, then, that their children develop and mature at a rate faster than the established norm.

Review Exercises

1.1   Correlation.

1.3 k-sample.

1.4   Correlation or two-sample (might also be considered total population).

1.6   Total population.

1.8   Two-sample.

1.9   One-sample.

1.12 Paired-data.

Appendix VI 311

CHAPTER 2

Questions

2.3.1 Tennessee: 10.7 suicides per 100,000.
Florida: 13.7 suicides per 100,000.
Florida has an older population than Tennessee. Since suicide rates are highest for the elderly (see Example 2.3.1), we would expect the Florida rate to be higher.

2.3.2 17.

2.4.2 6.9 leukemia deaths per 100,000.

2.5.1 Lower. Persons in underdeveloped countries tend to die at early ages, from causes other than cancer.

2.5.3 It would probably depend on who was asking the questions, and under what circumstances.

2.5.5 No.

2.5.6 It appears from the graph that about 40 out of every 10,000 pregnancies are complicated by tonsillitis. Therefore, about 14,000 of all the live births in the U.S. in 1967 fell into that category.

2.6.3 The "125–129" class really extends from 124.5 to 129.5; the "130–134" class from 129.5 to 134.5, and so on. But since all the observations are integers, it is not necessary to express the class limits to an extra decimal place.

2.6.4 The midpoint is more representative of a "typical" observation than either the lower class limit or the upper class limit.

2.6.5 Model Two.

2.6.7 The sample members are the 21 cities where the dental surveys were done.

2.6.8 Other factors involved here would include the socioeconomic backgrounds and the ages of the children being examined. Hopefully, as a group, the children in the 21 samples were as similar as possible, except with respect to the fluoride concentrations in their drinking water.

2.7.1 Women whose pregnancies were expected to have complications normally would be sent to a hospital. As a result, those women constituted a higher risk group than the ones delivering their babies at home.

2.7.2 The spreads of the observations, as indicated by the first and last bars, were not symmetric with respect to the *true* fetal heart rate. When the true FHR was very slow, the estimates tended to be much faster; but when the true FHR was very fast, the estimates tended to be much slower.

2.7.3 Age, sex, whether or not the person worked or lived in a certain area, etc.

2.7.4 The percentages in that age group are small because of losses sustained in World War II.

2.8.1 1919.

Review Exercises

2.2 139.8 deaths per 1,000.

Appendix VI

2.5 (a) 34.7 deaths per 10,000.
(b) 43.6 male deaths per 10,000.
25.3 female deaths per 10,000.
(c) 34.3 deaths per 10,000.

2.7 (a) Nominal.

2.8 (a) 149.2 deaths per 100,000.
(b) 4540 expected deaths.
(c) 149.4 deaths per 100,000.

CHAPTER 3

Questions

3.3.1 (a) $\sum_{i=1}^{4} x_i^3 = 289$.

(b) $\left(\sum_{i=1}^{4} x_i\right)^3 = (13)^3 = 2197$.

3.3.2 (a) 464.
(b) 272.
(c) 400.
(d) 24.
(e) 24.

3.4.1 $\bar{x} = 638{,}140$ bacteria per sq in.
$\tilde{x} = 140{,}750$ bacteria per sq in.

3.5.2 $\sum_{i=1}^{8} x_i = 266; \sum_{i=1}^{8} x_i^2 = 10{,}900; s = 17.1$.

3.5.3 $|x_i - \bar{x}|$, where $|x|$ denotes the absolute value of x.

3.5.4 $\bar{x} = 143.8$ mm; $s = 6.0$ mm.

3.6.1 Possible sample means: 10, 13, 14, 12, 12, 7, 8, 6, 6, 11, 9, 9, 10, 10, 8.

Response	Frequency
6– 7	3
8– 9	4
10–11	4
12–13	3
14–15	1
	15

3.7.1 No. Convicting an innocent person probably would be considered a more "serious" error than acquitting a guilty person. That is, a Type I error would be worse than a Type II error.

3.7.2 No.

Appendix VI 313

3.8.1 Out of the 24 blood samples tested, a total of 4 showed a platelet count less than 150,000 per mm^3. Therefore, in the absence of any additional information, we would estimate that the probability is 4/24, or 0.167, that a newly-admitted resident would fall into this category.

3.9.1 (1) $1 - 0.4325 = 0.5675$.
(2) $0.8365 - 0.0455 = 0.7910$.
(3) 1.0000

3.9.2 $P\{-2.00 < Z < 2.00\} = 0.9772 - 0.0228 = 0.9544$.
$P\{-1.00 < Z < 1.00\} = 0.8413 - 0.1587 = 0.6826$.

3.9.3 $P\{104 < X < 122\} = P\{0.25 < Z < 1.38\} = 0.3175$.
$P\{99 < X < 101\} = P\{-0.06 < Z < 0.06\} = 0.0478$.
$P\{X < 60\} = P\{Z < -2.50\} = 0.0062$
$P\{X < 75 \text{ or } X > 125\} = P\{Z < -1.56 \text{ or } Z > 1.56\}$
$= 0.0594 + 0.0594 = 0.1188$

3.9.4 133.

3.9.6 $P\{X > 18.1\} = P\{Z > 2.05\} = 1 - 0.9798 = 0.0202$

Review Exercises

3.1 $P\{X > 310\} = P\{Z > 2.75\} = 1 - 0.9970 = 0.0030$.
$.0030 \times 318{,}000 = 954$.

3.3 $P\{X > 150\} = P\{Z > 2.50\} = 0.0062$.
$P\{X < 115\} = P\{Z < -0.42\} = 0.3372$.
$P\{110 < X < 130\} = P\{-0.83 < Z < 0.83\} = 0.5934$.

3.4 $x_{90} = 135.4$; x_{50} is the median.

3.5 $Q = 16.0$; dispersion.

3.6 $\sum_{i=1}^{10} x_i = 4.84$; $\sum_{i=1}^{10} x_i^2 = 2.8602$; $\bar{x} = 0.48$; $s = 0.24$.

3.7 (a) 7.
(b) -5.
(c) -8.
(d) 2.6.
(e) 36,863,997.

3.8 $\sum_{i=1}^{9} x_i = 73.6$; $\sum_{i=1}^{9} x^2 = 603.68$; $\bar{x} = 8.18$; $s = 0.47$. Let X denote the 3rd molar length of a randomly selected member of the genus *Papio*.

$$P\{X > 9.0\} \approx P\left\{Z > \frac{9.0 - 8.18}{0.47}\right\}$$

$$= P\{Z > 1.75\} = 0.0401$$

The chances are somewhat remote (4 out of 100) that a member of the *Papio* genus would have a 3rd molar length as long or longer than 9.0 mm.

3.11 (a) $P\{7.1 < X < 7.6\} = P\{-1.33 < Z < 0.33\} = 0.5375$.
(b) $P\{X < 7.0 \text{ or } 7.4 < X < 7.6\} = P\{Z < -1.67 \text{ or } -0.33 < Z < 0.33\} =$
$0.0475 + (0.6293 - 0.3707) = 0.3061$.
(c) $(7.4 - 7.5)/0.3 = 0.33$.

CHAPTER 4

Questions

4.2.1 As n increases, the probability that the sample mean, $\bar{X}$, lies within a fixed interval of the true mean, μ, increases. In this sense, $\bar{x}$ is a more accurate estimator when n is large.

4.2.2 When $P = .10$, $\bar{X}' = \mu_o + 1.28(s/\sqrt{n})$.
When $P = .025$, $\bar{X}' = \mu_o + 1.96(s/\sqrt{n})$

4.2.3 No.

4.2.4 Yes.

4.2.5 When $P = .01$, $\bar{X}' = 7.39 - 2.33(0.17/\sqrt{44}) = 7.33$. Reject H.

4.2.6 $\bar{X}'_1 = 250,000 - 3.3(15,300) = 199,500$.
$\bar{X}'_2 = 250,000 + 3.3(15,300) = 300,500$. Reject H.

4.3.1 There is no reason for believing that an exposure of this sort would *improve* a person's air-flow rate.

4.3.2 $\bar{X}' = 0.80 - 1.71(0.086/\sqrt{25}) = 0.77$. But $\bar{x} = 0.77$, which implies that H should be rejected.

4.3.4 $\bar{X}'_1 = 15 - 2.26(5.8/\sqrt{10}) = 10.9$.
$\bar{X}'_2 = 15 + 2.26(5.8/\sqrt{10}) = 19.1$. But $\bar{x} = 17.4$ so H is accepted.

4.4.1 Longer.

4.4.3 A 90% confidence interval would be $[0.015 - 1.77(0.008/\sqrt{14}), 0.015 + 1.77(0.008/\sqrt{14})] = (0.011, 0.019)$. A 99% confidence interval would be $[0.015 - 3.01(0.008/\sqrt{14}), 0.015 + 3.01(0.008/\sqrt{14})] = (0.009, 0.021)$. Yes.

4.4.4 Confidence intervals, by virtue of their length, provide an indication of the precision with which μ is being estimated. That information is not contained in a point estimate.

4.5.1 The standard deviation of the sampling distribution of X/n decreases with increasing n.

4.5.2 $P\{X/n > 0.208\} = P\{Z > 4.91\} = 0.0000$.

4.5.3 $(0.13 - 2.58\sqrt{[(0.13)(0.87)]/1171}, 0.13 + 2.58\sqrt{[(0.13)(0.87)]/1171}) = (0.11, 0.15)$.

4.6.1 $P\{\text{Type II error}\} = P\{210,500 < \bar{X} < 289,500, \text{ when } \mu = 300,000\} \approx P\{\bar{X} < 289,500, \text{ when } \mu = 300,000\} = P\{Z < -0.69\} = 0.2451$.

4.6.2 As n increases, the standard deviation of the $\bar{X}$ distribution decreases and the overlap between the null and alternative distributions is reduced.

Review Exercises

4.1 $(0.81 - 1.96\sqrt{[(0.81)(0.19)]/220}, 0.81 + 1.96\sqrt{[(0.81)(0.19)]/220}) = (0.76, 0.86)$.

4.2 The $\bar{X}$ distribution would be bell-shaped with a mean of 500 and a standard deviation of $100/\sqrt{64} = 12.5$.
$P\{\bar{X} > 510\} = P\{Z > 0.80\} = 1 - 0.7881 = 0.2119$.
$P\{X > 510\} = P\{Z > 0.10\} = 1 - 0.5398 = 0.4602$.

4.3 $[0.48 - 3.25(0.24/\sqrt{10}), 0.48 + 3.25(0.24/\sqrt{10})] = (0.23, 0.73)$.

4.5 $x_1 = 2.9$, $x_2 = 3.4$, $x_3 = 5.2$, $x_4 = 6.2$, $x_5 = 5.9$. $\sum_{i=1}^{5} x_i = 23.6$; $\sum_{i=1}^{5} x_i^2 = 120.26$;
$\bar{x} = 4.7$; $s = 1.49$. $[4.7 - 2.13(1.49/\sqrt{5}), 4.7 + 2.13(1.49/\sqrt{5})] = (3.3, 6.1)$.

4.6 Test H: $\mu = 50$ versus A: $\mu \neq 50$.
$\sum_{i=1}^{7} x_i = 284$; $\sum_{i=1}^{7} x_i^2 = 11{,}736$; $s = 6.0$.
$\bar{X}_1' = 50 - 2.45(6.0/\sqrt{7}) = 44.4$.
$\bar{X}_2' = 50 + 2.45(6.0/\sqrt{7}) = 55.6$. Since $\bar{x} = 40.6$, reject H.

4.9 $\sum_{i=1}^{11} x_i = 532$; $\sum_{i=1}^{11} x_i^2 = 29{,}000$; $\bar{x} = 48.4$; $s = 18.1$.
$[48.4 - 2.23(18.1/\sqrt{11}), 48.4 + 2.23(18.1/\sqrt{11})] = (36.2, 60.6)$.

CHAPTER 5

Questions

5.2.1 $(\bar{X} - \bar{Y}_1)' = -1.76(3.0)\sqrt{(1/8) + (1/8)} = -2.64$
$(\bar{X} - \bar{Y}_2)' = 1.76(3.0)\sqrt{(1/8) + (1/8)} = 2.64$
But $\bar{x} - \bar{y} = 1.4$ so H: $\mu_X = \mu_Y$ is accepted at the $P = .10$ level of significance.

5.2.2 Given that $P = .05$ is to be the level of significance, that particular probability expression indicates the range of values for $(\bar{x} - \bar{y})/[s_p\sqrt{(1/8) + (1/8)}]$ that would be compatible with the null hypothesis. By "inverting" that expression, the two critical values for $\bar{X} - \bar{Y}$ can be determined.

5.2.3 No — the unfavorable relationship could be the effect, rather than the cause.

5.3.1 As the two sample sizes increase, the estimates s_X and s_Y become more precise. Therefore, if H: $\sigma_X = \sigma_Y$ is, in fact, true, we would expect the sampling distribution of s_X^2/s_Y^2 to become more and more concentrated around the value 1.

5.3.2 $(s_X^2/s_Y^2)_1' \simeq 0.28$, $(s_X^2/s_Y^2)_2' \simeq 4.1$.
(These values are interpolations between the F-distributions with $N = 20$ and $D = 15$ and $N = 20$ and $D = 12$. Among the curves tabulated in Appendix III, these are the two most similar to the one we actually want — the F-distribution with $N = 20$ and $D = 14$.)
Since $s_X^2/s_Y^2 = 4.70$, H should be rejected at the $P = .01$ level of significance.

5.3.3 A t-distribution with 31 degrees of freedom has a smaller variance than one with 11 degrees of freedom. This implies that a test of H: $\mu_X = \mu_Y$ based on 31 degrees of freedom will be more "precise" than one based on 11 degrees of freedom, in the sense that smaller $\bar{x} - \bar{y}$ differences will result in the rejection of the null hypothesis.

5.4.1 The denominator would be $s_u = \sqrt{(s_X^2/n_X) + (s_Y^2/n_Y)}$ instead of $s_p\sqrt{(1/n_X) + (1/n_Y)}$. Also, the expression

$$\frac{\bar{x} - \bar{y} - (\mu_X - \mu_Y)}{s_u}$$

has f degrees of freedom (as given in Theorem 5.3.1) rather than $n_X + n_Y - 2$.

5.4.2 $N = 7$ and $D = 7$. Therefore, $(s_X^2/s_Y^2)_1' = 0.113$ and $(s_X^2/s_Y^2)_2' = 8.89$. But $s_X^2/s_Y^2 = 0.55/0.58 = 0.95$, so H: $\sigma_X = \sigma_Y$ is accepted at the $P = .01$ level of significance.

5.4.3 H and A could also be written
$$\text{H:} \quad \mu_X - \mu_Y = 2 \quad \text{versus} \quad \text{A:} \quad \mu_X - \mu_Y \neq 2$$
The test statistic, under the null hypothesis, would be
$$\frac{\bar{X} - \bar{Y} - 2}{s_p\sqrt{\dfrac{1}{n_X} + \dfrac{1}{n_Y}}}$$
in which case the critical values would be
$$(\bar{X} - \bar{Y})_1' = 2 - t \cdot s_p\sqrt{\dfrac{1}{n_X} + \dfrac{1}{n_Y}}$$
$$(\bar{X} - \bar{Y})_2' = 2 + t \cdot s_p\sqrt{\dfrac{1}{n_X} + \dfrac{1}{n_Y}}$$
where t has $n_X + n_Y - 2$ degrees of freedom. Of course, if σ_X were not equal to σ_Y, s_u would replace $s_p\sqrt{(1/n_X) + (1/n_Y)}$.

5.4.4 $\bar{x} = 2.11$; $s_{\bar{X}}^2 = 0.136$; $\bar{y} = 0.62$; $s_{\bar{Y}}^2 = 0.039$; $s_p = 0.30$. The 99% confidence interval has the form
$$\left(2.11 - 0.62 - 2.88(0.30)\sqrt{\dfrac{1}{10} + \dfrac{1}{10}},\ 2.11 - 0.62 + 2.88(0.30)\sqrt{\dfrac{1}{10} + \dfrac{1}{10}}\right)$$
$$= (1.10,\ 1.88)$$

Review Exercises

5.1 (b) $\sum_{i=1}^{6} x_i = 51$; $\sum_{i=1}^{6} x_i^2 = 443$; $s_X^2 = 1.90$

$\sum_{i=1}^{6} y_i = 132$; $\sum_{i=1}^{6} y_i^2 = 3232$; $s_Y^2 = 65.6$

With 5 and 5 degrees of freedom,
$$\left(\dfrac{s_X^2}{s_Y^2}\right)_1' = 0.067 \quad \text{and} \quad \left(\dfrac{s_X^2}{s_Y^2}\right)_2' = 14.9$$
But $s_X^2/s_Y^2 = 1.90/65.6 = 0.029$ so H: $\sigma_X = \sigma_Y$ is rejected.

(c) $s_u = 3.35$; $f = 6$.
$(\bar{X} - \bar{Y})' = -1.94(3.35) = -6.50$.
Since $\bar{x} - \bar{y} = 8.5 - 22.0 = -13.50$, the null hypothesis is rejected.

5.2 $s_X^2 = 3145$; $s_Y^2 = 2494$; $s_p = 51.4$.
$(\bar{X} - \bar{Y})_1' = -2.11(51.4)\sqrt{(1/5) + (1/14)} = -56.5$.
$(\bar{X} - \bar{Y})_2' = 2.11(51.4)\sqrt{(1/5) + (1/14)} = 56.5$.
But $\bar{x} - \bar{y} = 113.0 - 159.0 = -46.0$. Accept H.

5.3 (b) Yes. To guard against the introduction of biases that might invalidate the results, every aspect of the experimental procedure should be kept as similar as possible in the two groups, except for the treatment itself.

5.4 In forming a pooled standard deviation, it would not make sense to give equal weight to s_X^2 and s_Y^2 if the two sample sizes were very different. For example, if the X-sample were larger than the Y-sample, s_X^2 would be a more reliable estimator than s_Y^2 and the information it contains should be emphasized accordingly.

5.5 (b) $s_X^2 = 137.36$; $s_Y^2 = 340.27$; $s_p = 14.9$.

$$\left(63.2 - 44.7 - 2.18(14.9)\sqrt{\frac{1}{8} + \frac{1}{6}},\ 63.2 - 44.7 + 2.18(14.9)\sqrt{\frac{1}{8} + \frac{1}{6}}\right)$$

$$= (0.9, 36.0)$$

5.8 (b) Let μ_X = true intradiscal pH of persons having a herniated disc
μ_Y = true intradiscal pH of persons not having a herniated disc
Test

$$H: \quad \mu_X = \mu_Y \quad \text{versus} \quad A: \quad \mu_X \neq \mu_Y$$

at the $P = .05$ level of significance. $s_X^2 = 0.084$; $s_Y^2 = 0.388$; $s_p = 0.41$.
$(\bar{X} - \bar{Y})_1' = -2.04(0.41)\sqrt{(1/22) + (1/9)} = -0.33$
$(\bar{X} - \bar{Y})_2' = 2.04(.41)\sqrt{(1/22) + (1/9)} = 0.33$
Therefore, we accept H, since $\bar{x} - \bar{y} = 6.98 - 6.70 = 0.28$.

CHAPTER 6

Questions

6.2.1 $[12.0 - 2.26(10.6/\sqrt{10}),\ 12.0 + 2.26(10.6/\sqrt{10})] = (4.4, 19.6)$.

6.2.2 There might be a residual learning effect in this experiment. That is, children might tend to do better on the test the second time they take it, whether or not any treatment had been involved. If this was the case, the benefits of ethosuximide would be overestimated if all 10 children were first tested while on the placebo.

6.2.3 $\bar{D}_1' = -2.36(10.7/\sqrt{8}) = -8.9$.
$\bar{D}_2' = 2.36(10.7/\sqrt{8}) = 8.9$.
Accept H, since $\bar{d} = 4.0$.

6.2.4 To make a comparison of this sort using Model Three, it would be necessary to select two groups of people — those in the first group would have "normal" eyes; those in the second group, glaucoma. The results would be analyzed using the two-sample t-test of Section 5.2 (or 5.3). Individual variation is likely to be an important factor in measurements like these, so Model Four would probably be better than Model Three.

6.3.1 $[0.80275 - 2.31(0.45154/\sqrt{9}),\ 0.80275 + 2.31(0.45154/\sqrt{9})] = (0.45506, 1.15044)$.

This interval could be expressed in terms of actual titers by taking the antilogs of .45506 and 1.15044.

6.3.2 No.

Review Exercises

6.1 Let μ_D = True average difference between ESP scores when sender and student are hypnotized and when sender and student are awake.

Appendix VI

Test
$$H: \mu_D = 0 \quad \text{versus} \quad A: \mu_D > 0$$
Let $P = .05$.
$\sum_{i=1}^{15} d_i = 43; \sum_{i=1}^{15} d_i^2 = 363; s_d = 4.1.$
$\overline{D}' = 1.76(4.1/\sqrt{15}) = 1.86.$
$\bar{d} = 43/15 = 2.87$. Reject H.

6.3 From the graph, the six before and after scores are approximately {(4.8, 1.3), (4.3, 1.3), (3.1, 1.3), (2.7, 1.3), (2.7, 1.6), (2.8, 1.4)} so the pair differences are {3.5, 3.0, 1.8, 1.4, 1.1, 1.4}. Therefore,
$\sum_{i=1}^{6} d_i = 12.20; \sum_{i=1}^{6} d_i^2 = 29.62; s_d = 0.98.$
$[2.0 - 2.57(0.98/\sqrt{6}), 2.0 + 2.57(0.98/\sqrt{6})] = (1.0, 3.0)$

6.4 Let μ_D = True average difference in prothrombin times (after − before).
Test
$$H: \mu_D = 0 \quad \text{versus} \quad A: \mu_D \neq 0$$
Let $P = .05$.
$\sum_{i=1}^{12} d_i = -1.3; \sum_{i=1}^{12} d_i^2 = 2.97; s_d = 0.51.$
$\overline{D}'_1 = -2.20(0.51/\sqrt{12}) = -0.32.$
$\overline{D}'_2 = 2.20(0.51/\sqrt{12}) = 0.32.$
But $\bar{d} = -0.11$, so H is accepted.

6.5 Two independent groups of subjects might have been selected. The first group would not be given any aspirin and their prothrombin times would act as a control. The second group *would* be given the prescribed dosage and would have their prothrombin times measured three hours later. Because of the considerable subject-to-subject variability evident in these data, Model Four would probably be a better experimental design than Model Three.

6.7 Let $d_i = y_i - x_i$. Test
$$H: \mu_D = 0 \quad \text{versus} \quad A: \mu_D < 0$$
$\sum_{i=1}^{11} d_i = -11.5; \bar{d} = -1.0; \sum_{i=1}^{11} d_i^2 = 37.25; s_d = 1.59.$
$D' = -1.81(1.59/\sqrt{11}) = -0.87.$
Reject H.

6.9 If the subject-to-subject variability did not strongly influence the measured responses, the larger number of degrees of freedom available for a two-sample t-test would make it preferable to a paired-data t-test (assuming the same number of observations would be taken for both models). Also, in some situations, the treatments have a definite residual effect, in which case it would be better to measure each subject only once — that is, use a Model Three format.

CHAPTER 7

Questions

7.2.1 Estimated blood pressure = $89.8 + 5.83(22) = 218.1$.

7.2.2 No.

7.2.3 $Y = 0.5 + 0.5X$.

7.2.4 $\bar{x} = 5/3$; $\bar{y} = 4/3$. Also, $4/3$ *does* equal $0.5 + 0.5(5/3) = 8/6 = 4/3$.

7.3.1 For the three points given, the least squares line is $Y = (1/2) + (3/4)X$. Also, $\bar{y} = 1.0$, so that

$$\sum_{i=1}^{3}\left[y_i - \left(\frac{1}{2} + \frac{3}{4}x_i\right)\right]^2 = \frac{1}{2}$$

$$\sum_{i=1}^{3}(y_i - 1.0)^2 = 2$$

It follows, then, that

$$r = +\sqrt{1 - \tfrac{1}{2}/2} = \sqrt{0.75} = 0.87$$

7.3.2 $\sum_{i=1}^{3} x_i y_i = 4$; $\sum_{i=1}^{3} x_i = 2$; $\sum_{i=1}^{3} y_i = 3$; $\sum_{i=1}^{3} x_i^2 = 4$

$\sum_{i=1}^{3} y_i^2 = 5$; $r = 6/(\sqrt{8}\sqrt{6}) = 0.87$.

7.3.3 $\bar{y} = 1.0$; $Y = (1/2) + (3/4)X$. Therefore,

$$\sum_{i=1}^{3}(y_i - 1.0)^2 = 2$$

$$\sum_{i=1}^{3}\left[y_i - \left(\frac{1}{2} + \frac{3}{4}x_i\right)\right]^2 = \frac{1}{2}$$

$$\sum_{i=1}^{3}\left[\frac{1}{2} + \frac{3}{4}x_i - 1.0\right]^2 = \frac{3}{2}$$

showing that, for these data, the equation holds.

7.3.4 For the heart weight–blood pressure data, $r = 0.70$ and $r^2 = 0.49$. For the smoking-CHD data, $r = 0.73$ and $r^2 = 0.53$. Since $0.53/0.49 = 1.1$, we would say that the linear relationship in the smoking data is 1.1 times as strong as the linear relationship in the heart weight data.

7.4.1 $r = 0.70$ (from Example 7.3.2). Therefore,

$$r' = 1.74\sqrt{\left(\frac{1 - (0.70)^2}{17}\right)} = 0.30$$

Reject H.

7.5.1 $55/160 = 0.34$ and $60/192 = 0.31$.

7.5.2 Let p_{CC} = True proportion of Catholics who are compliers.
p_{PC} = True proportion of Protestants who are compliers.
Test
        H: $p_{CC} = p_{PC}$ versus   A: $p_{CC} \neq p_{PC}$
Let $P = .05$.

320 Appendix VI

	Cath.	Prot.	
Compliers	10 (7.5)	15 (17.5)	25
Noncompliers	7 (9.5)	25 (22.5)	32
	17	40	57

$$\sum \frac{(obs - exp)^2}{exp} = 2.13$$

Since the appropriate critical value is 3.84, H is accepted.

7.5.3 The first table will have a larger χ^2 value than the second table.

7.6.1

	I	II	III	IV	
Yes	42 (38.1)	38 (32.3)	34 (32.9)	6 (16.7)	120
No	24 (27.9)	18 (23.7)	23 (24.1)	23 (12.3)	88
	66	56	57	29	208

$$\sum \frac{(obs - exp)^2}{exp} = 19.57$$

At the $P = .01$ level of significance, the critical value (with 3 degrees of freedom) is 11.3. Therefore, we should reject the null hypothesis and conclude that drinking habits and socioeconomic status are not independent factors for women.

7.6.2 No.

7.6.3 One way would be to distinguish only two diagnoses — for example, "hebephrenia" and "other."

	Heb.	Other	
Heb.	49	11	60
Other	31	69	100
	80	80	160

Review Exercises

7.1 (a)

	Dec., 1967–May, 1968	June, 1968–Nov., 1968	Dec., 1968–May, 1969	
Survived Yes three months	3 (5.9)	30 (24.2)	8 (10.9)	41
No	16 (13.1)	48 (53.8)	27 (24.1)	91
	19	78	35	132

$$\sum \frac{(obs - exp)^2}{exp} = 5.20$$

Let $P = .05$. The χ^2 critical value (with 2 degrees of freedom) is 5.99. Therefore, we should accept the null hypothesis that date of operation and success of operation are independent.

7.2 Let

p_{DD} = True proportion of persons on a similar diet who would die of an infarction after eight years.

p_{ND} = True proportion of persons not on a special diet who would die of an infarction after eight years.

We want to test

$$H: \quad p_{DD} = p_{ND} \quad \text{versus} \quad A: \quad p_{DD} \neq p_{ND}$$

at the $P = .05$ level of significance.

	Diet	No diet	
Died	66 (79.5)	93 (79.5)	159
Lived	357 (343.5)	330 (343.5)	687
	423	423	846

$$\sum \frac{(obs - exp)^2}{exp} = 5.65$$

Reject H.

7.4 (a) $Y = -0.98 + 1.14X$
(b) Estimated Barnhard value $= -0.98 + 1.14(5.70) = 5.52$

7.5 $Y = 114.72 + 9.23X$.

7.6 $r = 0.93$.
$r' = 1.90\sqrt{(1 - (0.93)^2)/7} = 0.26$.
Reject the null hypothesis.

7.7 $\sum (obs - exp)^2/exp = 3.90$. At the $P = .05$ level of significance, the appropriate critical value is 9.49. Therefore, we accept the null hypothesis.

7.9 Let

p_{SW} = True proportion of patients who would survive if the amputation was performed *with* carbolic acid.

p_{SW_o} = True proportion of patients who would survive if the amputation was performed *without* carbolic acid.

Test

H: $p_{SW} = p_{SW_o}$ versus A: $p_{SW} \neq p_{SW_o}$

Let $P = .01$.

		Carbolic acid		
		Yes	No	
Survived	Yes	34 (28.3)	19 (24.7)	53
	No	6 (11.7)	16 (10.3)	22
		40	35	75

$\sum (obs - exp)^2/exp = 8.39$. With 1 degree of freedom and for $P = .01$, the appropriate critical value is 6.63. Therefore, we should reject H.

CHAPTER 8

Questions

8.2.1 (a) 24
(b) 7
(c) 1.75
(d) 2.0
(e) 2

8.2.2 $\sqrt{[1/(n_i - 1)] \sum_{j=1}^{n_i} (x_{ij} - \bar{x}_{i.})^2}$

8.2.3 The second expression includes not only all the squares (x_{ij}^2) contained in the first expression, but, also, all the possible cross products $(x_{ij}x_{1m})$.

8.3.1 Let μ_1 and μ_2 denote the true average bacterial counts for carpeted and uncarpeted rooms, respectively. Test

H: $\mu_1 = \mu_2$ versus A: $\mu_1 \neq \mu_2$

at the $P = .05$ level of significance. Let x_{1j} denote the bacterial count recorded for the jth carpeted room and x_{2j}, for the jth uncarpeted room.

$\sum_{j=1}^{8} x_{1j} = 89.6; \bar{x}_{1.} = 11.2; \sum_{j=1}^{8} x_{2j} = 78.3; \bar{x}_{2.} = 9.8$

$\bar{x}_{..} = 10.5; \sum_{i=1}^{2} (\bar{x}_{i.} - \bar{x}_{..})^2 = 0.98$

$\sum_{i=1}^{2} \sum_{j=1}^{8} (x_{ij} - \bar{x}_{i.})^2 = 122.31$

Therefore, $[\hat{\sigma}^2(\text{between})]/[\hat{\sigma}^2(\text{within})] = 0.90$. For 1 and 14 degrees of freedom, the $P = .05$ critical value is 4.60. Since $0.90 < 4.60$, we should accept H.

8.4.1 Yes (see Question 8.3.1).

Review Exercises

8.1 (b) Accept the null hypothesis. $MS(\text{between}) = 66.125$, $MS(\text{within}) = 70.98$, and $F = 0.93$. For 2 and 14 degrees of freedom, the $P = .05$ critical value is 3.74.

(c) The effects of dieldrin are cumulative.

8.4 (a) (1) 7.39 (2) 6.25 (3) 6.11 (4) 0.065 (5) 24.45

(b) (1) $\sum_{i=1}^{5} \sum_{j=1}^{4} \sum_{k=1}^{3} (x_{ijk} - \bar{x}_{...})^2$

(2) $\sqrt{\frac{1}{2} \sum_{k=1}^{3} (x_{ijk} - \bar{x}_{ij.})^2}$

8.5 $\sum_{i=1}^{4} \sum_{j=1}^{3} x_{ij} = 96; \sum_{i=1}^{4} \sum_{j=1}^{3} x_{ij}^2 = 868; c = 768.0$

Source	df	SS	MS	F
Therapies	3	65.33	21.78	4.0
Error	8	34.67	4.33	
Total	11	100.0		

8.7 Let μ_1, μ_2, and μ_3 be the true average mercury concentrations in Lake Erie walleyed pike for the three different age groupings being considered. Test

H: $\mu_1 = \mu_2 = \mu_3$ versus   A: not all the μ_i's are equal

Let $P = .05$.

$\sum_{i=1}^{3} \sum_{j=1}^{4} x_{ij} = 9.11; \sum_{i=1}^{3} \sum_{j=1}^{4} x_{ij}^2 = 7.2625.$

Source	df	SS	MS	F
Age	2	.205	.102	6.38
Error	9	.141	.016	
Total	11	.346		

For 2 and 9 degrees of freedom, the critical value is 4.26. Since $MS(\text{age})/MS(\text{error})$ is greater than 4.26, we should reject the null hypothesis.

INDEX

Acute serum, 216, 222
Adjusted rate, 44–47, 68–69, 70
Alternative hypothesis, 97–101, 117–18
  one-sided, 99, 118, 133–39
  two-sided, 99, 119, 142–43
Analysis of variance:
  ANOVA table, 278–84
  assumptions, 274
  computing formulas, 278–82
  degrees of freedom, 274
  derivation, 271–74
  notation, 266–69
  test statistic, 273–74
Area, 103–16
  related to probability, 103–5, 110–11
  under histograms, 103–7
  under normal curves, 108–16, 130, 133–34, 164–69
Arithmetic mean, 78, 81, 84–89, 92–95, 97, 117, 119, 170
  as a measure of location, 81, 84–86, 97
  formula for, 83
Arithmetic scale, 65, 70
  comparison to logarithmic scale, 65
Average (*see* Arithmetic mean)

Bar graph, 38, 49–52, 68, 70
Bell-shape, 79, 84, 108, 118
  as an assumption, 153, 180, 191
Between-treatment variation, 278–82, 285–87
Binomial data, 126, 159–64, 171–72
  confidence intervals, 163–64
  hypothesis tests, 160–63
  point estimates, 159
Binomial distribution, 159–64
  mean, 159–60
  normal approximation, 160–64
  standard deviation, 160
Bivariate normal distribution, 241–42

Cell, 247
Central limit theorem, 126–29, 159–60, 172
Chi square distribution, 247–48, 251
  tables, 304–5
Chi square statistic, 247, 251–52
  approximate distribution, 247, 251–52
  degrees of freedom, 247, 251–52
Chi square test, 245–58
  for 2×2 contingency tables, 245–50
  for $R \times C$ contingency tables, 251–57
Class, 53–54, 56–58, 70
  frequency, 53
  limits, 53–54, 56, 58
  midpoint, 56–57
  ways of labeling, 54–58
Confidence interval, 125–26, 153–59, 163–64, 170, 172
  for p, 163–64
  for μ, 153–59
  for $\mu_X - \mu_Y$, 194–98
  interpretation of, 154–55, 164, 195
Contingency table, 245–46, 257, 259
Control group, 15, 27
Convalescent serum, 216, 222
Correlation, 20, 228–29, 244, 257, 259
  interpretation, 20, 244
  negative, 229
  positive, 228
  relationship to χ^2 test, 245
  spurious, 244
Correlation coefficient, 235–44
  as a test for independence, 240–44
  assumptions, 241
  interpretation, 239–40
  sample, 236–38
  true, 240–41
Correlation problems, 19–23, 27, 227–29
Critical value, 133–37, 172
Crude rate, 41–42, 68, 70

Index

Cumulative frequency polygon, 74–75
Curvilinear relationship, 228

Data, 5, 38–40, 47–61
   interval, 40, 52–61, 70
   nominal, 38–39, 47–52, 71, 159
   ordinal, 39, 47–52, 71
   qualitative, 5, 40, 245
   quantitative, 5, 40, 245
Decision rule, 134, 172
   in correlation problems, 241–43, 252–53
   in k-sample problems, 274, 280–81
   in one-sample problems, 134–37, 142–43, 160–61
   in paired-data problems, 211–13
   in two-sample problems, 179–80, 187–88, 193–94
Degrees of freedom, 172
   in analysis of variance, 274–75, 279
   in chi square test, 247, 251–52
   in one-sample t-test, 146, 148
   in paired t-test, 210–11
   in two-sample F-test, 187
   in two-sample t-test, 180, 191–94
Descriptive statistics, 37–38, 70
   for qualitative data, 47–52
   for quantitative data, 52–61
Difference between means, 177–86, 193–98
   confidence intervals, 194–98
   tests of hypotheses, 177–86, 193–94
Dispersion (*see* Standard deviation)
Distribution, 5, 28
   binomial, 159–64
   cumulative frequency, 74–75
   frequency, 47–49, 70
   normal, 108–18, 127–46, 160–70
   population, 5, 28
   probability, 102–3, 118
   sample, 5–7, 28
   sampling, 92–96, 119, 125–37
Double blind, 19, 27

Empirical probability, 102–3
Epidemic curve, 62–63, 68, 70
Equality of variances, 180, 186–92
   effect on two-sample t-test, 186
   test for, 187–92
Expected frequency, 246
Experimental error, 208, 220–22
Extreme values, 84–87

F-distribution, 187–88, 199–200
   for testing the equality of two variances, 187–91
   in analysis of variance, 274–75
   tables, 301–3, 306–8
Fitting a normal curve, 109
Frequency distribution, 38, 47–49, 68, 70
   conventions, 53
   weakness as a descriptive technique, 49
Frequency polygon, 38, 53, 57–59, 68
   advantages, 53

Geometric mean, 85, 216–18
   application to titers, 216–20, 222
Grand mean, 268
Graphical descriptive statistics, 37–38, 49–52, 54–68
   bar graph, 38, 49–52, 70
   epidemic curve, 62–63, 70
   histogram, 38, 53–56, 68, 70
   population pyramid, 63–64, 71
   scatterdiagram, 38, 59–61, 71, 228–30
Grouped mean, 122
Grouped standard deviation, 122

Histogram, 38, 53–56, 68, 70, 103–4
   relation to frequency distribution, 53
Hypothesis, 97–99
   alternative, 97, 117
   null, 97, 117
   one-sided, 99, 118
   two-sided, 99, 119
Hypothesis testing, 96–99, 118, 125–26, 170
   in correlation problems, 240–42, 247–48, 251–53
   in k-sample problems, 269–75, 278–81
   in one-sample problems, 137–40, 143–46, 160–62
   in paired-data problems, 210–11, 219–20
   in two-sample problems, 177–81, 186–88, 191–94

Independence, 257
   testing for, qualitative data, 245–48, 251–55
   testing for, quantitative data, 240–44
Independent samples, 14, 23, 27, 179–80, 266, 274
Independent trials, 159–60
Index of summation, 81–83, 266–69
Inference, 12, 77–78, 96–99, 125–26
Interval scale, 40, 52–61, 70

J-shaped distribution, 108
   effect on sample mean, 84–85

k-sample problems, 23–25, 27

Large sample test, 125–46, 160
Least squares criterion, 231, 234
Least squares regression line, 229–35, 257, 259
   computing formulas, 231
   relation to correlation coefficient, 257
Level of significance, 134, 142–43, 164–69, 172
   relationship with Type II error, 164–69
Linear relationship, 20, 27, 228–32, 235–40
Location, 79, 87
   alternate measures of, 85–87
   sample mean as a measure of, 84
Logarithmic scale, 65–68, 70
Logarithms, 66–68, 218
   in computing geometric mean, 218

Matched samples, 15, 28
Mathematical model, 108, 117–18
Mean (*see also* Arithmetic mean):
   confidence intervals, 153–59
   deviation from, 87–89, 236–40, 273
   for grouped data, 122–23
   geometric, 85, 217–18, 222
   grand, 268
   population, 96–99, 118
   sample, 78–80, 83, 85, 97, 117, 119
   sampling distribution of, 92–95, 119
Mean square, 279–80, 285–87
Measurement, 5
   dissimilar, 19
   similar, 14, 16
Measures of dispersion, 78–80, 87–92, 180–81, 210, 271–73
Measures of location, 79, 84–87
Median, 85–87, 119
Method of least squares, 229, 259
Midpoint, 56–57, 70
Modified relative frequency, 101, 104–7, 117–18
Morbidity rates, 41, 70
Mortality rates, 41, 70

Natality rates, 41, 71
Negative correlation, 228
Nominal data, 38–39, 71, 159–64
   ways to graph, 47–52
Nonlinear relationship, 20, 28, 228–29
Normal curve, 108–18, 126–29
   approximation to bell-shaped histograms, 108
   approximation to binomial, 160
   areas under, 110–17, 130–34
   tables, 297–98
   Z-transformation, 113–14, 117, 145–46, 160, 166
Null hypothesis, 97–99, 117–18

Observed frequency, 246–47
One-sample problems, 12–13, 28, 125–26
One-sided alternative, 99, 118
Operating characteristic curve, 126, 167–71, 172
   relationship with sample size, 169
Ordinal data, 39–40, 71
   ways to graph, 47–52

Paired-data problems, 16–19, 28, 207–9
Parameter, 96–99, 117–18, 159–61
Percentile, 121
Point estimate, 132, 162
Pooled standard deviation, 180–81, 200
Population, 4–5, 28
Population correlation coefficient, 229, 240–42
Population distribution, 5, 28
Population mean, 96–99
Population pyramid, 63–64, 68, 71
Population standard deviation, 96, 118
Positive correlation, 228
Posttiter, 216, 222
Pretiter, 216, 222

Probability, 102–3, 118
   definition, 102
   of committing Type I error, 165
   of committing Type II error, 165–70
   properties of, 102
   relationship to area, 105
Probability distribution, 102, 113, 118
Proportions, 159
   confidence intervals, 163–64
   hypothesis tests, 160–63
   sampling distribution, 160

Qualitative data, 5–6, 28, 40, 257
Quantitative data, 5, 28, 40, 258

Random sample, 28, 146, 180, 274
Random variable, 93, 107, 155
Rates, 40–47, 68, 71
   adjusted, 44–47, 68, 70
   crude, 41, 68, 70
   specific, 42–44, 68
   ways of expressing, 41
Regression, 227–35
   formula for slope, 231
   formula for Y-intercept, 231
   line, 230–31
   method of least squares, 229–31
   scatterdiagrams, 38, 59–61, 68, 71, 228
Relative frequency, 101–2, 119
   modified, 101, 104, 118
   relationship with probability, 102
Retrospective study, 61, 71

Sample, 4–5, 9, 28
Sample correlation coefficient, 229, 235–40, 257, 259
Sample distribution, 5, 28
Sample mean (*see* Mean)
Sample median, 85–87, 119
Sample size, 4, 28, 126
Sample standard deviation, 78, 87–92, 117, 119, 170
Sample variance, 90, 119
Sample-population structure, 4, 9–10, 26, 28
Sampling distribution, 92–95, 170, 187
   of χ^2 statistic, 247, 252
   of $\overline{D}$, 210–11
   of F ratio, 187, 274
   of r, 242
   of $\overline{X}$, 92–95, 117, 119, 126–29, 170
   of $\overline{X} - \overline{Y}$, 180, 191
Scale, 38–40, 65, 71
   interval, 40
   nominal, 38–39
   ordinal, 39
Scatterdiagram, 38, 59–60, 68, 71, 228
Sigma notation, 81–83, 117, 119, 266–69

Significance level, 124, 139, 142–43, 145, 165, 172
Slope, 230–31, 237, 239
Source of variation, 220–22, 278–79
Specific rate, 42–44, 71
Standard deviation, 78, 87–92, 117–19, 170
   computing formula, 89, 91
   defining formula, 89
   pooled, 180–81, 200
   population, 96, 108, 113, 118, 180
Standard error of the mean, 132, 172
Standard normal distribution, 110–17, 119, 160
   areas under, 110–13
   transformation to, 113–14, 117, 160
Statistic, 96, 117, 119
Statistical inference, 5, 28, 77–78, 96–99
Subject effect, 208–9, 220–22
Subscript notation, 9, 81–83, 266–69
Sum of squares, 231–35, 239–40, 278–84
Summation notation, 81–83, 117, 119, 266–69

t-distribution, 126, 146–48, 170, 172
   comparison with the normal distribution, 148
   degrees of freedom, 146–48
   for the correlation problem, 242
   for the one-sample problem, 146–48, 153–54
   for the paired-data problem, 210–11, 219
   for the two-sample problem, 180–81, 186, 191, 194–95
   tables, 299–300
Titer, 30, 216–20, 222
Total variation, 239–40, 278–79, 287
Total-population problems, 10–12, 28
Treatment effect, 208–9, 220–22, 278–81
Two-sample problems, 14–16, 28, 177–79
   confidence intervals, 194–98
   hypothesis tests, 179–94, 200
Two-sided alternative, 99, 119, 142–43
Type I error, 99, 117, 119, 164–70
Type II error, 99, 117, 119, 164–70

U-shaped distribution, 84, 108

Variance, 90, 119
   for the binomial distribution, 160
Variation, 92–93
   explained by regression line, 239–40
   not explained by regression line, 239–40
   partitioning, 239–40, 278–79

Within-treatment variation, 278–82, 285–87

Y-intercept, 230–32

Z-transformation, 113–14, 117, 145–46, 160, 166